CLINICAL APPLICATION OF RESPIRATORY CARE

CLINICAL APPLICATION OF
RESPIRATORY CARE

SECOND EDITION

BARRY A. SHAPIRO, M.D.
Associate Professor of Clinical Anesthesia and Physical
Medicine, Northwestern University Medical School; Director,
Division of Critical Care, Department of Anesthesia,
Northwestern University Medical School; Medical Director,
Department of Respiratory Therapy, Northwestern Memorial
Hospital; Associate Medical Director, Pulmonary Rehabilitation,
Rehabilitation Institute of Chicago; Medical Director,
Programs in Respiratory Therapy, Northwestern University
Medical School

RONALD A. HARRISON, M.D.
Associate Professor of Clinical Anesthesia, Northwestern
University Medical School; Associate Director, Division of
Critical Care, Department of Anesthesia, Northwestern
University Medical School; Associate Medical Director,
Department of Respiratory Therapy, Northwestern Memorial
Hospital; Associate Medical Director, Medical Intensive Care
Area, Northwestern Memorial Hospital

CAROLE A. TROUT, R.N., R.R.T.
Associate in Clinical Anesthesia, Northwestern University
Medical School; Respiratory Care Coordinator, Department of
Respiratory Therapy, Northwestern Memorial Hospital

YEAR BOOK MEDICAL PUBLISHERS, INC.
CHICAGO • LONDON

Reprinted, August 1982

Reprinted, June 1983

Library of Congress Cataloging in Publication Data
Shapiro, Barry A
    Clinical application of respiratory care.

    Includes index.
    1. Inhalation therapy.   I. Harrison, Ronald A.,
joint author.   II. Trout, Carole A., joint author.
III. Title.
RM161.S5   1979   616.2'004'636   79-13483
ISBN 0-8151-7635-X

To Leslie, David, Nancy, and Web

PREFACE TO THE SECOND EDITION

THE SECOND EDITION OF *Clinical Application of Respiratory Care* has been undertaken because of rapid advancements in the field of respiratory care. The general acceptance of augmented modes of ventilation, the universal acceptance of positive end expiratory pressure as a therapeutic mode, and the improved capability of bedside hemodynamic monitoring via the Swan Ganz catheter have created major and rapid changes in the care of the critically ill patient. Thus, the last 16 chapters of this edition include 3 chapters that define acute respiratory failure, its pathogenesis and clinical assessment; 5 chapters that discuss "airway pressure therapy," including the up-to-date concepts of ventilator care and PEEP therapy; and 3 chapters that are devoted to cardiovascular monitoring and supportive therapy in respiratory care. The first 17 chapters have been updated, with major revisions in the discussion of intermittent positive pressure breathing therapy and incentive spirometry.

The text maintains its basic nontechnical orientation and expands the pathophysiologic discussion of specific entities in respiratory care. These include specific discussions of pulmonary edema, the Adult Respiratory Distress Syndrome, the postsurgical patient, chronic obstructive pulmonary disease, and aspiration pneumonitis.

Individuals involved in the acute care of critically ill patients have been challenged by the rapid technologic and medical advancements of respiratory care. This new edition places these advancements in an overall perspective and provides a foundation upon which the understanding of future advancements can be placed.

ACKNOWLEDGMENTS

The advanced concepts of respiratory care contained in this text would not be possible without the constant vigilance and enthusiastic participation of the members of the Respiratory Therapy Department of Northwestern Memorial Hospital. Our humble thanks to them and to the Intensive Care Nursing Staff of Northwestern Memorial Hospital.

The consistent support of Dr. Edward Brunner, Dr. James Eckenhoff, and Dr. Roy Cane is warmly acknowledged. A special thanks to

our physician respiratory care colleagues in Pulmonary Medicine —
Dr. John Buehler and Dr. James Webster. Above all, our deepest
appreciation to our closest colleague in critical care medicine — Dr.
Richard Davison.

The originality and excellence of the illustrations is due entirely to
the talents of Jennifer Giancarlo. The overwhelming task of manu-
script development and preparation was superbly accomplished by
Judith Stutz and Patti Hara.

B. Shapiro
R. Harrison
C. Trout

TABLE OF CONTENTS

Section II: Oxygen Therapy

SECTION I
FOUNDATIONS OF
RESPIRATORY CARE

1 • PULMONARY ANATOMY AND PHYSIOLOGY

CLINICAL MEDICINE is predicated on the basic sciences of anatomy, pharmacology, physiology, and biochemistry. The following is an overview of the *functional* anatomy and physiology of the pulmonary system. It is not a definitive treatise, but rather a useful and up-to-date presentation of anatomy and function as related to respiratory care.

The pulmonary system is separated into two major portions: the upper and lower airways. The *upper airway* is composed of the nose, nasopharynx, oropharynx, oral cavity, laryngopharynx, and larynx. The *lower airway* is composed of the tracheobronchial tree and the lung parenchyma. The *tracheobronchial tree* is considered to be two distinct portions: the large and small airways.

The Upper Airway

The upper airway is composed of the nose, mouth, and pharynx. The larynx is the transition from the upper to lower airway. We shall consider the larynx to be anatomically the lower airway but to have functions consistent with classification as part of the upper airway. Among other factors, the upper airway: (1) acts as a conducting system for air to enter the lower airway; (2) acts as a protective mechanism to prevent foreign material from entering the pulmonary tree; (3) constitutes a considerable portion (30–50%) of the anatomic deadspace; (4) acts as an "air conditioner" of the inspired gases; and (5) plays an important role in the processes of speech and smell.

The Nose

The nose is an organ that possesses skeletal rigidity. This rigidity serves to prevent collapse when a subatmospheric pressure is present during spontaneous inspiration. The nose has a small inlet, a large outlet, and is shaped to produce an airflow pattern allowing maximum exposure of inhaled gas molecules with the mucosal surface.

The upper third of the nose is bony; the lower two-thirds is composed of cartilage. The nasal septum is cartilage in its anterior portion and divides the nose into two nasal fossae whose lateral boundaries are the *alae* (Fig 1–1). Although straight at birth, the nasal septum often becomes deviated in later life. The opening between the septum

3

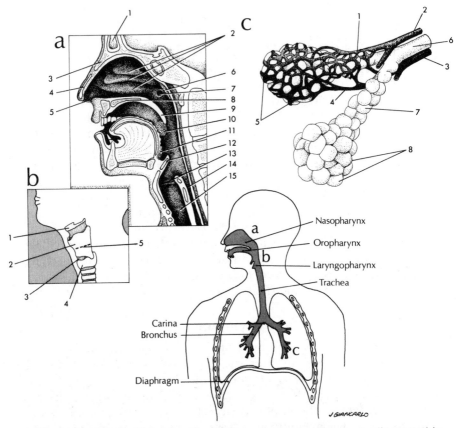

Fig 1–1.—Anatomic landmarks of the pulmonary system, as discussed in the text. Numbered structures are **A,** *1,* frontal bone and sinuses; *2,* turbinates; *3,* bony structure to upper third of nose; *4,* cartilaginous structure to lower two thirds of nose; *5,* vibrissae and nasal vestibule; *6,* pharyngeal tonsils ("the adenoids"); *7,* eustachian tube stoma (taurus tubarus); *8,* hard palate; *9,* soft palate; *10,* faucial tonsils ("the tonsils"); *11,* lingual tonsils; *12,* epiglottis; *13,* vocal cords; *14,* esophagus; and *15,* trachea. **B,** *1,* hyoid bone; *2,* thyroid cartilage; *3,* cricothyroid membrane; *4,* cricoid cartilage; and *5,* area of larynx and vocal cords. **C,** *1,* pulmonary venule; *2,* small pulmonary vein; *3,* small pulmonary artery; *4,* pulmonary arteriole; *5,* pulmonary capillaries; *6,* terminal respiratory bronchiole; *7,* alveolar duct; and *8,* alveolar sacs.

and the alae is called the *naris* (nostril). The channel leading from the nares to the nasopharynx is called the *choana.* The anterior portion of the nasal cavity (the vestibule) is lined with skin and contains hair follicles (vibrissae), which are the first defense mechanisms of the pulmonary system.

Three major projections *(turbinates)* arise from the lateral nasal walls. Airflow is separated into ribbonlike streams by these turbinates, allowing very close contact between the inspired air and the nasal mucosa. The nasal sinuses of the skull drain into the nose through openings which lie beneath the turbinates.

The anterior third of the nose is lined with squamous, nonciliated epithelium. The posterior two-thirds is covered with a *ciliated, pseudostratified epithelium* containing many serous and mucous glands. The mucosal blood flow is very "plush"; increased blood flow results in congestion and swelling which may totally obstruct the nasal passages. Topical vasoconstrictors are extremely efficient in decreasing such congestion.

The *olfactory area* is located in the region of the superior turbinates and is yellowish brown in color, in contrast to the pink color of the normal nasal mucosa. A "sniffing" action of the nose causes peripheral air currents to rise to the olfactory region, facilitating the smelling process. The sense of smell is poorly developed in man compared with other mammals.

The internal and external carotid arteries provide arterial blood supply to the nose. Most of the venous drainage is via the anterior facial veins; a small portion of this venous drainage leads to the cavernous sinus. The lymphatic flow follows the general pattern of the venous drainage. The seventh cranial nerve provides the motor innervation to the muscles of the external nose; the mucosal sensory nerve supply is via the fifth cranial nerve.

The primary functions of the nose are to *humidify, heat,* and *filter* the inspired air. Two significant secondary functions are the sense of smell and a resonance chamber for phonation. The copious capillary blood flow allows for transfer of heat to the inspired air. The copious mucous and serous secretions add as much as 1,000 ml of water per day to inspired air. The intimate contact between inspired air molecules and the nasal mucosa assures that the relative humidity of the inspired gas will be as high as 75–80% by the time the air reaches the nasopharynx.[1]

The filtering action of the nose is accomplished by the large hair follicles in the vestibule and the thick mucous layer covering the mucosa. This sticky substance tends to capture foreign particles in the inspired air and mobilize them toward the outlet of the nose.

The Pharynx

The pharynx is the space behind the oral and nasal cavities (see Fig 1–1). It is subdivided into a nasopharynx, oropharynx, and laryngopharynx. The *nasopharynx* is that portion that lies above the soft palate; the *oropharynx* is the portion from the soft palate to the base of the tongue; the *laryngopharynx* is that portion below the base of the tongue.

The nasopharynx is lined with ciliated, pseudostratified epithelium. The middle ear chamber is connected with the nasopharynx by a channel called the *eustachian tube*. The eustachian tubes have the function of maintaining proper air pressures in the middle ear; this allows the tympanic membranes to function properly. These tubes play a large role in the normal drainage of fluid from the middle ear. Nasopharyngeal inflammation can result in swelling and closure of these tubes, leading to middle ear disease (otitis media) and hearing deficits.

The *pharyngeal tonsils* are located in the superior nasopharynx. This tonsillar tissue is called "the adenoids" and is particularly large in children. When enlarged, the adenoids may block the openings of the eustachian tubes and cause middle ear infection. The abundant lymphoid tissue located in the pharynx is an important defense mechanism of the pulmonary system.

The oropharynx extends from the soft palate to the base of the tongue. It receives air from the mouth and nasopharynx, and receives food from the oral cavity. The anterolateral borders of the oropharynx contain lymphoid tissue called the faucial tonsils, which may be extremely large in children. The *faucial tonsils* are commonly referred to as "the tonsils." The base of the tongue contains lymphoid tissue called the *lingual tonsils*.

The laryngopharynx extends from the base of the tongue to the opening of the esophagus. Important landmarks of endotracheal intubation, such as the epiglottis, aryepiglottic folds, and arytenoid cartilages, are contained within the laryngopharynx.

The pharyngeal musculature is composed of complex layers whose motor innervation is the tenth cranial nerve (vagus); the sensory supply is via the ninth cranial nerve (glossopharyngeal). The primary function of the pharyngeal musculature is to provide for the act of swallowing. The mucosa of the oropharynx and laryngopharynx is composed of stratified, squamous epithelium without cilia.

Significant enlargement of pharyngeal lymphoid tissue can cause partial or complete airway obstruction. The base of the tongue can obstruct the airway by "falling back" to the posterior pharyngeal wall. The process of assuring that the base of the tongue does not touch the posterior pharynx is one of the cardinal maneuvers in establishing and maintaining a patent airway.

The Larynx

The larynx is the connection between the upper and lower airways. It lies in the anterior portion of the neck at the level of the fourth, fifth, and sixth cervical vertebrae. The opening to the larynx is called the *glottis*.

Cartilages

The larynx is composed of a number of cartilages connected to one another by muscles and membranes. The major cartilages are the thyroid, cricoid, arytenoid, and epiglottis. The largest laryngeal cartilage is the *thyroid cartilage,* commonly referred to as the "Adam's apple." It is more protuberant in males than females and consists of two flat sections that are joined together. Below the thyroid cartilage is the *cricoid cartilage.* An avascular structure, the *cricothyroid membrane,* connects the thyroid and cricoid cartilages. Since this cricothyroid membrane is below the level of the vocal cords, it is the site of choice for emergency surgical entrance into the lower airway (cricothyroidotomy).

The cricoid cartilage forms a complete ring — the only tracheal ring that is complete. The cricoid cartilage is the narrowest portion of the upper airway in the infant and small child. In the older child and adult, however, the glottic opening is the narrowest portion of the upper airway.

The two *arytenoid cartilages* play a significant role in vocal cord movement. The vocal cords are composed of ligamentous and cartilaginous tissues that extend from the arytenoid cartilages to the thyroid cartilage.

Mucosa

The laryngeal mucosa is composed of stratified, squamous epithelium above the vocal cords and pseudostratified, columnar epithelium below. No cilia are present in the larynx. The sensory innervation to the anterior surface of the epiglottis is the ninth cranial nerve; the remainder of the innervation to the larynx is the tenth cranial nerve (vagus). The primary motor innervation of the larynx is the tenth cranial nerve via the recurrent laryngeal nerve.

The Epiglottis

The epiglottis is a leaf-shaped elastic cartilage that attaches to the thyroid cartilage. The epiglottis is flexible and lies flat against the anterior pharyngeal wall. The primary function of the epiglottis is to cover the glottic opening during swallowing, thus preventing entrance of foreign substance into the airway.

Laryngeal Function

There are four prime functions of the larynx: (1) to act as a gas-conducting channel connecting the upper and the lower airways; (2) to protect the lower airway from foreign substances; (3) to participate in the cough mechanism; and (4) to participate in speech.[2]

The larynx serves a protective function for the lower airway by closing off the glottis during the swallowing mechanism. This prevents food, when it is being mobilized from the oropharynx to the esophagus, from entering the tracheobronchial tree.

An essential defense mechanism of the pulmonary system is the cough. The cough mechanism (see Chapter 8) depends on the ability of the false cords, aryepiglottic folds, true vocal cords, and epiglottis to establish an airtight laryngeal closure. The degree of tensing of the vocal cords is responsible for the pitch and quality of sound produced in the process of speech.

The Tracheobronchial Tree

The lower airway is separated into two sections: the tracheobronchial tree and the lung parenchyma. The tracheobronchial tree functions as a system of conducting tubes, allowing passage of gas to and from the lung parenchyma, where molecular exchange takes place between blood and alveolar gas. The tracheobronchial tree can be further subdivided into two portions: the central airways (bronchi) and the transitional airways (bronchioles).

Histology

As the tracheobronchial tree branches, the diameters become progressively smaller (Table 1–1). The tracheobronchial wall is composed of three major layers (Fig 1–2): (1) an epithelial lining, (2) the lamina propria, and (3) the cartilaginous layer.

The *epithelium* is composed of pseudostratified, ciliated, columnar epithelium with numerous mucous and serous secreting glands. The epithelium has a well-defined basement membrane with some mucous glands extending beneath the basement membrane. The *lamina propria* (submucosa) is composed of loose, fibrous tissue containing numerous small blood vessels, lymphatic vessels, and nerves. A complex network of longitudinal and circular (geodesic) elastic fibers ex-

TABLE 1-1.—SIZE RELATIONSHIPS IN TRACHEOBRONCHIAL TREE

STRUCTURE	AVERAGE DIAMETERS		
	CM	MM	MICRONS
Trachea	2	20	20,000
Main stem bronchus (1st generation)	1	10	10,000
Large bronchiole (11th generation)	0.1	1	1,000
Terminal bronchiole (16th generation)	0.05	0.5	500

Oxygen atom is approximately 1 angstrom (Å) in diameter. Ultrasonic droplet is approximately 1 micron (μ) in diameter.

$1,000 \text{ Å} = 1 \mu$
$1,000 \mu = 1 \text{ mm}$
$10 \text{ mm} = 1 \text{ cm}$
$1,000 \text{ mm} = 1 \text{ meter}$

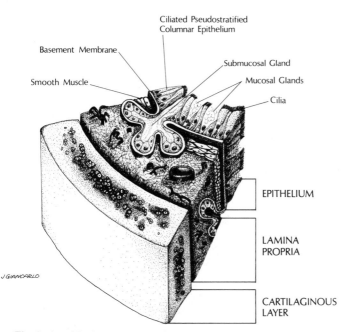

Fig 1-2.—Model concept of the three major layers of the tracheobronchial wall (see text).

ists in relation to a reticular network of smooth muscle. This bronchial smooth muscle may contract, resulting in an acute increase in airway resistance; such "bronchospasm" is a common disease entity. In respiratory care, a great deal of effort and concern is concentrated on the prevention and relief of bronchospasm. The *cartilaginous layer* is composed of varying amounts of cartilage, which completely disappears in the tubes of less than 1 mm in diameter.

The contents and functional significance of these layers change as the diameters of the tubes become smaller.

The Trachea

In the adult the trachea is a tube 11–13 cm in length and 1.5–2.5 cm in diameter.[1] It extends from the larynx to its bifurcation at the level of the second costal cartilage (fifth thoracic vertebra). The area where the trachea branches into two main stem bronchi is called the *carina*. The trachea lies directly in front of the esophagus and is flanked by the great vessels of the neck. A portion of the thyroid gland crosses the anterior surface of the trachea in the neck.

The trachea is supported by 16–20 C-shaped cartilages.[22] The posterior wall is composed of a flat membrane which is devoid of cartilage. This membrane is separated from the anterior esophageal wall by loose connective tissue.

Main Stem Bronchi

The trachea bifurcates into a right and left main stem bronchus which are histologically similar to the trachea. The right main stem bronchus is wider and shorter than the left, and appears to be an extension of the trachea; the left main stem bronchus appears to be a branch of the trachea. In the adult, the right main stem bronchus forms an approximately 25° angle with the vertical axis; the left main stem bronchus, a 40°–60° angle.[3] In the infant, both main stem bronchi form equal angles of approximately 55°.

Lobar Bronchi

The right main stem bronchus divides into three lobar branches named the upper, middle, and lower lobar bronchi. The left main stem bronchus divides into the upper and lower lobar bronchi. Here, the cartilages lose their horseshoe-shape characteristic that distinguishes them in the trachea and main stem bronchi. Although the rings are far from complete, they tend to provide circumferential rigidity to the tubes under most circumstances.[4]

Segmental Bronchi

The lobar bronchi give rise to various branches which are called segmental bronchi and are named according to the lung segments they supply. These segmental bronchi are very important to the application of bronchial hygiene and chest physical therapy (see Chapter 12).

Small Bronchi (Subsegmental)

Every branching in the tracheobronchial tree produces a new "generation" of tubes. Thus, the main stem bronchi are first generation, the lobar bronchi are second generation, and segmental bronchi are third

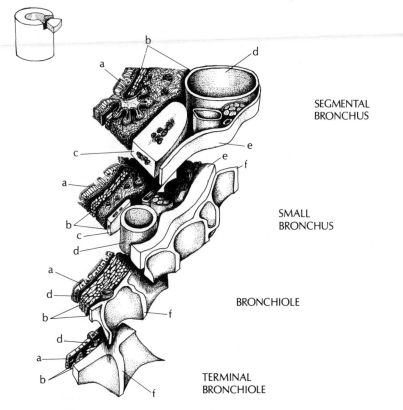

SEGMENTAL
BRONCHUS

SMALL
BRONCHUS

BRONCHIOLE

TERMINAL
BRONCHIOLE

J GIANCARLO

Fig 1–3.—Relationship of tracheobronchial wall components at various levels: *a,* pulmonary mucosa; *b,* lamina propria (smooth muscle component); *c,* cartilage; *d,* blood vessels; *e,* peribronchial connective tissue; *f,* lung parenchyma.

generation. The fourth through approximately the ninth generation are referred to as the small bronchi. In these "subsegmental" bronchi, the diameters decrease from approximately 4 mm to 1 mm. Since the number of bronchi increases with each generation, the total cross-sectional area at that level increases with each generation. The eleventh generation has approximately seven times the cross-sectional area that exists at the level of the lobar bronchi.

The bronchi are surrounded by peribronchial connective tissue which contains the bronchial arteries, lymphatics, and nerves (Fig 1–3). This connective tissue sheath surrounds all tubes through the ninth to eleventh generation, where diameters become 1 mm or less.[4] At this point, the connective tissue sheaths end and the walls of the tubes become continuous with the lung parenchyma.

Tubes greater than 1 mm diameter with connective tissue sheaths are called *bronchi;* these central airways are responsible for 80% of normal airway resistance.[5] Tubes less than 1 mm diameter *without* connective tissue sheaths are called *bronchioles*.

Bronchioles (Transitional Airways)

In the bronchioles, beginning with the ninth to eleventh generation from the trachea: (1) diameters become less than 1 mm; (2) cartilage is completely absent; and (3) lamina propria is directly imbedded in lung parenchyma. The patency of the airways no longer depends on structural rigidity; airway patency here is primarily dependent upon elastic recoil formed by the surrounding tissues. At this level, airway patency is influenced less by intrathoracic pressure and influenced more by alveolar pressure and alveolar geometric changes.

Since the number of bronchioles increases with each generation, the total cross-sectional area of these airways increases greatly. The net effect is that resistance to airflow in these smaller airways is individually greater, although the over-all airway resistance in these smaller airways represents only 10–20% of the *normal* total airway resistance.[6]

The bronchioles have spiral muscle bands and a cuboidal epithelium. Blood supply for the entire tracheobronchial tree is via the bronchial-arterial circulation. The tracheobronchial tree ends at approximately the sixteenth generation from the trachea. These final generations are known as terminal bronchioles.

Terminal Bronchioles

In terminal bronchioles the average diameter is approximately 0.5 mm; the epithelium becomes flattened; mucous glands and cilia disappear. Although mucus can be found at this level, its origin is uncertain. It may come from secretory cells called *clara cells* which are found in the terminal and preterminal bronchioles. There is some evidence to support the belief that these clara cells are responsible in part for surfactant production and not mucus production.[7] In any case, both mucus and surfactantlike substances are found at the level of the terminal bronchioles.

Lung Parenchyma

The function of the tracheobronchial tree is to conduct, humidify, and heat inspired air. Distal to terminal bronchioles, the function is to allow molecular gas exchange between blood and alveolar air. The bronchial-arterial system ends at the terminal bronchiole.[6] Nutrient blood supply distal to this point must be via the pulmonary-arterial system.

Respiratory Bronchioles

Flat alveolar epithelium, void of cilia, mucus, and serous glands, is present in respiratory bronchioles. The respiratory bronchioles continue for approximately three generations and serve as a transition to pure alveolar epithelium possessing maximum gas-exchange capability.

Primary Lobules (See Fig 1–1)

The alveolar epithelium lines all of the lung parenchyma. This parenchyma is actually composed of numerous primary lobules or functional units. Although anatomists disagree about this concept of primary lobules, the popular view is that the primary lobule is the unit supplied by a first-order alveolar duct. There are approximately 130,000 primary lobules in the lung. Each lobule has a diameter of about 3.5 mm and contains approximately 2,200 alveoli. A primary lobule is believed to be supplied by a single pulmonary arteriole.[6]

Alveolar Ducts

The alveolar ducts arise from the respiratory bronchiole. The walls of the alveolar duct are composed of alveoli separated by "septal walls."[6] The septa contain smooth muscle and are believed to be capable of contracting and narrowing the lumen of the duct. About one half of the total lung alveoli arise directly from the alveolar ducts and are responsible for about 35% of alveolar gas exchange.

Alveolar Sacs

Alveolar sacs are the last generation of the airways and are functionally the same as alveolar ducts except that they are completely blind passages. These alveolar sacs exist in clusters of 15 to 20 and have common walls between them. This mechanism greatly increases the surface area of the lung and plays a great role in the elastic recoil of the lung parenchyma. The alveolar sacs are responsible for approximately 65% of alveolar gas exchange.

Alveolar Epithelium (Fig 1–4)

The precise nature of the lung gas-tissue interface has been a subject of controversy for many years. The advent of electron microscopy has added great knowledge about the nature and substance of the alveolar epithelium. Although the exact make-up of this epithelium is still not completely known, generalizations can be stated beyond reasonable doubt.

Ninety-five percent of the total alveolar surface is composed of alveolar type I pneumocytes.[8] These cells have a relatively flat nucleus from which the cytoplasm extends in a disk-like fashion for a significant distance. This very thin (0.1 μ) cytoplasm provides the surface area for gas diffusion.[9] The metabolic activity of these cells is believed

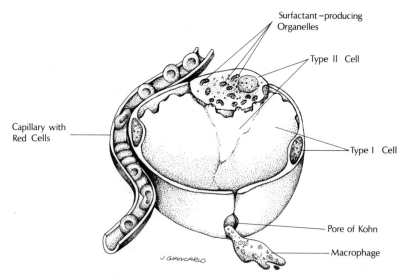

Fig 1–4.—Schematic representation of alveolar epithelium (see text). Note the majority of surface is the cytoplasmic extension of type I cells.

minimal. The intercytoplasmic junctions are very "tight"[10] between all the epithelial cells.

The most numerous alveolar pneumocyte is the type II cell, which undergoes mitotic division and is believed to give rise to the type I cell. These pneumocytes are cuboidal secretory type cells, with microvilli on the alveolar surface, and have profound metabolic activity.[11] The cytoplasmic lamellar bodies are the site of production of pulmonary *surfactant*, whereas the microvilli are responsible for secreting the fluid lining of the alveolar epithelium. It is obvious that nuclear and cytoplasmic biochemical functions are numerous.[12]

Lung Interstitium

The space interposed between alveolar epithelium and capillary endothelium is composed of collagen and elastic elements, water, and electrolytes. This space is very narrow between alveolar septa and relatively larger around alveolar ducts. Smooth muscle and nervous tissue abound in this space. Perhaps the most important element within the interstitium is the *lymphatic system.*

Since pulmonary interstitial pressure is below atmospheric, whereas right atrial pressure is above atmospheric, lymphatic flow cannot be passive. The active propulsion involves both extrinsic forces (e.g., respiratory movements, arterial pulsations) and intrinsic lymphatic peristalsis.[13-15] Most probably the lymphatic smooth muscle is under autonomic regulation.[16] Mechanisms responsible for transporting fluid to the lymphatic ostia are controversial.

Lung Endothelium

Compared to most systemic endothelia, the pulmonary endothelium is "leaky."[18] This means that fluid and some colloid molecules normally pass from plasma to interstitium. The fact that capillaries are leaky, and readily made more so by disease, and the epithelial junctions tight is a crucial relationship to remember.[19]

Intracellular biochemical activity of pulmonary endothelial cells appear similar to systemic endothelial cells. Pulmonary endothelial cells are known to be responsible for production and/or destruction of catecholamines, bradykinin, acetylcholine, serotonin, histamine, and prostaglandins. Undoubtedly others will be discovered in the future.

The Mucous Blanket

The lung has always been recognized as an organ vulnerable to disease. Throughout the recorded history of man, plagues of pneumonia and pneumonialike diseases have resulted in countless deaths. Infectious pneumonia was the greatest killer in the United States prior to the advent of antibiotics. As early as 1930, there were serious investigative efforts made to delineate the normal defense mechanisms of the lung. Numerous theories were developed over the next several decades concerning the normal defense mechanisms and their resultant alterations in disease. The advent of the electron microscope in the 1950s resulted in a rapid increase in knowledge of the pulmonary defense mechanisms. Of great importance to the field of respiratory care is the discovery of the existence and functioning of a normal defense mechanism of the pulmonary tree known as the *mucociliary escalator* or *mucous blanket.*

Mucus

The tracheobronchial tree epithelium contains numerous serous and mucous glands. Mucous glands in the epithelium are called *surface goblet cells* and react to irritation by becoming enlarged and chronically inflamed. The submucosal glands (Fig 1–5) produce bronchial secretions in the healthy adult estimated at 100 ml per day. The composition of this normal mucus is 95% water, 2% glycoprotein, 1% carbohydrate, trace amounts of lipid and DNA, in addition to cellular debris and other foreign elements. The mucus forms a continuous, uninterrupted covering of the epithelium of the tracheobronchial tree. The characteristics of this *mucous blanket* have been studied in great detail.[20] Its properties of viscosity and elasticity are greatly dependent upon the water content, mucin, and serous elements present.

There is a progressive decrease in the water content of mucus from its formation at the mucosal surface to the inner luminal surface (see Fig 1–5). This continuum has been arbitrarily subdivided into two distinct layers: the layer adjacent to the mucosal surface (the sol layer) and the more viscous layer (the gel layer).

Cilia (See Fig 1–5)

The *cilia* lie almost entirely within the fluid sol layer. The ciliary control mechanisms are unknown, but their "beating" action has been well studied. The forward movement of the cilia makes the upper end of the hairlike projection extend into the viscous gel layer and pulls it forward. During its backward motion, the cilia folds upon itself. Thus, the backward motion is entirely within the sol layer and has little backward pull on the mucous blanket. Because of the viscous and elastic properties of the gel layer, this intermittent ciliary "pull" is transformed into a continuous movement toward the larynx.

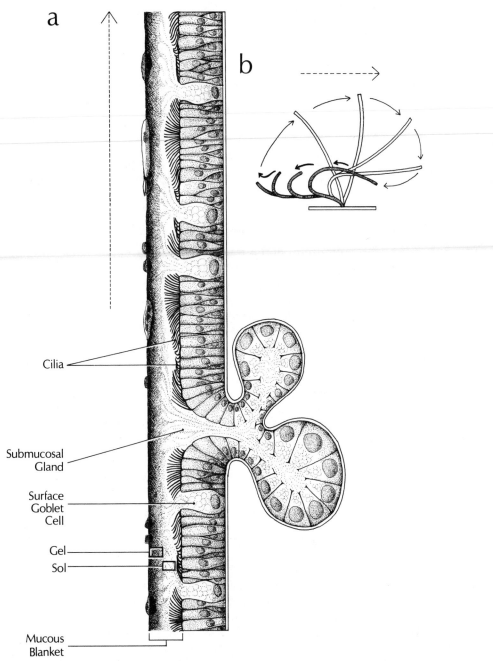

a

b

Cilia

Submucosal
Gland

Surface
Goblet
Cell

Gel

Sol

Mucous
Blanket

Fig 1–5. — A, the mucociliary escalator (see text). **B,** conceptual scheme of ciliary movement, allowing forward motion to move viscous gel layer and backward motion to take place entirely within more fluid sol layer.

Function

The mucous blanket moves at an average rate of 2 cm per minute and is claimed to be an efficient self-cleansing mechanism of the normal lung.[20] Inhaled foreign materials stick to the mucus and are mobilized toward the larynx. The mucous blanket is an important element in the cough mechanism since it is the mucous blanket that is mobilized by the high-velocity airflow.

Sputum is the substance that is mobilized by the cough mechanism. It is composed not only of the mucus from the tracheobronchial tree, but also of nasal secretions and salivary gland secretions.

The Alveolar Fluid Lining

Like the epithelium of the tracheobronchial tree, alveolar epithelium is normally lined with a fluid. The origin of this fluid is the alveolar type II cell. It is generally believed to be mobilized in the direction of the bronchioles where it becomes part of the mucous blanket; the mechanisms for such mobilization are unknown.

Macrophages

The fluid lining contains numerous free cells, the most important of which are *macrophages*, often referred to as type III alveolar cells. The origin of the macrophage cells has been debated for many years and has been claimed to arise from (1) endothelial cells of alveolar capillaries; (2) bronchial epithelium; (3) peribronchial lymphoid tissue; and (4) pulmonary surface epithelium.

Electron microscopy and other modern investigative techniques, however, have not supported these theories. At the present time, it is believed that these macrophages arise from the bone marrow. Whatever their origin, macrophages are important to respiratory care because they *do exist* in the lung parenchyma and because they are a significant part of the normal defense mechanism.[21]

Surfactant

If the epithelial fluid were composed only of water, the surface tension would be so great that the lungs would remain collapsed. However, the fluid lining the alveolar epithelium contains a "detergent-like" phospholipid substance referred to as *pulmonary surfactant.* This substance reduces the surface tension of the fluid lining the alveolar epithelium in such a way that the alveolus can function normally. The surfactant is believed to form a film about 50 angstroms in thickness on the surface of the alveolar lining fluid.[6] Although highly insoluble, this lipoprotein is freely permeable to all gases.

The origin of this surface active material is the alveolar type II cells. It is also believed that the substance is constantly produced and extruded onto the surface lining and that this surface lining fluid is continuously being mobilized and/or destroyed. This means that normal alveolar function is greatly dependent upon the *continuous* production and secretion of this surface active material.

The Thorax (Fig 1–6)

The lungs are the organ of external respiration and, in the adult, provide over 70 square meters of epithelial surface and capillary networks through which external respiration takes place. The lungs lie free in their pleural cavities and attach only at the *hilus,* where various structures enter and leave.

The liver pushes the right hemidiaphragm up, resulting in the right lung being shorter and broader than the left lung; however, the left lung has a smaller volume because the heart occupies a portion of the left thorax. The two lungs are separated by the *mediastinum,* which lies in the midline and contains the heart, great vessels, trachea, esophagus, thymus gland, lymphatic structures, and numerous nerves.

The *thoracic cage* is composed of the sternum in the midline anteriorly and thoracic vertebrae in the midline posteriorly. These two bony structures are connected by C-shaped ribs which join directly to the vertebral bodies and indirectly to the sternum by cartilage. The thorax is cone-shaped, with the smaller end of the cone near the head. The thorax houses and protects the vital organs of the cardiopulmonary system and gives support to the shoulder girdle of the skeleton. It provides attachment for many extrinisc muscles of the upper limb, the vertebral column, and the skull.

The sternum is composed of three flat, elongated bones. The *manubrium* is the superior portion; the *body* is the midportion; and the *xiphoid process* is the inferior portion. The lower third of the body of the sternum is reasonably mobile; it is this portion which is compressed for closed chest cardiac massage.

There are twelve pairs of ribs and costal cartilages. The first seven ribs are called the "true ribs," since they articulate through costal cartilages directly with the sternum. The last five pairs of ribs articulate with the rib above through costal cartilages but are not directly connected with the sternum.

The thoracic vertebral column is composed of twelve bony verte-

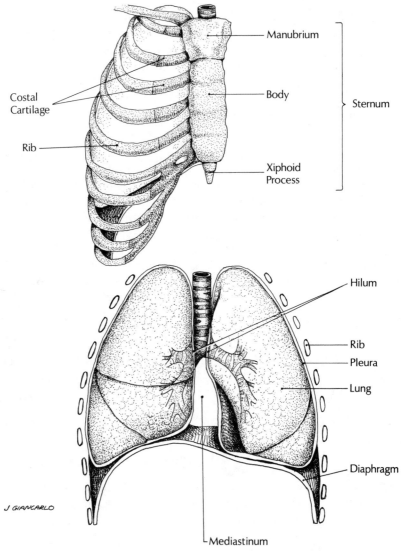

Fig 1–6. — Significant structural relationships of the thorax.

brae separated by intervertebral disks of a spongy nature. These disks act as "shock absorbers" and protect the numerous nerves entering and leaving the spinal canal.

Muscles of Ventilation

Air is moved in and out of the lungs as the volume of the thoracic cavity increases and decreases. This volume change is accomplished by the action of muscles on the bony structures of the thorax. There are three major groups of muscles of ventilation: the diaphragm, the intercostal muscles, and the accessory muscles of ventilation.

The Diaphragm

The *diaphragm* separates the thoracic cavity from the abdominal cavity. It is composed of two muscular hemidiaphragms connected by a membranous portion in the midline. Its origin and insertion is on the interior surface of the lower ribs. Normally, the center portion of the hemidiaphragms is domed upward, toward the head, because of the greater intra-abdominal pressure in relation to the intrathoracic pressure.

The motor innervation of the diaphragm originates from the spinal cord via the third through fifth cervical roots, which combine to form the *phrenic nerve.* Contraction of the muscle fibers causes the domes of the diaphragm to be pulled down, thereby increasing the volume of the thoracic cavity.

The diaphragm is the major muscle of ventilation. The normal excursion of the diaphragm is approximately 1.5 cm, which can be increased to as much as 7 or 8 cm during deep breathing.[23] Although the diaphragm is the primary muscle in normal breathing, the other muscles of inspiration provide a great reserve. In some disease states, resting ventilation may be provided without significant diaphragm function.

Intercostal Muscles

The *intercostal muscles* are composed of two layers of muscle fibers connecting the ribs; these external and internal intercostals are innervated by nerves which leave the spinal cord at the levels of T_1 through T_{11}.

Contraction of the external intercostal muscles elevates the anterior end of each rib, causing the rib to be pulled upward and outward. This action increases the anteroposterior diameter of the thorax. The internal intercostals tend to pull the ribs down and in; they are believed to play a role in forceful expiration.

The intercostals are capable of maintaining a high level of ventilation on their own. These muscles do not play a major role in normal resting ventilation. It has been suggested, however, that they play a role in the normal, *smooth* transition from inspiration to expiration.

Accessory Muscles

Accessory muscles of ventilation elevate and stabilize the chest wall in its greatest diameters and thereby improve the efficiency of diaphragmatic movement. They are also capable of independently providing a reasonable degree of inspiratory activity. The major accessory muscles are the *scalene, sternocleidomastoid, trapezius,* and *pectoralis muscles.* They are not *normally* active during resting ventilation.[23]

Expiratory Muscles

Inspiration is always an active muscular event. Expiration is usually passive, depending primarily upon the elastic recoil of the lung and the chest wall. The abdominal muscles play a major part in *active* expiration. These muscles include the *external oblique,* the *rectus abdominis, internal oblique,* and *transverse abdominis* muscles. They are innervated by nerves originating from T_6 through L_1. Contraction of these muscles depresses the lower ribs, flexes the trunk, and forces the diaphragm up by increasing intra-abdominal pressure.

The Neurochemical Control of Ventilation

Since spontaneous ventilation is dependent upon the action of muscles, there must be a nervous system component to regulate ventilation. The breathing pattern can be affected both in health and disease by conscious levels of the central nervous system as well as unconscious levels. Knowledge of the *automatic* (unconscious) neurochemical control of the ventilatory cycle is essential. The primary components of this unconscious control are the central and peripheral chemoreceptors.

Central Chemoreceptors

The *respiratory center* in the midbrain contains a group of cells that will cause the nerves to the muscles of inspiration to transmit a signal. There is also a complex array of inhibitory cells affecting this "inspiratory center," and through a complex homeostatic mechanism the unconscious (automatic) regulation of inspiration and expiration occurs.

These central chemoreceptor cells are primarily influenced by the chemical composition of cerebrospinal fluid (C.S.F.). The cerebrospinal fluid differs from blood in its lack of hydrogen ion buffers (e.g., hemoglobin). Since carbon dioxide freely diffuses between blood and cerebrospinal fluid, a given PCO_2 change will result in a hydrogen ion concentration change in the cerebrospinal fluid. In response to an increase in hydrogen ion concentration (decrease in pH) of the cerebrospinal fluid, the central chemoreceptors stimulate the inspiratory center as well as the vasomotor center.[24]

Thus, *the normal neurochemical control of the ventilatory cycle is that of the arterial PCO_2 and its effect on the cerebrospinal fluid pH.* The normal response will be an increase in depth followed shortly by an increase in rate.[24] The vasomotor center is stimulated to increase cardiac output and increase peripheral vascular resistance.

Peripheral Chemoreceptors

There are chemoreceptors located on the aortic arch and at the bifurcation of the internal and external carotid arteries which are called the *aortic and carotid bodies.* These small, specialized neural bundles are extremely vascular and have a metabolic rate and oxygen consumption per gram of tissue far in excess of any other tissues in the body. This makes these tissues extremely sensitive to decreases in *oxygen supply.* When oxygen supply to this tissue decreases, the tissue PO_2 decreases and the central respiratory center is stimulated.[24]

The carotid and aortic bodies can be stimulated by low PO_2's, decreased blood flow, decreased hemoglobin content, decreased hemoglobin saturation, greatly increased PCO_2's, increased hydrogen ion concentrations, and methemoglobin. *For all practical clinical purposes one can think of the peripheral chemoreceptors as responding to decreased oxygen supply.*

Stimulation of these bodies causes (1) increased tidal volume and ventilatory rate; (2) tachycardia (increase in heart rate); (3) systemic arterial hypertension (increase in blood pressure); (4) increase in bronchial smooth muscle tone; (5) increase in pulmonary vascular resistance; (6) increase in the secretions of the adrenal gland; and (7) increase in activity of the cerebral cortex.[24] Some studies have reported constriction of lung vessels and, occasionally, bradycardia. Again, *for all practical purposes, it can be considered that stimulation of the peripheral chemoreceptors increases minute ventilation and cardiac output.*

It is essential that the differences and interrelationships of the peripheral and central chemoreceptors be understood. The central chemoreceptors will respond to changes in arterial carbon dioxide tension of 1 mm Hg, whereas peripheral chemoreceptors will not respond to carbon dioxide tension changes of less than 10 mm Hg.[24] Central chemoreceptors do not respond to low oxygen tensions in the arterial blood. If blood flow, pH, PCO_2, and hemoglobin content are normal, the PO_2 must fall below 60 mm Hg before the peripheral chemoreceptors will respond.[24] It takes from 2 to 3 minutes for the central chemoreceptors to show a response to an increase in CO_2 tension of 6 mm Hg, whereas a CO_2 increase of 15 mm Hg will elicit a response in 1 second. Excessively high carbon dioxide tension in the arterial blood eventually depresses rather than stimulates the central chemoreceptors.

The Autonomic Nervous System

The autonomic nervous system is that part of the total body homeostatic mechanism that is concerned with nonvoluntary (reflex) function. This system is divided into two antagonistic systems: the sympathetic and parasympathetic.

Sympathetic System

The sympathetic (adrenergic) nervous system is that portion of the autonomic nervous system that causes the "fright and flight" response. It can be thought of as the initial response of the body to stress. There are two adrenergic receptors: alpha and beta. These were named because if epinephrine (Adrenalin) is injected into a dog, the blood pressure response is at first an increase followed by a decrease. The increase in blood pressure was labeled the "alpha" response, and the decrease in blood pressure the "beta" response (see Fig 13–2).

ALPHA RESPONSE. — The alpha response is due to receptors in the smooth muscle of the arterioles causing constriction. In general, the alpha-adrenergic response is increased peripheral vascular resistance (see Chapter 2).

BETA RESPONSE. — The prime function of the beta-adrenergic system is on the heart and the lungs. Beta-1 activity causes an increased strength in the myocardial fibers along with an increase in cardiac rate; beta-2 response causes dilation of the bronchial smooth musculature (bronchodilation).

Parasympathetic System

The parasympathetic nervous system releases a chemical called *acetylcholine* at the nerve endings. There are two portions to the parasympathetic nervous system: the muscarinic and nicotinic systems.

MUSCARINIC SYSTEM. — The muscarinic effect is primarily seen in organ systems innervated by the tenth cranial nerve (the vagus nerve). It causes a slowing effect of the heart rate as well as increased muscular activity in the gastrointestinal tract and increased activity in salivary gland secretion. Its effects are blocked by the drug atropine.

NICOTINIC SYSTEM.—The nicotinic effect deals with the motor nerves to the skeletal muscles of the body. The skeletal muscles are the voluntary, consciously controlled muscles. The nicotinic effect is important because most of the pharmacologic muscle relaxants act upon the nicotinic receptors.

2 • CARDIOVASCULAR ANATOMY AND PHYSIOLOGY

ALTHOUGH MAN'S KNOWLEDGE is embarrassingly meager in the biochemical and biophysical phenomena of cellular life, it has been known for over two centuries that oxygen must be continuously supplied to the cell and carbon dioxide continuously removed from the cellular environment in order for life processes to continue. This process of gas exchanging across permeable cellular membranes is defined as *respiration*. Although the field of respiratory care is commonly thought of in terms of the pulmonary system, one cannot deal with respiratory processes without a thorough appreciation and understanding of the cardiovascular system. Since the purpose of this text is to provide a firm foundation for the practitioners of respiratory care, it becomes essential to deal with the function and physiology of the cardiovascular system in some detail. We may consider a general approach to the cardiovascular system as being concerned with three component parts: (1) the heart (cor); (2) the blood vessels (conduits); and (3) the intravascular volume (content). If one has a basic knowledge of these "three C's" (cor, conduits, content), the ability to deal with the cardiovascular system in relation to respiratory care is greatly enhanced.

The *heart* is an organ designed to impart energy to the blood in sufficient quantity to provide circulation throughout the vascular system. The heart should be considered as two pumps in a series. Two pumps are necessary since there are two capillary systems that must be dealt with: the systemic circulation and the pulmonary circulation. The systemic circulation services the vast majority of tissues and, therefore, requires a higher driving pressure. Thus, the left heart must produce enough energy to supply this far-reaching vascular system. On the other hand, the right heart must produce only enough energy to circulate the blood through the smaller pulmonary circuit; this requires a lower driving pressure.[25]

The *conduits* are a series of vessels allowing rapid transit of blood away from the heart and back again. The arterial portion of the circulation is defined as those conduits that carry blood *away* from the heart and toward the capillary beds. The capillaries (microcirculation) allow exchange of gases, water, salts, nutrients, metabolites, and other substances across permeable membranes. In the systemic circulation this exchange is between blood and tissues, and in the pulmonary circulation it is between the blood and the atmosphere. The venous circulation is essentially a collecting system which allows for the return of blood to the heart. It is the low-pressure portion of the conduit system and contains the bulk of the blood volume. Unlike arteries, the veins are capable of having great changes in volume with little change in pressure — they are referred to as "capacitance" vessels.[26]

The *content* of the vascular system is the blood, a liquid medium with a large assortment of particles ranging all the way from molecular to microscopic to just subvisual in size. The blood is involved in numerous complex functions and has numerous physical properties such as (1) osmotic factors; (2) ionic particles demanding a moment-to-moment state of electric neutrality; (3) various dissolved gases; (4) hydrostatic pressure relationships; and (5) permeability relationships, to mention a few.

The Heart

Anatomy

The heart is a hollow, muscular organ enclosed in a membrane called the *pericardium*. Three layers comprise the heart muscle wall: (1) an outer layer called the *epicardium;* (2) a middle layer called the *myocardium;* and (3) an inner layer called the *endocardium*. This inner layer is lined by squamous endothelial cells which are continuous with the endothelial lining of the major blood vessels attaching to the heart.

The heart is composed of four separate chambers (Fig 2–1). The two atria are thin, muscle wall structures which act as collecting chambers for the veins. In addition, the atria supplement the delivery of blood to the ventricles by contracting at the appropriate time. The two ventricles have thick, muscular walls and are the basic pumping chambers of the heart. The right and left heart — each composed of an atrium and ventricle — are separated by walls of fibrous and muscular tissue. The separating walls are called the intra-atrial and intraventricular septa.

Blood Supply

The nutrient supply of the heart is via the *coronary arteries,* which originate from the aorta at its junction with the left ventricle. The

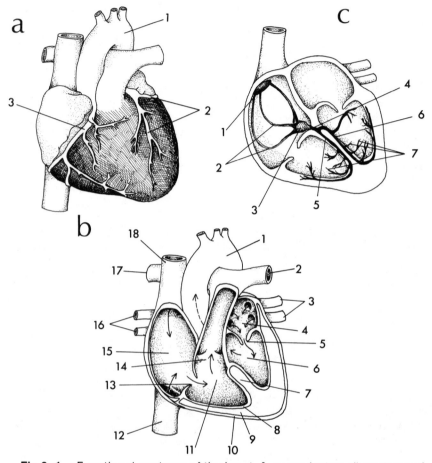

Fig 2–1. — Functional anatomy of the heart. **A,** gross (external) anatomy of the heart: *1,* aorta; *2,* left coronary artery; and *3,* right coronary artery. **B,** functional anatomy of the heart: *1,* aorta; *2,* left pulmonary artery; *3,* pulmonary veins from left lung; *4,* left atrium; *5,* mitral valve; *6,* left ventricle; *7,* intraventricular septum; *8,* endocardium; *9,* myocardium; *10,* epicardium; *11,* right ventricle; *12,* inferior vena cava; *13,* tricuspid valve; *14,* pulmonary semilunar valves; *15,* right atrium; *16,* pulmonary veins from right lung; *17,* right pulmonary artery; and *18,* superior vena cava. **C,** anatomy of the specialized myocardial conducting system: *1,* SA node; *2,* specialized atrial conducting tracts; *3,* AV node; *4,* bundle of His; *5,* right bundle branch; *6,* left bundle branch; and *7,* Purkinje's fibers.

openings to the coronary arteries lie within the cusps of the aortic valve and depend upon the pressure in the aorta, primarily during the diastolic period, for their perfusing pressure. This corresponds to the relaxed state, or diastolic period, of the heart, during which time most heart perfusion occurs. Major venous drainage empties into the *coronary sinus* which is located in the coronary sulcus separating the ventricles from the atria. The coronary sulcus also contains the left and right coronary arteries (see Fig 2–1, A). The coronary sinus empties into the right atrium. The minor venous drainage empties directly into the right and left ventricle and is known as the thebesian veins.

Nerve Supply

The autonomic nervous system has a role in regulating the heart rate. The *vagus nerve,* part of the parasympathetic system, slows the heart rate. The cardioaccelerator nerves, part of the sympathetic system, increase the rate and strength of contraction of both the atria and the ventricles.

Functional Anatomy

The functional anatomy of the heart can be described in terms of the normal transit of blood through its chambers (see Fig 2–1, B). Venous blood returns from the systemic circulation through two main channels: the superior and inferior venae cavae. Both of these structures empty into the right atrium. The right atrium is separated from the right ventricle by the *tricuspid valve.* The right ventricle empties into the pulmonary artery through the *pulmonary valve.* From the pulmonary artery, the blood flows through the pulmonary circulation, eventually reaching the pulmonary veins.

The left atrium contains the openings of the four pulmonary veins. The left atrium empties into the left ventricle through a bicuspid valve called the *mitral valve.* The outlet of the left ventricle is through the *aortic valve* into the aorta — the main artery of the body. The cusps of the aortic valve are important since this is where the right and left coronary arteries originate.

During contraction (systole), the tricuspid and mitral valves are closed while the pulmonary and aortic valves are open, allowing the ventricles to pump blood into the pulmonary artery and the aorta, respectively. During relaxation (diastole), the tricuspid and mitral valves are open while the pulmonary and aortic valves are closed, allowing blood to flow from the atria into the ventricle. During diastole the aortic pressure is responsible for supplying the majority of flow through the coronary arteries to the myocardial tissue.

Histology

In addition to ordinary connective tissue cells, there are two major types of heart cells that must be distinguished: (1) the myocardial contractile cells, which are the majority of heart muscle cells; and (2) myocardial conduction cells, which have nervelike properties.[27]

The basic myocardial contractile cell is a multinucleated cell whose length varies from 30 to 60 microns, and width from 10 to 15 microns. There are abundant organelles (mitochondria) found throughout the cell, denoting its high degree of metabolic activity. Electrochemical change in the cell activates intracellular components, leading to the activation of contractile proteins. Such activation causes interdigitation of these muscle cell elements, leading to mechanical shortening. This is an example whereby *electric stimulation results in mechanical activation.*

In addition to the myocardial contractile cells, there are special cells that can initiate and efficiently conduct electric impulses. These *myocardial conduction cells* have characteristics closely resembling nervous tissue and are the cells which normally spread impulses rapidly to all areas of the heart. A major collection of these specialized cells is located in the right atrium and is referred to as the *sinoatrial (SA) node* (pacemaker of the heart). From the SA node, a group of cells referred to as specialized atrial conducting tracts conduct the impulse to the next configuration of specialized tissue, called the *atrioventricular (AV) node.* This collection of cells is located at the base of the intra-atrial septum near the tricuspid valve. A function of the AV node is to facilitate a delay in transmission of the impulse from the atria to the ventricles, allowing the atrial muscle cells to contract and augment the volume of blood delivered to the ventricles.

From the AV node, the impulse travels along a specialized tract of tissue called the bundle of His – the initial conducting tract of the ventricular system. The tract then divides into structures that are called right and left bundle branches and which continue on to the respective ventricles, dividing and subdividing into a complex fiber network and eventually ending in what are called Purkinje's fibers.

The ventricular conduction system allows a rapid and uniform distribution of electric impulses to the myocardial contractile cells. The conducting activation of the heart is normally from the inside to the outside.

Electrophysiology

The concentration of sodium and potassium ions is extremely important to the function of the myocardial muscle cell. The resting

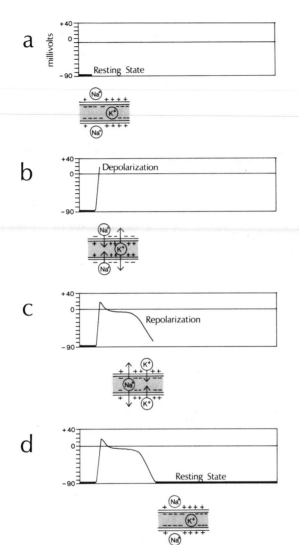

Fig 2–2. – Schematic diagram of the electrophysiology of a single myocardial cell, depicting both electrical activity and the electrolytic cellular environment. Note the horizontal axis represents time. **A** shows the resting state of repolarization – minus 90 millivolt intracellular state is primarily due to sodium (Na+) and potassium (K+) ion distribution (see text). Depolarization, **B,** occurs in response to appropriate stimulus – intracellular state becomes positive in relation to extracellular environment caused by ion changes. Repolarization, **C,** occurs as ionic distribution returns to pre-depolarization state. **D** indicates the resting state present – cell is capable of repeating process.

myocardial cell has a lesser concentration of sodium ions inside the cell than outside and a higher concentration of potassium ions inside the cell with respect to the outside (Fig 2–2). The primary cause of this distribution of ions is the active removal of sodium ions from the cell—a metabolic process referred to as the "sodium pump." Potassium ions migrate into the cell in an attempt to minimize the imbalance in intracellular electric charge. The final result of this distribution of sodium and potassium ions is still a net negative charge inside the cell with respect to the outside. This phenomenon can be measured and is termed the *negative resting membrane potential* of the cell.

When the cell membrane is stimulated, sodium ions enter at a faster rate than potassium ions leave. This results in a temporary net positive intracellular charge with respect to the outside of the cell. This process of changing the intracellular electric charge from negative to positive is called cellular *depolarization.*

After a period of time, the sodium ions are once again removed from inside the cell and the initial sodium and potassium relationships are restored. This process of changing from a positive intracellular charge to a negative one is called cellular *repolarization.*

If a sensing electrode is placed inside a cardiac muscle cell and compared with a reference electrode just outside the cell membrane, a measure of the electric charge across the cell membrane can be obtained. In this manner the process of depolarization and repolarization can be measured in terms of an electric voltage (millivolts). Such a measurement is illustrated in Figure 2–3. A resting membrane potential of a negative 90 millivolts is rapidly changed to a slightly positive charge of 20 millivolts during the process of depolarization. In order for a myocardial cell to respond maximally when stimulated, it must have a negative resting membrane potential of −80 to −90 millivolts.

Repolarization takes a longer time than depolarization and can be separated into two components: the absolute and the relative refractory periods. The *absolute refractory period* is the time in which effective depolarization cannot occur no matter how great the stimulus. The *relative refractory period* is when a greater than normal stimulus may cause depolarization; however, the cellular response is slower than usual.

The normal myocardial contractile cells remain at their resting membrane potential until stimulated by an adjacent cell. The baseline resting membrane potential in *specialized* myocardial conducting cells does not remain stable. The base line rises slowly (slow diastolic depolarization) and at a point called a *threshold potential,* the process

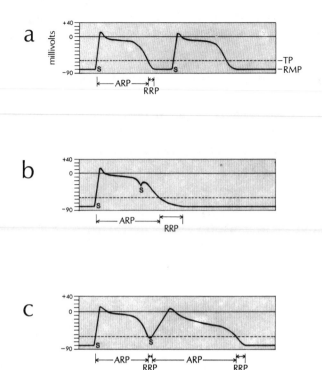

Fig 2–3. – Schematic representation of myocardial cell depolarization and repolarization patterns. The horizontal axis represents time; *ARP* is absolute refractory period; *RRP* is relative refractory period; *RMP* is resting membrane potential; *S* is point of cellular stimulus; *TP* is threshold potential. **A,** stimulation during RMP results in normal depolarization and repolarization pattern. **B,** stimulation during ARP results in absence of effective cellular response. **C,** stimulation during RRP results in a cellular response requiring a longer time period for both depolarization and repolarization.

of rapid depolarization occurs. The cell is then repolarized in a manner similar to the normal myocardial muscle cell. This process in which the cell undergoes spontaneous depolarization is defined as *automaticity*. The time interval required for the process of spontaneous depolarization and subsequent repolarization is known as the "latency interval." The shorter the latency interval, the greater the frequency with which the specialized myocardial cell depolarizes.

The cells in the SA node normally have the shortest latency interval and, therefore, become the normal pacemaker of the heart. Any specialized myocardial conduction cell in the heart has the potential of becoming a pacemaker and sometimes, under abnormal circumstances, will function in that manner.

Numerous factors determine the rate of the automatic cycle. Among these are (1) the level of the resting membrane potential; (2) the threshold potential; and (3) the time course of repolarization. Numerous pathophysiologic factors affect these variables, e.g., changes in temperature, pH, hypercarbia, hypoxia, ischemia, and stretch on the specialized tissues within the heart itself.[28]

If a sensing electrode is placed on one end of a heart muscle cell at rest and an indifferent reference electrode is placed near the other

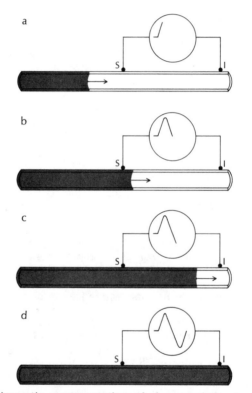

Fig 2–4.—Schematic representation of characteristic electrical response monitored by an externally applied sensing electrode *(S)* and indifferent electrode (I). Electrical potential differences between the two electrodes are graphically depicted as positive (upward) deflections and negative (downward) deflections. The shaded area represents a wave of depolarization.

In **A,** a wave of depolarization moving toward the sensing electrode produces a positive deflection on the ECG recording device. In **B** and **C,** the depolarization wave moves away from the sensing electrode, producing a negative deflection on the ECG recording device. Complete depolarization, **D,** results in a zero potential difference between the electrodes; thus the ECG recording device shows a zero reading.

side of the cell, zero potential will be recorded. When one end of the muscle cell is stimulated, a wave of depolarization will travel through the muscle cell and cause a deflection on the monitor (Fig 2–4). By convention, a deflection above the base line is considered positive and a deflection below the base line is considered negative. A wave of depolarization that is traveling toward the sensing electrode would cause a positive deflection, whereas a wave of depolarization going away from the sensing electrode would cause a negative deflection. If a wave of depolarization initially moves toward the sensing electrode and then away from the sensing electrode, it will create a positive followed by a negative deflection. This is termed a *biphasic deflection.*

Repolarization moving toward the sensing electrode will cause a negative deflection, whereas a wave of repolarization moving away from the sensing electrode will cause a positive deflection.[29]

The ECG

Standard deflections in the electric phases of the cardiac cycle are grouped in four categories: (1) ventricular depolarization; (2) ventricular repolarization; (3) atrial depolarization; and (4) atrial repolarization. The process of atrial repolarization is usually not seen since it occurs simultaneously with ventricular depolarization. As depicted in Figure 2–5, the P wave is a representation of atrial depolarization. The "QRS complex" characterizes the ventricular depolarization. By definition, the Q wave is the first negative deflection; the R wave is the first positive deflection; and the S wave is the second negative deflection. If a second positive deflection is present, it is called the R′ (R-prime) wave. It should be noted that every QRS complex does not necessarily have every individual deflection within the complex. The T wave is a reflection of ventricular repolarization.

Electrocardiographic deflections are recorded on a paper that is moving at a rate of 25 mm per second. Large divisions on the paper would represent 0.2 second, and each small division would then represent 0.04 second (see Fig 2–5). This makes it possible to look at the relationships of the electric phenomena with respect to time. The P–R interval includes both the P wave (atrial depolarization) and the P–R segment. The S–T interval includes the S–T segment and the T wave. These are the two most common intervals used in clinical electrocardiology.

It must be appreciated that the electric phenomenon recorded on the standard electrocardiogram represents the net summation of millions of myocardial fibers and their electric activity. It must be realized that *the electric activity of the heart is a related but separate enti-*

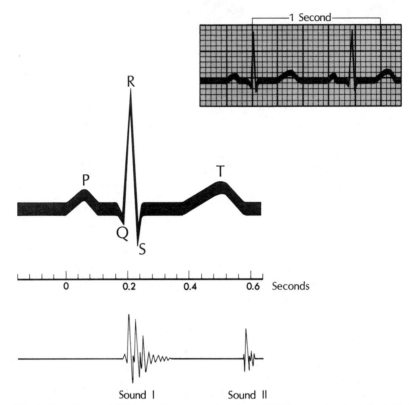

Fig 2–5.—Normal ECG pattern on standard ECG paper is depicted. Note each large square represents 0.2 second in the horizontal axis. Each small square represents 0.04 second. See text for description of normal ECG pattern.

The time relationships between electrical activity (ECG pattern) and mechanical activity (heart sounds) are depicted. Sound I (S_1) is the result of atrioventricular valve closures; sound II (S_2) is the result of the pulmonic and aortic valve closures.

ty from heart mechanics, which is evaluated by blood pressure, pulse, and heart sounds. The first heart sound (closure of the atrioventricular valves) follows the electric QRS complex, and the second heart sound (closure of the pulmonic and aortic valves) follows the T wave (see Fig 2–5). Since the electrocardiogram reflects only the electric activity of the heart, it must *not* be used as the sole assessment of the mechanical activity of the heart.

The ECG Monitor

In the field of respiratory care, the major use of the electrocardiogram is for continuous monitoring of heart rate and abnormal rhythms. The clinician involved in respiratory care must have a thorough knowledge of the use of the electrocardiographic monitor. It is strongly recommended that all respiratory care clinicians seek as much knowledge as possible in the field of electrocardiography. However, in this text, only the basics necessary for understanding the electrocardiographic monitor will be discussed.

Figure 2–6 illustrates sensing electrodes placed on the right arm, left arm, and left leg, with an indifferent electrode placed on the right leg. The interrelationship of these leads comprises the standard leads of the electrocardiogram (Einthoven's triangle). Lead I is frequently

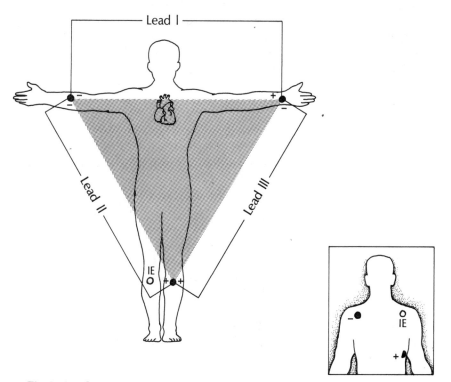

Fig 2–6.—Standard limb leads of the electrocardiogram. *IE* is the indifferent electrode. Insert demonstrates the simplified ECG monitoring used in acutely ill patients. These "chest leads" may be used in various positions to accomplish continuous ECG monitoring.

the standard ECG monitor lead, although any ECG lead is usable. In the clinical setting, the sensing electrodes are placed on the chest, since monitoring of the heart rate and rhythm is the primary requisite in respiratory care. Frequently in acutely ill patients, the leads are placed in appropriate chest positions to monitor specific myocardial rate and rhythm abnormalities.

Cardiac Arrhythmias

Cardiac arrhythmias are significant only in relation to their potential deleterious effects on the mechanical functioning of the heart. When monitoring the electrocardiogram in a critically ill patient, there are three major areas of consideration in the classification of cardiac rhythms: (1) the origin and rate of the rhythm; (2) the presence of any enhanced focus of automaticity competing with the basic rhythm; and (3) the interference with propagation and conduction of an impulse through the conduction system (conduction defects). This simplified classification of basic cardiac rhythms will be discussed in three major categories: (1) rhythms of supraventricular origin, (2) rhythms of ventricular origin, and (3) rhythms occurring in the presence of conduction defects.[30]

Supraventricular Rhythms (Fig 2–7)

Normal sinus rhythm is the rhythm found in healthy, normal people and is characterized by a proper sequence of activation of the atria and ventricles in a perfectly normal conduction system. The rate in normal

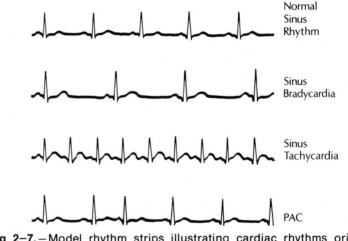

Normal
Sinus
Rhythm

Sinus
Bradycardia

Sinus
Tachycardia

PAC

Fig 2–7.—Model rhythm strips illustrating cardiac rhythms originating from above the ventricles in acutely ill patients (see text).

sinus rhythm is between 50 and 100 in adults. The term *sinus brady-cardia* is used when the ventricular rate is less than 50, but the origin and conduction of the beat are otherwise normal. The term *sinus tachy-cardia* is used when the ventricular response is greater than 100 per minute and the origin and conduction of the beat are normal. A situation called *sinus arrhythmia* occurs when there is a regular variation in the rate of sinus beats, a variation characterized by an increased rate during inspiration, and a decreased rate during expiration. Sinus arrhythmia is commonly present in children.

Atrial rhythms are characterized by abnormal P waves. The origin of the beat is not the sinus node but somewhere within the atria. A single beat from within the atria arising earlier than the normal SA beat is called a *premature atrial contraction (PAC)*. When this atrial focus gives rise to three or more beats in a row, occurring at a rapid rate, the rhythm is called an *atrial tachycardia*. A rhythm with extremely rapid atrial activity is called atrial fibrillation.

AV nodal or *junctional rhythms* originate from the area of the AV node. It was at first believed that the AV node was the actual origin, but this has subsequently been disproved. These rhythms are now referred to as junctional in origin. When this type of rhythm occurs, the atria are frequently depolarized in a reverse or retrograde fashion; therefore, the P wave often has a deflection opposite to that which would have occurred normally and is sometimes lost in the QRS complex.

Ventricular Rhythms (Fig 2–8)

Ventricular abnormal beats originate from some focus below the AV node and are characterized by a widened and bizarre-looking QRS complex. The T wave deflection is in the opposite direction to the major QRS deflection. In general, these beats are indicative of a severe state of physiologic stress. If the ventricular beat occurs prior to the expected time of a sinus beat, it is referred to as a *premature ventricular contraction (PVC)*. The frequency of these beats can be related to the severity of physiologic stress. The term *ventricular bigeminy* is used when an abnormal ventricular beat (PVC) is coupled to a normal sinus beat.

There may be several areas within the ventricles from which these abnormal beats are originating. If this occurs, the abnormal QRS complexes are different from one another. These phenomena are referred to as *multifocal premature ventricular contractions*. This is indicative of an even greater degree of physiologic stress. If these processes are allowed to continue, a situation referred to as *ventricular tachycardia*

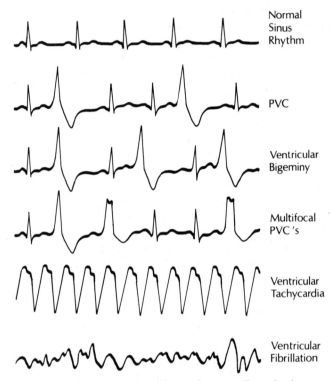

Normal Sinus Rhythm

PVC

Ventricular Bigeminy

Multifocal PVC's

Ventricular Tachycardia

Ventricular Fibrillation

Fig 2–8.—Model rhythm strips illustrating cardiac rhythms originating from the ventricles. Normal sinus rhythm is shown for reference and comparison (see text).

may eventually occur. This is defined as a ventricular rate of greater than 100, with all of the beats originating from the ventricles. By definition, three or more ventricular beats in a row are defined as "ventricular tachycardia." The major concern with ventricular tachycardia is that it can quickly deteriorate into a state called *ventricular fibrillation*. In ventricular fibrillation there is no longer any coordinated contraction of the ventricles and, thus, no mechanical output of the heart. This is immediately life threatening and requires external cardiac massage and electric defibrillation.

Conduction Defects

Technically, a conduction defect could occur anywhere along the entire conducting system. In respiratory care, we are primarily concerned with conduction defects interfering with the function of the ventricles. The interference with conduction at the AV node is referred to as "AV block." A *first degree AV block* can be thought of as requiring a prolonged time for propagation of the impulse through the AV node. This is seen in the electrocardiogram as a prolonged P–R interval; however, every single beat is conducted into the ventricles. Further progression of the abnormality results in a *second degree AV block* in which not every supraventricular beat is conducted through to the ventricles. The final degree in this abnormality is when none of the supraventricular beats are conducted through into the ventricles – a phenomenon termed *third degree AV block* (complete heart block). The atria in this situation are stimulated at their own rate. This basic rhythm is termed an idioventricular rhythm and the ventricular rate is very slow (30–50/min).

Cardiac Mechanics

The heart is functionally two pumps that are subject to the basic laws of mechanics. There are numerous physiologic variables determining how effectively the heart will respond to its workload. Extreme simplification of this complex subject results in two major factors that affect mechanical function as long as myocardial oxygenation is adequate: fiber length and the fiber contractility state.[31]

Within limits, the greater the initial fiber length, the greater is the muscle's ability to shorten. This means the muscle has a greater capability of contracting against a greater force. The individual cardiac muscle-cell fiber lengths must increase as the blood volume in the ventricle increases. The most important ventricular blood volume is that which is present at the end of diastole. Functionally, the greater the end-diastolic volume, the greater the ventricular muscle's ability to contract and pump the necessary volume. Of course, this mechanism has limits beyond which it can no longer be regarded as a compensation. This relationship of heart muscle function with respect to end-diastolic volume and ability to pump is called the Frank-Starling relationship.[32]

The capability of a heart muscle cell to contract against any given load can be compared by using the contractile state of the muscle as the theoretic zero load. *Positive inotropism* refers to an increase in the contractility state; *negative inotropism* refers to a decrease in the contractility state. Positive inotropism can be related to certain physiologic phenomena such as adequate tissue oxygen supply and appropriate acid-base environment. Pharmacologic agents, such as calcium ions, digitalis, epinephrine, and norepinephrine, can also create a state of increased inotropism. The net effect of these changes usually results in a greater volume output in a shorter period of time.

Negative inotropism usually results in less volume output over a longer period of time. It is caused by such pathophysiologic factors as hypoxia, acidemia, hypercarbia. In addition, pharmacologic agents such as propranolol (a beta blocker); anesthetic agents; and some pharmacologic antiarrhythmics can cause negative inotropism.

Considering the over-all function of the heart as a pump, the changes in ventricular end-diastolic volume and its effect on the stroke volume can be expressed in a concept known as *preload*. This can be thought of as an initial loading force, and it is influenced by such factors as (1) circulating blood volume; (2) state of venous tone; (3) the state of contractility of the ventricle; and (4) mechanical restriction to inflow.

Another factor affecting the heart's performance as a pump is the force against which the heart must work. This is commonly termed the *afterload*. The ventricles pump against a mechanical impedance, which is a function of both compliance and resistance properties of the vascular system and any mechanical restriction to outflow.

The Vascular System

Circulation can be defined as the dynamic process of circuital blood flow through the heart and blood vessels. The necessary energy for this process is derived from the heart. The vascular system may be considered as having two major subdivisions: the systemic and pulmonary circulations. The systemic circulation starts from the aorta (output vessel of the left ventricle) and ends in the right atrium; the pulmonary circulation starts from the pulmonary artery (output vessel of the right ventricle) and ends in the left atrium. Each circulatory system is composed of arteries, capillaries, and veins. Arteries are conduits that carry blood away from the heart. Capillaries are vessels in which gas exchange takes place. Veins are conduits that collect blood from the capillaries and carry it back to the heart.

The arterial systems are composed of a main artery (the aorta or pulmonary artery) which branches into large arteries, which subsequently branch into smaller arteries, which eventually branch into arterioles. The arterioles are the major *resistance* vessels. The arteries function as the major conducting vessels, and the arterioles regulate the distribution of blood to the various capillary beds.

The capillary beds are the portions of the circulatory system where gas exchange (respiration) takes place. This gas exchange in the systemic circulation is called *internal respiration* (exchange between tissue and blood). The gas exchange in the pulmonary circulation is called *external respiration* (exchange between blood and air). The capillary bed is a complex network of vessels and is referred to as the *microcirculation*. The flow within the capillary bed is primarily regulated by metarterioles, blood vessel channels containing muscle tissue called precapillary sphincters. It is these sphincters that control the actual distribution of blood flow within the capillary beds. Certain capillary channels within the network receive a more consistent flow and are commonly referred to as "preferential channels." *True capillaries* are believed to be vessels without muscle tone, existing solely to allow gas exchange.

Unlike the arteries, the veins are capable of large volume changes without great changes in pressure; thus, they are called *capacitance* vessels. The initial collecting vessels (venules) join to form small veins, which in turn join to form larger veins. The large veins join to form the major veins leading to the heart: the venae cavae and pulmonary veins. The venous system is capable of changing muscle tone within the vessels. The greatest percentage (up to 70%) of the total blood volume is contained within these capacitance vessels, underlining their important role in circulation.

Histology (Fig 2-9)

The conduits are composed of from one layer to many layers of tissue, depending upon the location of the vessel within the circulation. All vessels have an *endothelial* lining which consists of a single layer of flattened cells providing a smooth inner surface. This is the only layer of the capillaries, and it is capable of selective permeability to substances such as water, electrolytes, sugars, and gases.

Elastic fibers are found in all vessels except the capillaries. These elastic fibers form a layer just under the endothelial lining and resist the distending force of the intraluminal pressure, producing a tension within the vessel wall. *Collagen fibers* are found primarily in the arterial system. They also produce a tension in the vessel wall but are stiff, rigid, and resist stress many times that of the elastic fibers.

A circumferential layer of *smooth muscle* that can produce active tension is found in the arterial system. This smooth muscle layer is under the control of the sympathetic nervous system. There are both alpha and beta receptors on these muscle cells. Stimulation of the alpha receptors causes vascular constriction; stimulation of the beta receptors causes vascular dilatation.

The tension produced by the smooth muscle layer in the arterial system is referred to as *vasomotor tone*. A similar phenomenon is pres-

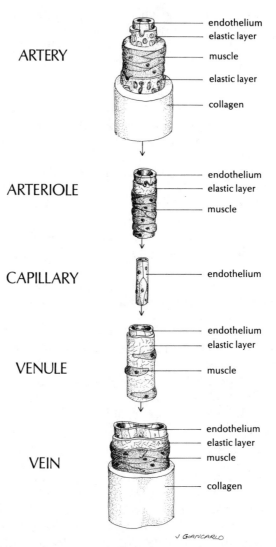

Fig 2–9.—Schematic representation of anatomic structures and relationships of components of major types of blood vessels (see text).

ent to a lesser degree in the venous system and is termed *venomotor tone*. The maintenance of proper blood vessel tone is dependent upon the degree of tension developed by the elastic and collagen fibers within the vessel wall and the degree of active smooth muscle tone in the vessel.

Arterial Blood Pressure

The right and left ventricles supply the energy to push blood through the conduit system. There is a progressive loss of energy as blood flows through the circulating vessels. The factor that causes this loss of energy is frictional resistance between blood and the vessel walls. This is demonstrated by a progressive drop in pressure. Therefore, in order for blood to flow through the vascular system and back to the heart, an adequate force must be developed (driving pressure). Without an adequate driving pressure, the frictional resistance of the system would not be overcome and circulation would cease. A significant factor determining frictional resistance through a given length of vessel is the radius of the vessel. According to Poiseuille's law, if we decrease the radius by one-half, we will increase the resistance to flow through that vessel by a factor of 16. The resistance increases by the fourth power of the radius.

The physical laws of hydrostatics must be appreciated to understand the concept of "blood pressure."[33] Pascal's first law of hydrostatics states that at every point in a fluid system there is a force which acts equally in all directions. This force is known as *hydrostatic pressure.* Pascal's second law of hydrostatics states that the pressure is the same at all points at the same level. His third law states that all fluids are affected by gravity—the pressure increases with depth and decreases with height above a known reference point.

These relationships are extremely important in clinical practice, since changes in posture will affect blood pressure measurements as related to predetermined reference points. This becomes even more important when the blood pressure measurements are assumed to estimate the blood flow.

As shown in Figure 2–10, when a patient lies in a supine (flat) position, the middle cerebral artery, aortic root, and dorsalis pedis artery will be at the same level. The pressure at the aortic root is illustrated as being 100 mm Hg, and the blood pressure at both the middle cerebral artery and the dorsalis pedis artery is 90 mm Hg. The drop in blood pressure is due to frictional resistance—there is no gravitation difference. When the patient is placed in a sitting position, the vascular reflexes cause changes in vascular tone. This allows the same distribution of blood flow as in the supine position. The pressure at the aortic root remains 100 mm Hg; however, the middle cerebral artery pressure is 70 mm Hg. This represents a real drop of 10 mm Hg as a result of frictional resistance and 20 mm Hg because of gravity. The dorsalis pedis pressure is higher than that at the aortic root. It lies 70

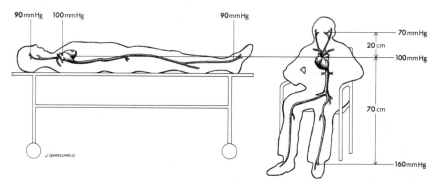

Fig 2–10.—Driving pressure interrelationships and the effect of gravity on measured blood pressure (see text). Measured blood pressures are shown at the middle cerebral artery, aortic root, and dorsalis pedis artery in both the supine and sitting person.

cm below the reference point and, therefore, has a 70 mm Hg gain in measured lateral wall pressure because of gravity. A 10 mm Hg loss in pressure caused by frictional resistance results in a pressure of 160 mm Hg.

It must be kept clearly in mind that lateral wall pressures are not to be confused with driving pressures. In all of the examples just given, the driving pressures have dropped 10 mm Hg from the aortic root to either the middle cerebral or dorsalis pedis arteries. The measurement of lateral wall pressures is very much dependent upon gravity and the basilar reference point. However, blood flow does not result from differences measured in lateral wall pressures, but rather from differences in driving pressures.

When dealing with the measurements of blood pressure, we must keep in mind the differences between the measurements of lateral wall pressures and driving pressures. Lateral wall pressures are obtained in the classic fashion by occluding a vessel with an external pressure and gradually releasing it until the vessel pressure reasserts its dominance and flow is reestablished. To be meaningful, lateral wall pressures must be expressed in terms from a known reference point.

Driving pressure has to do with the direction of blood flow and refers to changes in total pressure energy. This includes the effects of gravitation and the kinetic energy, along with lateral wall pressures.

Capillary Blood Flow

Transmural pressure is defined as the difference between intraluminal pressure and the tissue pressure immediately surrounding the vessel. Transmural pressure is of academic interest in arteries and veins. But it is of vital importance in the microcirculatory system because the capillaries are permeable to many elements of blood and there must be concern about the factors that maintain the vascular volume within the vascular space in these vessels.

The arterioles represent the greatest area of resistance in the vascular system. Thus, a great drop in pressure is observed distal to the arterioles. This, then, allows us to assume that there would be a relatively low intraluminal pressure in the capillaries. This assumption is borne out by the observation that the arterial side of the capillary bed demonstrates an intraluminal hydrostatic pressure of 30–35 mm Hg, whereas the venous side of the capillary bed demonstrates an intraluminal hydrostatic pressure of 15–20 mm Hg. Thus, the driving pressure through the systemic capillary beds is approximately 15–20 mm Hg.

These intraluminal pressures present in the capillaries are far in excess of normal tissue hydrostatic pressures. This fact raises an essential question that must be answered satisfactorily: What are the factors that maintain the vascular volume within the capillaries in spite of intracapillary pressures far exceeding the tissue pressures?

Hydrostatic pressure tends to force blood contents from the capillaries into the tissues. There are three factors that play a role in countering the forces of hydrostatic pressure: (1) blood osmotic pressure; (2) capillary membrane stability; and (3) tissue pressure in the systemic capillaries and alveolar pressure in the pulmonary capillaries.

The microcirculation must have a means of regulating blood flow, since various tissues demand different degrees of perfusion at various times. This ability of the microcirculation to regulate blood flow is an extremely important mechanism, one that is consistently challenged in the critically ill patient. Figure 2–11 depicts a model unit in the capillary system showing the existence of arteriovenous (A-V) anastomoses. This is essentially a short-circuiting device in which blood may flow directly from the arterial to the venous system without entering the microcirculation. This process is often referred to as *peripheral arterial-to-venous shunting.*

The *metarteriole* is a vessel with active sphincters having the capability of regulating blood flow through the capillary bed. A thoroughfare channel is the main capillary, and it is the basic path of blood flow when there is only a small or moderate need for flow through that particular tissue. When greater tissue perfusion is needed, the true capillaries are perfused by changes in capillary sphincter tone. The regulation of blood through the microcirculatory system is an extremely complex process and incompletely understood at the present time.

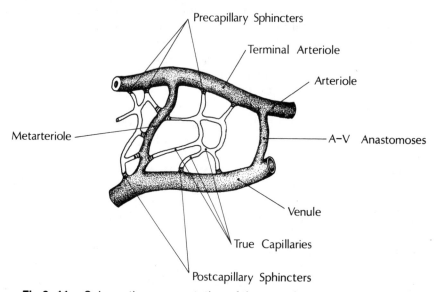

Fig 2–11. – Schematic representation of the vascular components involved in the regulation of blood flow through the systemic capillary beds (the microcirculation). See text for discussion.

What is understood is that it is basically a self-regulating system that allows the essential exchange of nutrients and metabolites in the capillary bed while maintaining the essential relationship between vascular volume and vascular space. This self-regulating system is termed *microcirculatory vasomotion* and is mediated primarily by blood components such as amines, polypeptides, proteolytic enzymes, and tissue metabolites.

Venous Blood Flow

The collecting portion of the vascular system is composed of *capacitance vessels*, i.e., vessels that can accept great changes in blood volume without extreme changes in lateral wall pressure. Venous blood flow to the heart from portions of the body that lie above the heart is primarily accomplished by gravity. However, in the erect or sitting position, the majority of arterial blood flow is to gravity-dependent areas of the body. The venous system is capable of exerting a certain degree of venomotor tone, but venous blood flow to the heart from gravity-dependent areas of the body is regulated by three factors: (1) tissue pressures, (2) the venous valvular system, and (3) body cavity pressures.

Venous return from the legs is primarily provided by extraluminal pressure of tissues, since the deep veins of the legs are surrounded by muscular structures. In addition, these veins have one-way valves which do not allow retrograde flow. When these valves are competent, the muscular movements of the lower extremities provide a "milking" action which forces blood toward the heart. If these valves become incompetent, they cause blood flow to stagnate and the veins to dilate; such veins are called varicose veins.

Upon entering the pelvic and abdominal region, venous blood flow depends primarily upon intra-abdominal pressures exceeding intra-thoracic pressures.

It should be obvious that in order for these mechanisms of venous return to the heart to act appropriately, there must be an adequate blood volume filling the venous vascular space. *These factors of vascular volume-to-vascular space relationships, and intra-abdominal-to-intrathoracic pressures are extremely significant factors in the field of respiratory care.*

It is extremely important to realize that 65–70% of the blood volume is contained within the venous systems. Thus, the arteries provide the resistance vessels and play a great role in the distribution of the blood flow; the capillaries are responsible for carrying out respiration itself; the venous systems contain the greatest portion of blood in the vascular system. The venous systems are extremely important in effective circulation.

The Blood

We have thus far considered the pump (cor) and the vascular system (conduits). We must now consider the third element in the cardiovascular system—the blood (content).[34] Total body fluid is generally divided into two compartments: intracellular and extracellular. Extracellular fluid is, in turn, divided into (1) interstitial fluid (fluid outside cells and outside the vascular system) and (2) intravascular fluid (blood volume).

The blood is defined as the body fluid that is contained within the vascular system. Approximately 13% of the total blood volume is contained in the heart, spleen, liver, and other undefined reservoirs. The remaining portion of the total blood volume is contained within the vascular system itself. Of this vascular volume, approximately 30% is contained in the pulmonary circulation and 70% in the systemic circulation.

In the adult, the blood volume is equal to 5.5–7.5% of total body weight in kilograms. In other words, there is approximately 55–75 ml of blood per kilogram of normal body weight. This relationship is somewhat decreased in females and obese people, and increased in children, infants, and muscular or thin people.

The function of the blood is to transport vital nutrients to tissues and to transport metabolic waste products away from tissues. It is through the blood that the cells of the body are maintained in a milieu allowing normal metabolic processes to proceed. In general, we may list some of the more important elements of transport, such as oxygen, carbon dioxide, carbohydrates, fats, and proteins. In addition, the blood is responsible for the transport of water, electrolytes, and metabolites such as urea nitrogen and creatinines.

The blood is composed of formed elements and liquid elements. These are commonly referred to as "fractions" of the blood. The formed elements are primarily cellular, e.g., the red blood cells and white blood cells. The *hematocrit* is defined as the percentage of the blood that is occupied by cellular elements.

If the cellular elements are removed, the remaining liquid is called *plasma*. If blood is allowed to clot, the liquid portion that remains after the clot has formed is called *serum*. Serum is essentially plasma from which fibrinogen, platelets, and other clotting components have been removed.

When measured by weight, plasma is composed of 90% water, 7% plasma proteins, and 3% organic and inorganic substances. It contains cations (sodium, potassium, calcium, and magnesium) as well as anions (chloride, bicarbonate, and phosphate). All of these ions are important in the maintenance of cellular homeostasis and are referred to as *electrolytes*.

Plasma proteins are too large to pass freely through the permeable walls of capillaries and, therefore, are the main determinant of the *colloid osmotic pressure*. As discussed previously, this is the basic force that maintains the balance of water between the intravascular and the extravascular (interstitial) space. The proteins are composed of albumins, which have molecular weights of about 69,000; globulins, which are larger molecules; fibrinogen, which is a very large molecule; and lipoproteins.

The primary agent for maintaining colloid osmotic pressure is the serum albumin. Total osmotic pressure (in contradistinction to colloid osmotic pressure) is a function not only of the plasma proteins but of electrolytes and other substances, such as sugar and urea.

The red blood cell is a biconcave disk which is just slightly smaller than the true capillary. It measures approximately 8.5 microns in length by 2 microns in width. It originates in the bone marrow and has an average life span of approximately 100–120 days. The red blood cell contains *hemoglobin*, which is principally responsible for the oxygen reserve in blood and one of the major buffering mechanisms for carbon dioxide and hydrogen ions.[35]

3 • THE MECHANICS OF VENTILATION

THERE CAN BE NO ARGUMENT that the lungs exist solely for the purpose of exchanging gases between the blood and the atmosphere—a process known as *external respiration*. The evaluation and support of external respiration is the basis of all respiratory care. The goal is to assure proper interrelationship between the two requisites for external respiration: pulmonary blood flow and gas movement in and out of the lungs. *The process of gas movement in and out of the pulmonary system is defined as ventilation.* To apply the principles of respiratory care one must understand the mechanics of ventilation and what is involved in its artificial support.

In general, medical disciplines approach the process of ventilation from a physiologic and pathophysiologic viewpoint. Although this knowledge is essential in respiratory care, it is not adequate in and of itself. The respiratory care clinician must be concerned with the *mechanics* of ventilation as well as the physiology. To approach this broad and complex subject, we have chosen to discuss the subject in five sections: (1) the lung-thorax relationship; (2) the physics of ventilation; (3) the pulmonary function studies; (4) the work of breathing; and (5) the mechanical support of ventilation.

The Lung-Thorax Relationship

At the very root of understanding the mechanics of ventilation is the necessity for a thorough knowledge of the manner in which muscular energy exerted on the thoracic cage is transmitted into molecular movement of gases in and out of the thoracic cavity via the pulmonary tree. The entire mechanism is based on the simple fact that *there exist elastic forces in lung tissue and chest wall tissue.*

Elasticity is the property of matter causing it to return to its resting state after deformation by some external force. At the end of a normal expiration there are chest wall elastic forces tending to expand the intrathoracic volume. These forces are balanced by lung tissue elastic forces tending to reduce the intrathoracic volume (Fig 3–1). The communication linking these two opposing forces is the *pleura,* its visceral layer attached to lung and its parietal layer attached to the

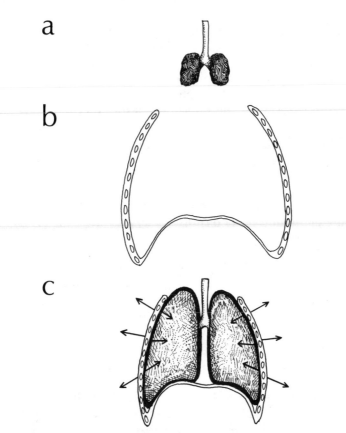

Fig 3–1.—**A** represents resting state of normal lungs when removed from the chest cavity; i.e., elasticity causes total collapse. **B** represents resting state of normal chest wall and diaphragm when apex is open to atmosphere and the thoracic contents removed. **C** represents end expiration in the normal, intact thorax. Note that elastic forces of lung and chest wall are in opposite directions. The pleural surfaces link these two opposing forces (see text).

chest wall. The visceral and parietal pleurae are held together by a film of fluid in a manner similar to two glass microscope slides that are wet and stuck together. The slides can readily move back and forth but resist being pulled apart.

The "pleural space" is in reality a *potential* space between two layers of pleura that is normally occupied by a small amount of fluid. This pleural fluid acts as a lubricant to decrease friction as the pleural layers slide along one another. The parietal pleura is attached to the interior wall of the thorax and moves with the chest wall. The visceral pleura (lining the lung) moves along the thoracic wall because of its adherence to the parietal pleura. The same mechanism is simultaneously expanding lung tissue as the diaphragm descends.

The average resting intrapleural pressure is approximately 4–5 cm of water less than the atmospheric pressure. This subatmospheric pressure is a result of the opposing elastic forces of the thorax and lung. During a strong inspiratory effort against a closed glottis, the average intrapleural pressure can drop to as low as negative 50 cm of water subatmospheric. On the other hand, during a forced expiration, the intrapleural pressure may rise to as high as positive 70 cm of water above atmospheric.[36]

Gas flows in response to pressure gradients (ΔP). In the lung this pressure gradient is termed *transairway pressure* – the pressure difference between mouth and alveolus.

$$\Delta P \text{ (transpulmonary pressure)} = P_{mouth} - P_{alveoli}$$

Transairway pressures must equal zero at end inspiration and end expiration, since flow has stopped at both these points in time.

Transpulmonary pressure (see Fig 21–1) is the pressure difference between mouth and intrapleural pressure. In the spontaneously breathing patient, inspiration occurs when the normal resting balance of equal and opposite forces exerted by the thorax and the lungs is changed. The muscles of ventilation upset this balance and cause the thorax to enlarge and the diaphragm to descend. Since the two pleural layers normally are not separated, some increase in subatmospheric pressure in the intrapleural space results. This increased transpulmonary pressure is associated with a decreased intra-alveolar pressure (below atmospheric), creating a positive transairway pressure. Assuming a patent airway, air flows into the lung until transairway pressure equals zero. With the cessation of active muscle effort at the end of inspiration, the elastic forces in the lung and chest dominate and result in supra-atmospheric alveolar pressure, creating a negative transairway pressure. Thus, gas flows out of the lungs until once again transairway pressure equals zero.

Physics of Ventilation

The Principle of Elastance

Elastic forces can most simply be defined as the forces acting to return a substance to its resting state. A substance that manifests this property is called an elastic substance. For instance, a rubber band may be stretched by active forces, but when released, the forces within the rubber band act to restore it to the resting state. Those forces acting to return the rubber band to its resting state are called the elastic forces.

The lung is an elastic organ; i.e., it has many forces acting to return it to its resting (collapsed) state. The two primary elastic forces are the interstitial elastic fibers and the fluid lining the alveolar surface. Thus, we may think of an alveolus as a semisphere that is highly elastic. Since all elastic spheres behave according to the physical law of Laplace, this becomes an essential physical law to understand in respiratory care.

Law of Laplace

The Laplace equation, as applied to geometric spheres, states: $P = 2 \times T/R$. "P" represents the distending pressure within the alveolus (dynes per sq cm); "T" is surface tension of the alveolar fluid (dynes per cm); and "R" is the radius of the alveolus (cm).

This relationship indicates that the distending pressure necessary to expand the alveolus is determined by (1) the surface tension properties of the liquid substance lining the sphere; and (2) the radius of curvature of the sphere. Inherent in this relationship is the fact that if surface tension remains unchanged, the smaller the radius, the greater the distending pressure must become to maintain the alveolar volume.

If such a situation truly existed in the lung, all alveoli would have to be the same size so that the smaller alveoli would not empty their air into the larger ones. However, all alveoli are not the same size. In fact, some alveoli are four to five times larger than others. If surface tension remained constant, the inspiratory airflow would preferentially inflate the larger alveoli, while little or no air entered the smaller alveoli. The end result would obviously be one huge, extended alveolus, with all of the others totally collapsed.

Surfactant

The obvious reconciliation of this mechanical dilemma would be the capability of altering the surface tension of the alveolar fluid lining so that a state of equilibrium could be maintained. As early as 1929, it was concluded that the active surface forces in the alveolar lining fluid must be less than that of water or plasma.[37] It was also suspected that the surface tension must be variable, depending upon the size of the alveolus. Recent studies have shown that the surface tension of the alveolar lining fluid is indeed variable and decreases as the alveolar surface area is reduced.[38] The substance *surfactant* is responsible for this variability.

Surface tension is the molecular force present on the surface of a liquid that tends to make the surface area exposed to the atmosphere as small as possible. Simply stated, the molecules on the surface of water are much closer together than elsewhere in the fluid. In an elastic sphere, surface tension would play a very major role in the tendency for that sphere to collapse. Surfactant decreases surface tension.

Alveolar Critical Volume

All alveoli have a *critical volume,* i.e., a volume below which the elastic forces become overwhelming and cause complete collapse of the alveolus. One might think of the critical volume as the alveolar volume below which surface tension constantly exceeds the distending pressure. This causes the radius to become progressively smaller until ultimately the alveolus collapses.[39]

Alveolar Elastance

Keeping all these complex relationships in mind, and yet attempting to simplify the concepts to a workable level, we may generalize the application of the law of Laplace to the functioning of alveoli in the following way: There is a critical volume at which the potential internal expanding forces can equal or exceed the external elastic forces which are tending to collapse the alveolus. Below this critical volume, these external forces are overwhelming and total collapse eventually ensues. Above the critical volume, the surface-acting substances work in such a way as to maintain a dynamic state of equilibrium. This is accomplished by a balance between the expanding pressures tending to inflate the alveolus and the surface tension properties tending to collapse the alveolus.

The Principle of Compliance

The lung is an elastic organ with inherent forces constantly tending to make it collapse. It is obvious that these forces function as elastic forces during the process of expiration. However, part of the time the lung must be inspiring, and, therefore, the elastic forces tending to collapse the lung must be overcome. In other words, *a force greater than the elastic forces must be applied in the opposite direction before the lungs can expand.* Instead of considering the elastic forces as those tending to collapse the lung, we may consider them as forces which must be overcome to expand the lung. Forces opposing expansion of the lung are referred to in terms of *compliance.* Mathematically, compliance is the reciprocal of elastance.

To use our previously stated example of the rubber band, the force that is needed to stretch the rubber band will be dependent upon the elastic forces tending to return the rubber band to its resting state. A highly compliant substance would be one in which there were few elastic forces; therefore, it would take little force to stretch the substance. In other words, a substance with a high compliance is one with few elastic forces. A substance with a low compliance would be one possessing great elastic forces and, therefore, could be stretched only with great difficulty.

Compliance can be defined as the volume change in the lung per unit of pressure change in the lung:

$$C = \frac{\Delta V}{\Delta P}$$

C equals compliance, V equals change in volume, and P equals change in pressure. In simple terms, the greater the pressure that is needed to allow a given volume change, the less compliant the lung.

The Principle of Airway Resistance

Gas flows from a region of higher pressure to one of lower pressure. Obviously, the rate at which a volume of gas is displaced (flow) is a function of the pressure gradient and the resistances to that gas flow. Thus, we may make the following statement: Resistance equals pressure gradient divided by flow ($R = \Delta P/F$). A more exact relationship between pressure difference and gas flow can be derived if we know the nature of the flow, i.e., whether it is laminar or turbulent.

Laminar Flow

Laminar gas flow refers to a streamlined molecular flow in which there is little friction between the molecules of gas themselves and mostly friction between the molecules and the sides of the tube. Therefore, laminar flow through a tube would have a cone-shaped pattern; i.e., the gas molecules near the side of the tube would be subject to friction with that surface and would tend to travel slower than the gas molecules in the center of the tube (Fig 3–2). This phenomenon was first theorized in 1915 and demonstrated to be present in the pulmonary tree in 1954. The phenomenon undoubtedly plays a great role in the respiratory process of the obtunded and intubated patient with small tidal volumes in that it helps explain why tidal volumes of less than the patient's theoretical anatomic deadspace may provide gas delivery to the alveoli.[40]

Laminar flow follows the general *law of Poiseuille* which states that at a constant driving pressure, the flow rate of a gas will vary directly

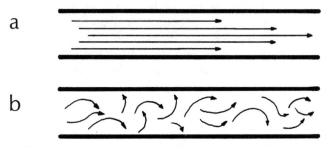

Fig 3–2.—Schematic concept of laminar gas flow, **A,** and turbulent gas flow, **B.**

with the fourth power of the radius of the airway. Thus, we can see how small changes in airway caliber can greatly affect the delivery of air to the alveoli.

Turbulent Flow

Turbulent flow is present when gas molecules are inter-reacting in a random manner and the resistances are not only at the sides of the tube but also caused by molecular collision. High flow rates, especially through irregular tubes, result in a breakdown of laminar flow. With turbulent flow, the viscosity of the gas is not critical, but, rather, the density of the gas is the major factor. All other factors being equal, resistance to flow is greater when the flow is turbulent as opposed to laminar.

Tracheobronchial Flow

Tracheobronchial flow is a descriptive term given to the mixture of laminar and turbulent flows that are normally found in the pulmonary tree. This circumstance makes accurate measurements of airway resistance extremely difficult. In respiratory care, we must always be aware that external apparatus connected to the airway can be sites of tremendously increased airway resistances.

Airway Patency

The upper airway is normally responsible for 45% of the total airway resistance and, of course, this can be tremendously increased by such factors as obstruction caused by foreign material, swelling of the upper airway, etc. In the lower airway, the resistance is markedly affected by the patency of the airways. The large airways have a significant amount of structural rigidity, whereas the bronchioles are dependent primarily on transmural pressure gradients for their patency.

Pulmonary Function Studies

It should be appreciated that any consideration of pulmonary function testing applied to respiratory care is not as extensive as it is when applied to the clinical aspects of pulmonary disease. The discipline of pulmonary medicine uses pulmonary function studies to measure lung volumes, analyze flow rates, study diffusion capacities, and study the distribution of ventilation. Multiple lung function studies are required to provide a complete, quantitative evaluation of lung disease.

In respiratory care, we use pulmonary function tests to evaluate *mechanical* ability, *mechanical* efficiency, and gross *mechanical* abnormalities in the ventilatory system. We are concerned not only with the mechanical function of the pulmonary system at the time of testing, but also in assessing the ability of that system to meet stress by increasing its work. Because of these circumstances, we feel justified in discussing pulmonary function solely in terms of mechanics, and we remind the reader that what follows is not meant to be a treatise on diagnostic pulmonary function testing. Rather, its purpose is to provide basic information for the application of pulmonary function measurements to the field of respiratory care.

Total Lung Capacity and Lung Volumes (Fig 3-3)

The *total lung capacity* (TLC) is defined as the maximum volume of gas the lungs can contain. As applied to clinical practice, this is defined as the volume of gas contained within the lungs at the end of a maximal inspiratory effort. The total lung capacity is divided into four *lung volumes:* inspiratory reserve volume (IRV); tidal volume (VT); expiratory reserve volume (ERV); and residual volume (RV).

When the thorax is intact, the lungs will contain gas even after a maximal expiratory effort has been accomplished. The gas remaining in the lungs after a maximal expiratory effort is defined as the *residual volume* (RV). All individuals have a basal ventilatory pattern at rest. The measurement of the amount of gas that is expired during normal ventilation is defined as the tidal volume (VT). The normal ventilatory pattern occurs at a volume significantly above the residual volume and, therefore, the gas volume between the tidal volume and the residual volume is defined as the *expiratory reserve volume*. This is a portion of the volume of gas available for increasing the tidal volume, but is not utilized during normal resting ventilation. The volume of gas between the tidal volume and the upper limits of the total lung capacity is defined as the *inspiratory reserve volume*. This is the other volume of gas that is available for increasing the tidal volume but that is not utilized in normal resting ventilation.

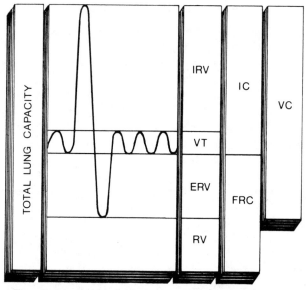

Fig 3–3.—The divisions of total lung capacity. Total lung capacity (TLC) is the maximum amount of air the lungs can hold. The total lung capacity is divided into four primary volumes: inspiratory reserve volume (IRV); tidal volume (VT); expiratory reserve volume (ERV); and residual volume (RV). Capacities are combinations of two or more lung volumes. They are inspiratory capacity (IC), functional residual capacity (FRC), and vital capacity (VC). (From Shapiro, B. A., Harrison, R. A., and Walton, J. R.: *Clinical Application of Blood Gases* [2d ed.; Chicago: Year Book Medical Publishers, 1977].)

In a normal male with a total lung capacity of 6 liters, the tidal volume is ideally 0.5 liter; the inspiratory reserve volume 3.1 liters; the expiratory reserve volume 1.2 liters; and the residual volume 1.2 liters.[41] A rule of thumb in the normal adult lung is that the inspiratory reserve volume is as large or larger than the other three volumes combined, and that expiratory reserve volume and residual volume are close to equal.

Lung volumes are static quantities and, therefore, not readily measurable in a dynamic ventilatory system. To make clinical measurements more practical, we speak in terms of lung capacities, i.e., combinations of two or more lung volumes. There are three lung capacities that must be understood in the field of respiratory care: *vital capacity, functional residual capacity,* and *inspiratory capacity.*

Functional Residual Capacity

The functional residual capacity (FRC) is defined as the combination of the residual volume and the expiratory reserve volume (FRC =

RV + ERV). In essence, *this measurement represents the content of gas remaining in the lungs at the end of a normal expiration!* Over the past decade it has become apparent that arterial blood oxygenation is very much dependent upon, and affected by, changes in the functional residual capacity. Although this measurement is not easily available in acutely ill patients, the concept of functional residual capacity and its effect on gas exchange and work of breathing in the critically ill patient is paramount.

The principles of measuring residual air were first elicited more than 170 years ago. These principles have been sophisticated over the last 40 years to become an extremely sensitive and reliable measurement. The basic principle is that an *inert gas* (such as helium) will not significantly diffuse into the pulmonary blood. Thus, as illustrated in Figure 3–4, we start out with a known volume of breathable gas containing a known concentration of helium and allow the patient to breathe this atmosphere. The helium will equilibrate throughout the total space, i.e., the lungs and the breathing box. After equilibration of the helium has taken place, the patient is disconnected from the

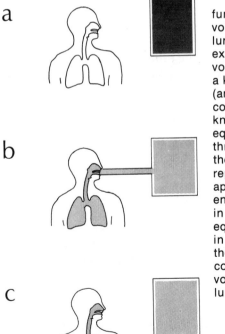

Fig 3–4. — Principle of measuring functional residual capacity (the volume of gas remaining in the lungs at the end of a normal expiration). **A** represents a known volume of breathable gas containing a known concentration of helium (an inert gas). **B** represents connection of the airway to the known gas and allowing equilibration of the helium throughout the entire system, i.e., the lungs and the apparatus. **C** represents disconnection of the apparatus from the airway at the end of a normal expiration (volume in the lungs = FRC) after helium equilibration. The measured change in the concentration of inert gas in the apparatus will allow computation of the total lung volume of gas remaining in the lungs by using the gas laws.

breathing box at the end of a normal expiration. Having kept temperature and volume constant, the change in helium concentration can be converted into a volume measurement via the ideal gas law. Thus, by measuring the change in helium concentration, we can calculate the volume of gas left in the lungs after a normal expiration.[41]

Helium is the most commonly used gas for this measurement since it can easily be measured by a thermal conductivity meter. Although other methods are available for measuring functional residual capacity, they are attempts to make the measurements faster and more practical, rather than more reliable.

The basic disadvantage of the helium method of measuring functional residual capacity is that only areas of lung that are reasonably ventilated will be included in the calculation. Thus, if a patient has very large lung "blebs" that do not ventilate well, this gas-containing space will not be included in the calculated functional residual capacity by the helium method. Measurements in the body plethysmograph will include these unventilated spaces, and disparity between FRC as measured in the body plethysmograph and by the helium method is often used as a way of detecting large, nonventilating blebs.[41]

Inspiratory Capacity

The inspiratory capacity (IC) is defined as the combination of the tidal volume and inspiratory reserve volume (IC = V_T + IRV). In essence, *this measurement represents the ability to take a deep breath from FRC*. Normally, the inspiratory capacity is 75% of the vital capacity.

Expiratory Spirogram

Vital Capacity

The vital capacity is defined as the combination of inspiratory reserve volume, tidal volume, and expiratory reserve volume (VC = IRV + V_T + ERV). In other words, the vital capacity is the total lung capacity minus the residual volume! *The vital capacity represents the patient's maximum breathing ability*. Its measurement is simple since it requires only that the patient take the deepest inspiration possible and then expire as completely as possible. The measured exhaled air is the vital capacity.

Forced Vital Capacity

A piece of equipment that measures gas volumes is called a *spirometer*. A recording spirometer is one that will record a tracing on pa-

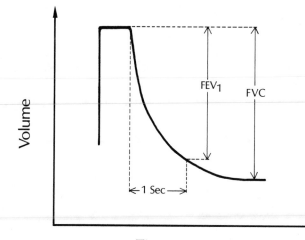

Time

Fig 3–5.—Schematic representation of a forced expiratory spirogram. Moving from left to right, a maximum inspiration is depicted by the rapid increase in volume (this represents inspiratory capacity). The patient holds his breath at maximum inspiration and then forces the air out as fast as possible. The total air expelled is the forced vital capacity (FVC); the volume expelled in the first second is the FEV_1 (see text).

per. Vital capacities can be measured with the patient forcing or not forcing his expiration. Utilizing a recording spirometer, one can exhibit the forced vital capacity and have what is called the *forced expiratory spirogram* (Fig 3–5). This is an extremely important measurement in respiratory care since numerous measurements can be obtained from this one simple maneuver. In addition, the forced expiratory spirogram can be obtained at the bedside; i.e., it does not require moving the patient to a pulmonary function laboratory.

The measurement of a forced vital capacity (FVC) makes three important measurements readily available: (1) the actual vital capacity under stress; (2) the volume expired in the first second (FEV_1); and (3) the maximum mid-expiratory flow rate (MMEFR).

The forced vital capacity is a useful measurement in respiratory care because it represents *the maximum volume available to the patient for ventilation under conditions of stress.* The patient's measurement is then compared with the predicted normal based on sex, height, and age. The per cent of forced vital capacity (FVC%) reflects the patient's present capability for exchanging air in relation to his theoretically normal capability.

FEV$_1$

The forced expiratory volume in 1 second (FEV$_1$) is the measurement of the volume of air forcefully expired in the first second of a forced vital capacity maneuver. In a normal person between 20 and 30 years of age, it is expected that 83% of the total vital capacity will be expired in the first second. The forced expiratory volume in 1 second is usually compared with the *actual* forced vital capacity and referred to as FEV$_1$%.

MMEFR

The maximum mid-expiratory flow rate (MMEFR) is calculated by measuring the middle portion of the forced expiratory spirogram. This is believed by many experts to be the most accurate estimate of airway resistance that can be found in the forced expiratory spirogram. Many experts prefer to use the peak flow measurement for this purpose.

Flow-Volume Curve

Many experts in the field of pulmonary function studies believe that the flow-volume curve is a more useful single test than the traditional volume-time curve.[42] When flow-volume relationships are noted in graphic form (Fig 3-6), the nature of a pulmonary abnormality can be easily recognized simply by the shape of the curve. Only time will delineate whether or not the flow-volume curve will replace the traditional volume-time curve in spirometry. At the present time, it is important for all of those in respiratory care to be familiar with both methods.

Maximum Breathing Capacity (MBC)

The maximum breathing capacity or MBC (also called MVV — maximum voluntary ventilation) is the maximal volume of air that a patient can breathe per minute. It is usually measured by having the patient exert a maximum breathing effort for 10 – 15 seconds and then computing this to a minute. This measurement has been traditional in pulmonary function studies for many years, and, from its inception, has been recognized as a test with a number of limitations. Besides being dependent upon numerous intrinsic properties of the lungs, such as flow resistance, it is also influenced greatly by nonpulmonary factors, such as motivation, sensorium, muscular force, and endurance. For these and other reasons, the MBC has in large part been replaced in recent years by the single breath measurements previously described. Its traditional use as an indicator of ventilatory reserve has been widely disputed over the past several decades.

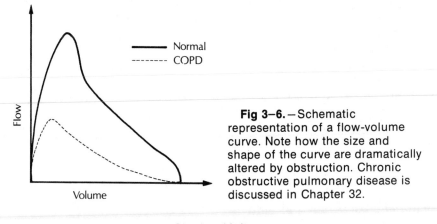

Fig 3–6. – Schematic representation of a flow-volume curve. Note how the size and shape of the curve are dramatically altered by obstruction. Chronic obstructive pulmonary disease is discussed in Chapter 32.

Closing Volume

The most commonly used method for closing volume measurement is the *single breath oxygen test*. The patient inspires pure oxygen from RV to TLC and then slowly exhales back to RV through an apparatus that measures expired nitrogen concentration. Figure 3–7 depicts a classic test. Phase I represents deadspace air devoid of nitrogen; phase II is believed to be a mixture of alveolar air and deadspace air; phase III is a slope representing a mixture of all alveolar gases with gradual-

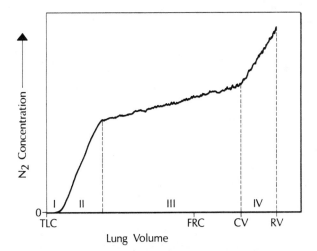

Fig 3–7. – Representative curve measuring expired nitrogen concentration following single maximal inhalation of 100% oxygen (see text). *TLC* = total lung capacity; *FRC* = functional residual capacity; *CV* = closing volume; *RV* = residual volume. Roman numerals *I – IV* represent the four phases of the curve. The closing volume occurs at the junction of phases *III* and *IV*.

ly more apical and less basilar alveolar gas; and phase IV is believed to represent sudden emptying of only apical alveoli.[43]

The junction of III and IV is attributed to sudden closure of dependent airways and is termed *closing volume,* expressed as a percentage of the vital capacity. The absolute volume at which phase IV begins is termed *closing capacity* (CC = CV + RV).

Theoretically, the basilar alveoli receive the greatest dilution of nitrogen, the apical alveoli the least dilution. This theory is complemented by repeatability with boluses of tracer gases. The reliability and meaning of closing volume measurements are not clear.

Pulmonary Function Screening in Respiratory Care

With the recent development of sensitive and portable spirometric equipment, a useful and important tool has become available to the respiratory care practitioner in the evaluation of ventilatory function at the bedside. These tests can readily be provided as a service of the respiratory therapy department, if the personnel are properly trained.

Minimal Requirements

In general, the requirements for bedside spirometry are: (1) the test must be simple for the patient to perform; (2) the test must be able to reliably distinguish normal from abnormal results within ranges of clinical significance; (3) the system must be portable to allow bedside testing; (4) the test must minimally provide the forced vital capacity, forced expiratory volume in 1 and 3 seconds, peak expiratory flow rate and/or maximum mid-expiratory flow rate. Ideally, the technique should provide a printed graph of the forced expiratory curve for later study and documentation. The technician performing the study must be well trained in maintaining and calibrating the equipment as well as properly performing the tests. It is important that the patient be properly instructed to expend maximal effort and that the level of cooperation be noted and evaluated by the technician. At least three separate tests should be performed with the best of the three then used to represent the study.

Interpretation

In respiratory care, abnormal spirometric studies are generally categorized as restrictive or obstructive abnormalities. A *restrictive abnormality* (restrictive component) implies a condition in which inspiratory capability is restricted to less than the predicted normal. This must be distinguished from the diagnosis of *restrictive disease* which necessitates the measurement of reduced total lung capacity.[41] Restrictive components are diagnosed by the presence of a reduced forced vital capacity in the presence of normal expiratory flow rates.

An *obstructive abnormality* (obstructive component) implies airway obstruction. This is characterized by a reduction in expiratory flow rates. This condition must be distinguished from *obstructive disease* in which the diagnosis necessitates the measurement of an increased total lung capacity.[41] The spirometric parameters generally used to interpret obstructive components are (1) the presence of reduced forced expiratory volumes in 1 second; (2) reduced maximum mid-expiratory flow rates; (3) reduced peak expiratory flow rates; and (4) reduced forced vital capacity in severe obstructive disease.

There still exists a great deal of controversy concerning the application of the expiratory spirogram in respiratory care. For example, there are those who feel the most helpful measurement in delineating the patient's ability to cough adequately is the forced vital capacity,[44, 45] whereas others feel that the peak expiratory flow rate is the most useful single test for this purpose.[46] Our experience has shown the FVC to be the most useful and reliable measurement.

Although the use of screening pulmonary function studies seem well founded in clinical practice, their use at present is generally limited. This is most likely due to lack of knowledge about their appropriate use and application. In general, spirometric pulmonary function testing can be used to (1) provide information concerning any functional impairment that may be present in the pulmonary system; (2) provide a base-line study for surgical patients; (3) provide a day-to-day evaluation of the effectiveness of medical and bronchial hygiene pulmonary regimens; and (4) serve as an initial screening procedure.

Available spirometric systems range from very simple screening devices to sensitive and accurate computerized programs that provide complete spirometric evaluation. The simplest screening devices have a bellows into which the patient forcefully exhales. A stylet moves across a graph paper and records the time-volume relationship. Electronic spirometers have become very popular in the past decade. These have a range of features that include digital and direct readouts; some provide graphic tracings of flow-volume curves. Some recently developed computerized systems are available to provide very complete spirometric studies by use of the telephone.

It should be emphasized that recently published articles have questioned the accuracy of some electronic units.[47] It is the responsibility of the department offering the testing service to assure that the performance characteristics of the unit being used are clearly defined and periodically checked. There is no question that the next decade will provide us with even more convenient and accurate spirometric studies.

The Work of Breathing

Definitions

Work

Mechanical work is accomplished when a force moves an object to which it is applied. The quantification of that work will be the result of the force multiplied by the distance moved (Work = Force × Distance). The spontaneous movement of air in and out of the lungs requires an expenditure of energy by the muscles of ventilation. The pulmonary pressures may be used as an expression of force and the pulmonary volumes involved may be used as an expression of distance. Thus, during steady-state breathing conditions, the mechanical work involved may be computed in terms of the pressure times the changes in volume (Work = Pressure × Volume).

Power

Power is a term that refers to the rate at which work is being done.[6] In clinical terms, the work of breathing actually refers to the power necessary to accomplish the ventilation.

To move air in and out of the lungs, the muscles of ventilation must expend enough energy to overcome two major factors: (1) the elastic recoil of lung and chest wall; and (2) the frictional resistance to gas flow in the airways. For completeness, factors such as the frictional resistance in the movement of lung and chest wall tissues and the very low component of inertia must also be mentioned.

Essential Clinical Factors

Four major clinical factors must be considered when assessing the work of breathing: (1) compliance, (2) resistance, (3) active expiration, and (4) ventilatory pattern. It would be a disservice to the reader if the impression were left that quantification of the work of breathing is simple and straightforward. If we consider the elastic recoil of the expiratory system as if it were a single entity exerted primarily by the lungs with some assist from the chest wall, the concepts become simple. The *true* interrelationships and complexities of these mechanical factors are fortunately of little clinical significance, especially when we are dealing with patients in respiratory distress and possibly in need of mechanical support of ventilation. Therefore, it is clinically acceptable to view these factors in their simplistic relationships.

Compliance

The process of moving gas into the lungs requires energy to overcome the elastic recoil properties of the lung and chest wall. It should be obvious that part of the energy expended for inspiration is "stored" in the elastic tissues of the chest and thorax as elastic recoil energy. This energy is normally used to provide most of the work of expiration.

In normal breathing at basal conditions, expiration is referred to as "passive" because it does not require active muscular work. The lower the compliance, the greater the elastic recoil energy available for expiration. More importantly, the lower the compliance, the greater will be the energy expended to provide a deeper inspiration.

Resistance

At the end of shallow inspiration, intrathoracic airways may remain narrower and, therefore, cause a greater resistance to gas flow than they normally would.[41] To overcome this potentially increased airway resistance, an increased expenditure of energy may be needed (active exhalation) during expiration. This increased expiratory energy can be reduced by deeper inspirations that allow less resistance and a greater degree of elastic recoil during expiration. This generally indicates that shallow breathing at a rapid rate demands a greater energy expenditure to overcome airway resistances than deep and slow breathing.

Active Expiration

Thus far, our discussion has assumed that expiration is entirely passive. As pointed out previously, this is the case in normal, resting ventilation. In fact, in healthy people, expiration is almost totally passive, even with minute volumes as high as 20 L per minute.[6] However, for very high minute volumes in patients with healthy lungs and for normal minute volumes in patients with diseased lungs, the expiratory muscles may be brought into play. That work must also be included in a total assessment of the work of breathing!

Ventilatory Pattern

If a constant minute volume is maintained, the work necessary to overcome elastic recoil is increased when breathing is deep and slow. On the other hand, the work expended to overcome airway resistance is increased when breathing is rapid and shallow. If we plot total work against ventilatory frequency (Fig 3–8), we see that *there is an opti-*

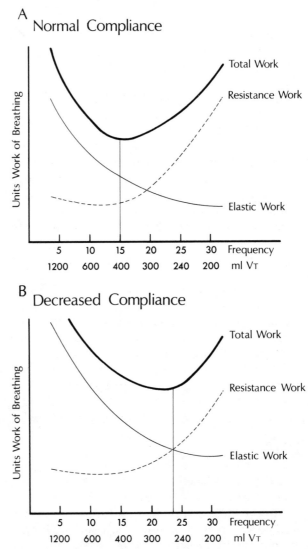

Fig 3–8.—A is a graphic representation of total work of breathing when minute ventilation is unchanged, but ventilatory pattern (tidal volume and frequency) is varied. Note that for any minute ventilation there is a ventilatory pattern that requires minimal work. Of course, total work is the summation of resistance work (airways) and elastic work (lung parenchymal and chest wall recoil forces).

If compliance is decreased, as in **B,** the graph shows that the pattern of ventilation at which the minute volume can be achieved with minimal work is dramatically altered.

This is a schematic representation of the principle that work of breathing is the major factor determining ventilatory pattern (see text).

70

mal ventilatory frequency at which the total work of breathing is minimal. Many investigators have noted that human subjects and animals tend to select ventilatory frequencies that correspond very closely to calculated frequencies for minimum work.[48] This response has also been well documented in patients with diseased pulmonary systems. When compliance is decreased, ventilatory frequency increases and tidal volumes decrease; when airway resistance increases, the ventilatory frequency decreases and tidal volumes increase. This is objective testimony to the clinical statement that *the ventilatory pattern present in a diseased patient is determined almost entirely by minimal expenditure of energy rather than by efficient physiologic ventilation!* The ventilatory pattern chosen by a physiologically stressed patient must never be assumed to be advantageous in terms of molecular gas exchange; rather, it should be assumed to be the pattern requiring the least expenditure of energy for that minute ventilation.

Ventilatory Reserve

A classic description of a healthy, resting adult denotes an oxygen consumption of approximately 250 ml per minute.[41] Oxygen consumption for the work of breathing is less than 5% of the total.[49] Even under these excellent physiologic conditions, the efficiency with which the energy is utilized for the actual mechanical aspects of ventilation is astoundingly poor.[50] In the resting state, about 90% of the energy expended for the work of breathing is lost as heat within the ventilatory muscles. This means that only 10% of the energy is used for moving gas in and out of the lungs. The efficiency is further reduced in the presence of pulmonary disease and with increased minute ventilation.[6] In severe disease states the system may become so inefficient that any oxygen potentially gained from increased ventilation is completely consumed by the increased muscular work.[51] This may progress to the point where an increase in ventilation results in net oxygen loss to the organism. In this circumstance, the alveolar gas improvement that can be accomplished by increased spontaneous ventilation is greatly limited. It is important to note that for a patient being mechanically ventilated the situation just described would not be true; the increased work in this case would be provided by the apparatus rather than the ventilatory muscles.

The limitation of active ventilatory efficiency is only reached at very high minute volumes in healthy patients. However, in the presence of significant disease, the efficiency level may be so low as to impose severe limitations to even minor degrees of physiologic stress. In respiratory care we are consistently confronted with the potential problem of the patient who may become unable to maintain adequate ventilation or meet increased physiologic stress. An appreciation of the fatigue process is so vitally important to the clinical support of the pulmonary system that an attempt must be made to assess the work of breathing and the reserves available to meet physiologic stress.[52]

Despite the difficulties and numerous complexities that have been elaborated here, clinical guidelines for assessing ventilatory reserve have been developed.[44] The guidelines are based on functional concepts and clinical realities of the work of breathing. The following concept produces obtainable, reproducible, and reliable information that can be applied in the clinical circumstance of supporting gas exchange in the critically ill patient.

Of the body's total oxygen consumption, the percentage that is used by the ventilatory muscles can be considered a reflection of the work of breathing.[51] If this is so, then the relationship depicted in Figure 3–9, A, exists. As minute volume is increased, the percentage of the total oxygen consumption that is used for breathing is increased exponentially. In other words, in the normal resting state, a person uses approximately 5% of his total oxygen consumption for ventilatory muscular work.[53] As the person increases mechanical ventilation, he must use more muscular power. The increased muscular work demands increased oxygen consumption, and so the amount of total oxygen consumption that is used for the work of breathing increases. As a matter of fact, this increase in oxygen consumption is not linear; therefore, not only the amount but the percentage of total oxygen consumption applied to the work of breathing increases. The untrained person has experienced this after running for a period of time; the work of breathing becomes so demanding that he must stop and, for a short period of time, concentrate on doing enough ventilatory muscular work to repay his oxygen debt.

Increasing minute ventilation causes an exponential increase in ventilatory oxygen consumption. If we add airway resistance, such as results from obstructive lung disease, the curve looks much like the dotted line in Figure 3–9, A. The work of breathing is far greater at the resting stage, and the increase in the percentage of oxygen consumption is far greater when there is increased airway resistance to overcome.[54]

Figure 3–9, B, shows the same curve plotted as a function of the vital capacity; i.e., the curve represents the ventilatory work as a function of the portion of the vital capacity being used as tidal volume. Suppose, for example, that a man with a vital capacity of 5,000 ml has a tidal volume of 500 ml. He is using 10% of his vital capacity as tidal volume (a). The percentage of oxygen consumption being used for

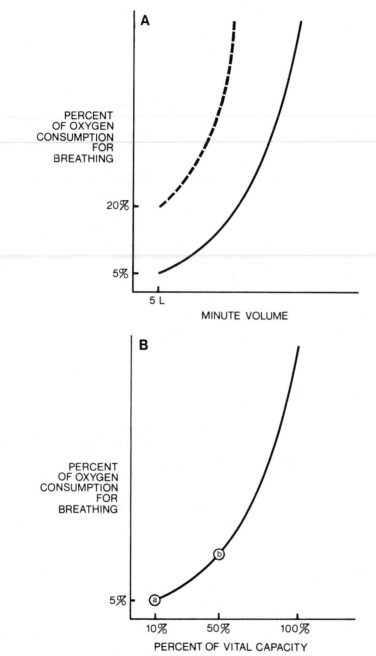

Fig 3–9 – A, the work of breathing in relation to vital capacity (see text). In **B,** point *a* represents a Vᴛ of 500 ml with a VC of 5 L; point *b* represents a Vᴛ of 500 ml with a VC of 1 L. (From Shapiro, B. A., Harrison, R. A., and Walton, J. R.: *Clinical Application of Blood Gases* [2d ed.; Chicago: Year Book Medical Publishers, 1977].)

breathing is low. A second man has a vital capacity of only 1,000 ml, but must maintain the same 500 ml tidal volume as the first man. He is using 50% of his vital capacity (b) and is consuming far more oxygen for breathing than the first man. It is important to note that even though the tidal volumes of both men are the same and the total body oxygen consumptions are the same, the percentage of oxygen consumed for the work of breathing is much higher for the second man.

In such an example, the second man has far less capability to increase his ventilation to meet stress. Because of his greatly diminished reserve, it is far more costly for him to increase his ventilatory work. *The greater the portion of the vital capacity that is being used for a tidal volume, the less the ability of the patient to increase his tidal volume to meet a stressful situation.*[55] *Therefore, vital capacity can be used as a gross indicator of ventilatory reserve.* Obviously, the degree of airway resistance must always be included in such an assessment.

Even though this is a greatly simplified and scientifically imprecise reflection of ventilatory reserve, it is a very useful clinical concept, since vital capacity and tidal volume are easily measured at the bedside. This concept of *ventilatory reserve* is basic to the understanding of clinical supportive measures for pulmonary disease, and it also plays an extremely important role in the predictable insult to the pulmonary system by surgical and anesthetic stress.

Mechanical Support of Ventilation

Static lung mechanics refers to the properties of the pulmonary system that relate to the interaction of forces *without* motion. An understanding of these static properties is essential before the principles of dynamic lung mechanics can be appreciated. *Dynamic lung mechanics* refers to the properties of the pulmonary system as they relate to the interaction of forces taking motion (kinetics) into account. Both of these properties must be dealt with in artificial ventilation.

Static Lung Mechanics

We stated earlier that the lung is an elastic organ and will manifest changes in pressure with changes in volume. Simply stated, within the elastic limits of the lung, the pressure measured will be proportional to the volume which is in the lung (P is proportional to V).

We have defined elastance as the forces tending to collapse the lung. Elastance may also be thought of as the summation of forces resisting distention of the lung. It must follow, then, that the pressure necessary to inflate the lung must be equal to the product of the elastance times the volume ($P = E \times V$). This intuitive relationship is obvious if one considers the pressure exerted within the lung as dependent upon the volume in the lung and the elastic forces resisting the pressure of that volume.

By definition, compliance is the reciprocal of elastance ($C = 1/E$). Compliance, therefore, is equal to the ease of distensibility of the lung. In other words, the more easily distensible the lung, the greater the compliance; the lesser the ease of distensibility of the lung, the lower the compliance.

Compliance can now be referred to in terms of the volume-pressure relationship by the following derivation:

1. $P = E \times V$
2. $C = 1/E$ — This may be rearranged to read:
3. $E = 1/C$ — Replacing E in equation 1 with equation 3:
4. $P = 1/C \times V$ — Rearranging this equation to solve for C:
5. $C = \dfrac{\Delta V \text{ (liters)}}{\Delta P \text{ (cm H}_2\text{O)}} \quad \dfrac{\text{Change in Volume}}{\text{Change in Pressure}}$

The volume-pressure relationship stated in Equation 5 is graphically depicted in Figure 3–10. Volume is represented as the lung volumes and pressure is represented as above- or below-atmospheric pressure. One can see that the volume-pressure relationship is indeed

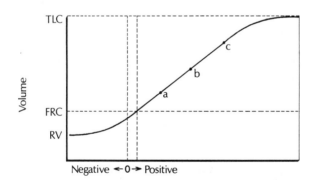

Transpulmonary Pressure

Fig 3–10. — The theoretic lung compliance curve (see text). TLC is total lung capacity; FRC is functional residual capacity; RV is residual volume. The 0 represents atmospheric pressure. Transpulmonary pressure is the difference between mouth pressure and pleural pressure. As transpulmonary pressure increases, the volume within the lung increases.

Volume-pressure relationships within the lung are linear as long as TLC or RV is not approached. Points a, b, and c depict that in appropriate lung volume ranges, a change in pressure results in a linear change in volume and vice versa. This represents theoretic static lung phenomena only!

a linear one until either (1) the total lung capacity is approached or (2) residual volume is approached. In other words, *in the normal lung, any static relationship of pressure and volume will be linear as long as the volumes are not at the extremes of approaching total lung capacity or residual volume.*

The volume-pressure relationship is true for the lung. However, we have previously stated that in artificial ventilation one must deal not only with the lung but with the chest wall as well. The term *total compliance* refers to the system compliance, i.e., lung compliance plus chest wall compliance. *Specific compliance* refers to a patient's lung compliance in relationship to the patient's actual lung volume. Specific compliance allows for more accurate measurements of compliance when the patient's size varies significantly from the normal adult — an expecially important factor in pediatrics.

Effective static compliance (ESC) is a method that has been described for approximating the total compliance of a patient on a ventilator (see Chapter 23). This is obviously not a true measurement of compliance since the definition requires static conditions, which are cumbersome to produce in the clinical setting. However, many clinicians feel that the ESC is a useful serial measurement of volume-pressure relationships within a particular patient, and it is used to reflect *gross* changes in lung compliance when chest wall compliance is controlled and remains relatively constant. This usually applies to the patient who is paralyzed or heavily sedated so that voluntary muscle activity is nonexistent. Of course, the airway, the ventilatory circuit, and the manner of delivering the volume must remain constant. Then a series of effective static compliance measurements made over a given time period can determine gross changes, when present, in lung compliance. The effective static compliance is calculated by dividing the expired tidal volume (ml) by the inspiratory pressure (cm H_2O).

Dynamic Lung Mechanics

Whereas static lung mechanics deals with the property of compliance, dynamic lung mechanics deals with the property of resistance. The force (driving pressure) of a gas will determine the flow through the system. Obviously, the other major factor that will affect the flow will be the forces impeding the movement of gas. This can be stated by the relationship that the driving pressure (ΔP) will equal flow times resistance ($\Delta P = F \times R$). Stated in terms of resistance: Resistance (R) will be equal to the driving pressure divided by the flow ($R = \Delta P/F$). Resistance is determined by numerous factors, including viscosity, length of tube, and the radius (Poiseuille's law). Recall that in the tracheobronchial tree both laminar and turbulent flow co-exist. Ninety-five percent of the total resistance is due to "airway resistance." It should be remembered that the resistance of the airways does not remain constant but changes, increasing as airways get smaller (exhalation) and decreasing as airways get larger (inspiration).

Driving pressure refers to the difference in pressure between the mouth and some other reference point. There are three common points of reference: (1) the alveolus, (2) the pleural space, and (3) pressure immediately surrounding the exterior chest wall. These pressure differences can be quantitatively defined in conditions giving static measurements (compliance) and dynamic measurements (resistance).

Transairway pressure is defined as the driving pressure between the mouth and the alveoli (see Fig 21−1). It represents the pressure drop along the entire airway and is reflected in the measurement of airway resistance. It is meaningless to refer to transairway pressure measurements in static lung mechanics since the pressures between the mouth and the alveoli are in equilibrium. Therefore, transairway pressures can only be meaningful when measurements of airway resistance or dynamic lung mechanics are ascertained.

Transpulmonary pressure has been defined as the pressure difference between the mouth and the intrapleural space. Intrapleural pressures are usually approximated by the pressure measurement in a balloon in the mid-esophagus. Transpulmonary pressure represents the drop in pressure from the mouth across the lung parenchyma. Its measurement is used in the calculation of pulmonary compliance under static conditions and pulmonary resistance under dynamic conditions.

Transthoracic pressure is defined as the pressure difference between the mouth and the area immediately surrounding the chest wall. This measurement must obviously be made in a rigidly controlled environment, such as a patient in a body plethysmograph. Transthoracic pressure is a reflection of the measurement of the total compliance and/or the total resistance (lung tissue and chest wall).

Lung Impedance

In providing inspiration, a mechanical ventilator or the muscles of ventilation must expend enough energy to overcome "lung impedance": (1) the elastic recoil properties of the lung and chest wall and (2) airway resistance. In other words, both static and dynamic forces must be overcome in order to deliver any given volume to the lung. Mathematically the total differential pressure (ΔP_{total}) is a reflection of the compliance and resistance characteristics of the lung-thorax system.

$$\Delta P_{total} = \Delta P_{compliance} + \Delta P_{resistance}$$

The equivalent values of ΔP compliance and ΔP resistance can be placed in the equation to illustrate more clearly their contribution to the total pressure difference.

$$^{\Delta P}total = \left(\frac{1}{C}\right) V + (R)(F)$$

In a patient with very stiff lungs, i.e., a low compliance ($\downarrow$ C), it may be seen that a greater component of $\Delta P_{compliance}$ and total pressure will result for any volume added. Also, if resistance is increased ($\uparrow$ R), it will also add a greater component to the total pressure. Once flow approaches or equals zero, the total pressure will be solely a reflection of the compliance characteristics of the system. It should be re-emphasized that this phenomenon exists whether the patient is on the ventilator or breathing spontaneously.

Negative-Pressure Ventilators

To create the movement of air into the lungs, it should be obvious that the basic essential is to develop a driving pressure between atmosphere and the alveoli. In normal, spontaneous ventilation, this driving pressure is produced through the work of the ventilatory muscles. When artificially supporting the ventilatory system, the driving pressure is provided by an external mechanical apparatus.

A *negative-pressure ventilator* is one in which the body is placed within a chamber that can produce a subatmospheric pressure. The head remains outside of the chamber and, therefore, when a subatmospheric pressure is produced around the chest wall, a driving pressure between ambient atmosphere and the alveoli is produced. The "iron lung" is a classic example of a negative-pressure ventilator. A newer type of negative-pressure ventilator is the chest cuirass; it is far more portable than the iron lung.

The prime advantage of a negative-pressure ventilator is that long-term ventilatory support is possible without an artificial airway (endotracheal tube or tracheostomy). This permits the patient to talk and eat, and it avoids the numerous discomforts and complications of artificial airways. This mode of ventilatory support proved extremely valuable in the days of poliomyelitis epidemics and is still frequently used for the long-term ventilatory support of neuromuscular diseases.

The main disadvantage of a negative-pressure ventilator is that the patient's body is not readily accessible for the nursing and monitoring needs of critical care medicine.[56, 57] Observation becomes nearly impossible, and availability of the trunk and extremities for measurements and administration of medication is most difficult. Another great disadvantage is that diseased lungs rarely manifest uniform changes in resistance and compliance. As early as 1947,[58] it became apparent that pulmonary gas exchange was maintained in *acutely* ill patients far better with positive-pressure machines than with negative-pressure machines.

In essence, then, negative-pressure ventilators can still be used for the long-term support of the chronic ventilator patient who has reasonably normal lungs. However, for the support of ventilation in acutely ill patients and in those with primary cardiopulmonary disease, negative-pressure ventilators are not satisfactory.

Positive-Pressure Ventilators

An inspiratory driving pressure may be provided by applying an above-atmospheric pressure to the mouth. Since the alveoli are at atmospheric pressure, this will allow inspiration to take place. By removing the positive pressure from the upper airway, expiration takes place in a manner similar to that of a patient breathing spontaneously. The lung and chest wall provide elastic recoil, creating a driving pressure from alveolus to mouth. This method of intermittent positive-pressure ventilation (IPPV) is the method presently used for the mechanical support of the ventilatory system in the acutely ill patient and for augmentation of bronchial hygiene.

Advantages

This technique of providing a driving pressure allows direct control of the driving pressure and, therefore, a greater chance of providing the desired ventilation.[58] In addition, attachment to the apparatus is accomplished through a small tube leading to the airway; the bulk of the apparatus is located a reasonable distance from the patient. This allows complete patient accessibility in the acute care setting.

Disadvantages

An artificial airway (endotracheal tube or tracheostomy tube) must be provided except when support of ventilation is for a very short term. This means that positive-pressure ventilation must carry with it the complications and risks of artificial airways.

Pressure dynamics of the thoracic cavity are dramatically altered by positive-pressure ventilation. Normal intrathoracic pressure in the spontaneously breathing patient is never above-atmospheric. Mean subatmospheric intrathoracic pressures play an important role in cardiac function. Under normal circumstances, intra-abdominal pressures are higher than intrathoracic pressures and, therefore, blood within the great veins is "milked" from the pelvis and abdominal region to the thorax. This mechanism is called the "intrathoracic pump" and plays a very important role in insuring adequate return of venous blood to the heart.

When intrathoracic pressures are increased to above-atmospheric, there is a potential embarrassment of blood return to the heart.

Classification of Positive-Pressure Ventilators

There are four *physical parameters* that must be dealt with whenever gas is moved in and out of the pulmonary tree: *volume, flow, pressure, and time.* Whenever a volume of gas is displaced over a period of time, a flow is developed. Since this flow moves through a series of tubes and into a second, confined space, a pressure is produced. Additionally, ventilation of the lungs entails a cyclical movement of air in a to-and-fro manner; therefore, the time component of the directional flow is important.

There are four *mechanical parameters* that must be dealt with whenever ventilation is to be provided by a machine. There must be a mechanism for *beginning the inspiratory cycle;* some means of *providing the force necessary to move the gas;* a method of providing for the *end of inspiration;* and a means of providing for the *expiratory phase.*

Ventilators are universally classified by the *physical parameter that ends the inspiratory cycle.*[58] In other words, a volume machine is one in which inspiration ends when a preset volume of gas is delivered; a pressure machine is one in which inspiration ends when a preset pressure is reached; a time machine is one in which inspiration ends when a preset time has elapsed; and a flow machine is one in which inspiration ends when a preset flow rate is delivered.

In the United States, it is reasonable to combine this basic classification of ventilators into two major types: *volume-time* and *pressure.*[59] Although there are numerous, sophisticated pieces of equipment which are combinations, it is clinically meaningful to separate the machines into these two basic categories.

Volume-Time Machines

For a machine to deliver a preset volume, it must have internal power sufficient to deliver the volume regardless of the presence of external forces. This is accomplished by building into the machine a high internal resistance which allows for the development of a high internal driving pressure. This makes the machine relatively insensitive to pressure changes on the patient end of the circuit. *This classification of volume-limited machines includes most of the time-cycled ventilators in use today.*

The advantages of volume-time machines are primarily: (1) the volume of gas delivered is reliably controlled; (2) volume delivery remains constant despite pathophysiologic changes; (3) they are far easier to adapt to various monitoring devices; (4) they are adaptable to most variations in airway pressure maneuvers; and (5) a consistent inspired oxygen atmosphere can be easily maintained. The disadvantages are primarily: (1) they may provide excessive intrathoracic and airway pressures and (2) they are expensive. In general, these are the machines of choice for long-term ventilatory support (see Chapters 22 and 23).

Pressure-Limited Ventilators

In order to readily respond to pressure changes at the patient end of the circuit, the pressure-limited ventilator must have a very low internal resistance. This classification of pressure-limited machines includes most of the flow-cycled machines.

The advantages of pressure-limited machines are primarily that (1) they are small, portable, and inexpensive; (2) they cannot deliver excessive pressures to the patient's airway; and (3) they are readily amenable to assisting ventilation.

The disadvantages of pressure-limited machines are that (1) they tend to provide an inconsistent ventilation, since the volume delivery is variable; and (2) they may not maintain a consistent oxygen atmosphere, since most of these machines adjust the FI_{O_2} on the basis of a Venturi mechanism (see Chapter 7).

The pressure-limited machine can be counted on for consistent ventilation only in patients who have no pre-existing pulmonary or thoracic disease and who will not resist mechanical support of ventilation. This type of machine is best suited for the patient in need of short-term support and who fulfills the criteria just discussed.

Expiratory Cycle

Most of today's ventilators provide the expiratory phase by opening the system — and thereby the patient's airway — to the atmosphere. By the process of elastic recoil, the chest wall and lungs provide the driving pressure to create airflow out of the lungs. This can be considered a constant atmospheric pressure generator, since the emptying of the patient's lungs has no real effect on the pressure in the atmosphere. Thus, we have a gradually decreasing intra-alveolar pressure within the patient's lungs providing the driving pressure between alveoli and atmosphere.

It is possible to place an injector type system to create a subatmospheric pressure within the circuit during the expiratory phase (negative pressure). Although this method was popular several decades ago, it is now known that this method of expiration causes early collapse of small airways and trapping of air within the alveoli.

A resistance may be placed at the exhalation port, resulting in prolonged airway pressures during expiration. This is known as "expiratory retard" (see Chapter 23).

A positive end-expiratory pressure (PEEP) can be placed on the expiratory port so that the airway pressure never returns to atmospheric pressure (see Chapter 24).

Inspiratory Driving Mechanism

Although it is desirable to keep the complexities of ventilator mechanics to a minimum, it is necessary to have a basic understanding of the two primary types of generators which are used in clinical practice today: the flow generator and the pressure generator.

The *constant flow generator* is the type most commonly found in volume- and time-limited machines. The mechanism provides a constant flow of gas as long as the inspiratory cycle lasts. The pattern of flow delivery is unchanged regardless of the lung and chest wall characteristics.

The *constant pressure generator* is essentially a mechanism whereby a constant pressure is produced throughout inspiration. The flow delivery will obviously be affected by the pressure being developed in the patient's thoracic cavity. The initial flow values are the highest and then progressively decrease in exponential fashion as the alveolar pressures increase. Thus, it is difficult to maintain consistent ventilation since the developed driving pressure of the apparatus is in the same magnitude of pressure range as the lung alveolar pressures. Any disease process causing decreased compliance or increased resistance will compromise the capability of the machine to deliver adequate volumes.

The pressure generator frequently utilizes a Venturi mechanism to provide various concentrations of oxygen. This makes the concentration of oxygen delivered variable with the flow rate.

For detailed information concerning ventilator function and physics, the reader is referred to several excellent reviews of the subject.[60, 61]

Applying Positive-Pressure Ventilation

Now that we have presented a basic description of pulmonary and ventilator mechanics, we are ready to take a simplified look at the complex interrelationships that occur when positive-pressure ventilation is applied. Table 3–1 states four essential relationships in mathematical form, as an aid to those who find the formulas helpful. We shall discuss these four relationships in nonmathematical terms.

1. Recall that compliance, a static phenomenon, is a description of the relationship of the volume delivered divided by the pressure developed because of elastic recoil. Resistance, a measurement of dynamic phenomenon, is dependent upon the driving pressure in relation to the flow.

2. The ventilator is a machine which provides a supra-atmospheric pressure at the mouth. The actual driving pressure during inspiration will be the result of the pressure being generated by the machine in relation to the pressure being developed in the alveoli.

3. Alveolar pressures increase as volume is delivered to the lung. The resultant alveolar pressure will be dependent upon the volume delivered in relation to the lung compliance.

4. The flow generated in the airways by positive-pressure ventilation is determined by the developed driving pressure in relation to the total resistance in the system. In other words, when no driving pressure exists there will be no flow. As the driving pressure increases, the flow will increase in relation to the resistances present to that flow.

With these four relationships clearly in mind, it becomes possible to consider the mechanical properties of the lung in relation to a ventilator. From this point on, reference to "the system" means the lungs and the ventilator.

TABLE 3–1.—POSITIVE PRESSURE AND LUNG MECHANICS

ΔP = Driving pressure
P_G = Pressure generated
P_{Alv} = Pressure in alveolus
$R_{Total} = R_{Airway} + R_{Ventilator}$

1. $\text{Compliance} = \dfrac{\Delta V}{\Delta P}$ $\qquad \text{Resistance} = \dfrac{\Delta P}{\text{Flow}}$

2. $\Delta P = P_G - P_{Alv}$

3. $P_{Alv} = \dfrac{\text{Volume}}{\text{Compliance}}$

4. $\text{Flow} = \dfrac{P_G - P_{Alv}}{R_{Total}}$

Figure 3–10 depicts compliance characteristics of the system in relation to volume and pressure. As previously stated, this is a linear relationship in the working range of the lung. The diagram demonstrates that the various changes in volume and pressure are proportional. The measurement of this change without regard to time is called compliance. If time relationships are taken into account, we are dealing not only with the ultimate volume delivered and its resulting pressures, but also with the moment-to-moment change in volume and pressure. This relationship of volume, pressure, and time would result in a curvilinear relationship as shown in Figure 3–11. This closed loop describes the dynamics of the system.

To make this point clearer, let us consider the delivery of a given volume of air into the lung in terms of both statics and dynamics. If the volume is delivered with enough time allowed for complete cessation of movement of air, the static relationship exists. Therefore, the pressure measured would be purely a resultant of the volume and elastic

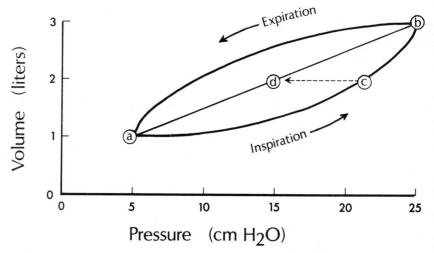

Fig 3–11. — Volume-pressure relationships secondary to the delivery of a volume of gas into a model lung. Point *a* represents zero flow at end expiration; point *b* represents zero flow at end inspiration. The curvilinear line *a-b* represents the inspiratory pressure-volume relationships which occur as the volume is being delivered; curvilinear line *b-a* represents the expiratory dynamic relationship.

If inspiratory flow is stopped at point *c*, the pressure-volume relationships will change from dynamic to static as the flow approaches zero. The dotted line *c-d* represents this change from dynamic to static state. Note that for the same volume at point *c* and *d*, the pressure is less in the static than the dynamic circumstance.

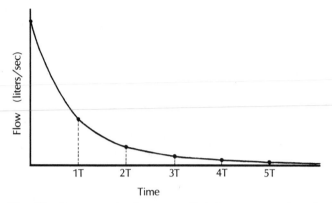

Fig 3–12.—The time constant exponential decay curve (see text). Flow-time curve obtained under the condition of a constant pressure generator. The length of the time constant intervals "T," plotted along the horizontal axis, is dependent upon the resistance and compliance characteristics of the lungs. "T" = R·C. The curve demonstrates that the initial flow at time "0T," the initial time, is highest—progressively decreasing in a predictable fashion (the exponential decay curve) as the driving pressure $\Delta P = P_{Generated} - P_{Alveolar}$ is reduced. In the same manner, the amount of volume delivered in each successive time constant interval also progressively decreases.

End of Time Constant	% Initial Flow	% Vol Delivered
0	100	0
1	37.0	63.0
2	13.5	86.5
3	5.0	95.0
4	1.8	98.2
5	0.7	99.3

recoil properties of the lung (compliance). However, if the pressure measurements are determined as the volume is being delivered, the resultant pressure measurement is a reflection of not only compliance properties, but also of the factor of resistance. In other words, since a static relationship is not present, there is a resistance factor related to flow in addition to the lung compliance factor. Thus, for the volume delivered at that point in time, the pressure measured is greater than it would be for the same volume once a static condition had been reached.

The clinical importance of describing these mechanical properties is that for a given driving pressure created by a ventilator, the volume delivered and the flow pattern will be the result of the resistance and compliance properties of the system. This interrelationship becomes important since it involves time and is characterized by a term known as a *time constant.* The actual numerical value of a time constant gives a measure of the time necessary to deliver a given volume into the patient's lung. The characteristic of the time constant relationship turns out to be an exponential decay curve, as seen in Figure 3–12. Using a pressure-limited ventilator, the relationship shows that the initial flow is greatest because driving pressure (mouth-to-alveolar pressure) is greatest. This flow will decrease with time since volume delivered to alveoli increases alveolar pressures and thereby decreases driving pressure. The rate of decreased flow is dependent upon the resistance and compliance properties of the lung. Quantitatively, 63% of the volume will be delivered in the first time constant. During the second time constant, less volume will be delivered (23.5%), with a total of 86.5% delivered by the end of 2 time constants. Ninety-five percent of the maximum volume which can be delivered will be delivered within 3 time constants.

The essential points to remember are (1) for a machine to deliver a given volume within a given time, a minimal driving pressure must be produced; (2) the driving pressure developed will determine the maximum volume that can be delivered to the patient; (3) the flow will progressively decrease with each instant in time, the rate of decrease determined by the compliance and resistance factors of the system; and (4) 95% of the maximum volume will be delivered within three time constants.

4 • PHYSIOLOGY OF EXTERNAL RESPIRATION

THE FOUNDATION of animal life is cellular metabolism. This metabolic system is dependent upon simple gas diffusion for its continuance, i.e., a continual supply of oxygen and a continuous removal of carbon dioxide. All organ systems depend upon the process of *homeostasis* for proper functioning. Homeostatic mechanisms invoke feedback systems that alter cellular and organ system function to maintain "physiologic normalcy."

Cardiopulmonary homeostasis involves the interrelationships and complexities of the pulmonary, cardiac, vascular, and blood systems[35] — all for one purpose — *appropriate gas exchange.*

The respiratory care practitioner must be concerned with the multiplicity of factors involved in oxygen and carbon dioxide exchange across *all* permeable membranes. A clear and concise understanding of these processes is essential to the application of proper respiratory care. The fundamental precept is that there are two distinct capillary beds where gas exchange takes place: systemic and pulmonary.

The Systemic Capillary Bed

The systemic capillary bed is commonly referred to as the *microcirculation,* and is composed of the vasculature between the systemic arterial and venous systems. These capillary beds provide the vehicle for gas exchange and nutrient supply for all cells except alveolar epithelium (respiratory bronchioles, alveolar ducts, alveoli).

Gas exchange across systemic capillaries is referred to as "internal respiration" — exchange between blood and tissue. Clinically, the measurement of this gas exchange is referred to as the *respiratory quotient* (R. Q.), the volume of carbon dioxide produced compared with the amount of oxygen consumed per unit time (R. Q. $= \dot{V}_{CO_2}/\dot{V}_{O_2}$). In the "normal" 70-kg (150-lb) man, approximately 200 ml of carbon dioxide is produced per minute while approximately 250 ml of oxygen is consumed. Using these numbers, the calculation of the respiratory quotient then becomes 200 ml of CO_2 divided by 250 ml of O_2, which is equal to 0.8. This relationship is assumed to be valid if all metabolism is taking place in the normal aerobic Krebs cycle and the patient is at a basal resting (steady state) condition.

The Ventilation-Perfusion Relationship

Gas exchange between blood and the external environment occurs in the pulmonary capillary bed – a process called *external respiration*. The quantities of carbon dioxide and oxygen exchanged must logically equal the exchange in the systemic capillaries, oxygen being added to the blood while carbon dioxide is being removed. This relationship of volumes of carbon dioxide and oxygen exchanged per minute by the lungs is the *respiratory exchange ratio* (RR).[6] The respiratory exchange ratio represents the *over-all* exchange capability of the lung, not individual variances occurring within different parts of the lung.[43]

The most efficient gas exchange would occur if there existed a perfect match between all lung ventilation and all pulmonary capillary blood flow. Theoretically, this would necessitate a lung constructed in such a way that a single large alveolar surface communicated directly with the atmosphere. All gas moving into such a lung would come into immediate contact with the alveolar surface. Additionally, it would be necessary to have a single capillary surface in immediate contact with the single alveolar surface. Presumably, all the blood passing through the single capillary would come in equal contact with the alveolar surface.

This ideal circumstance is impossible in man because the pulmonary system is constructed as a valveless to-and-fro pump necessitating a series of tubular structures through which gas must travel to reach the alveolar surface. Therefore, only a portion of the total ventilation comes into contact with the alveolar surface. The ventilation reaching the alveoli and having molecular exchange with blood is referred to as *alveolar ventilation* (physiologically effective ventilation). Using the example of our "normal" 70-kg (150-lb) man, the *minute ventilation* (total ventilation in one minute) could be approximated at 7 liters compared with a cardiac output of 5 liters in the same minute. At best, only 5 of the 7 liters can be alveolar ventilation. At the least, 2 liters must be "physiologically wasted" or *deadspace ventilation*.

A further characteristic of the pulmonary system that makes it less than ideal is that both gas and blood are affected by gravity. Therefore, dependent portions of the lung (for an upright patient, the base of the lung) will receive a greater portion of the ventilation and perfusion. However, because of the greater density of blood with respect to air, a mismatch of the ventilation-perfusion relationship is created; i.e., in the *gravity-dependent portion of the lung the blood flow exceeds the airflow*. On the other hand, in the nongravity-dependent portion of the lung, the airflow exceeds the blood flow. The mismatch between ventilation and perfusion is further complicated when areas in the lung exist where there is perfusion *without* ventilation, and where there is ventilation *without* perfusion. These two abnormal conditions are categorized under the concepts of shunting and deadspace.

An alternative method of expressing the effectiveness of pulmonary gas exchange is to consider the "matching" of ventilation and perfusion or, more precisely, the relationship between the volume of gas moving into an alveolus and the blood flow through the adjacent capillary.[62] The advantage of this approach is that it takes into account the *efficiency* of molecular gas exchange in all areas of the lung. It is difficult to fully comprehend the complex ventilation to perfusion relationship; however, a basic understanding of the concept is essential.

Distribution of Pulmonary Perfusion

The normal distribution of blood flow throughout the pulmonary vasculature is dependent upon two major factors: (1) gravity and (2) cardiac output.

Gravity

In normal man standing erect, there is a distance of approximately 30 cm from the *apex* (top) to the *base* (bottom) of the lung. Assuming the pulmonary artery enters the lung halfway between top and bottom, the pulmonary artery pressure would have to be great enough to overcome a gravitational force of 15 cm of water in order to supply flow to the apex; a similar gradient would be aiding flow to the lung base. A column of blood (essentially H_2O) 15 cm high exerts a pressure of approximately 11 mm Hg. *This gravitational effect on blood flow results in a lateral wall pulmonary artery pressure at the lung base of greater magnitude than the pulmonary artery pressure at the apex.*[62] Thus, blood will preferentially flow through the gravity-dependent areas of the lung (Fig 4–1).

Under normal circumstances, *alveolar* pressures are equal throughout the lung. Theoretically, the least gravity-dependent areas of the lung (the apex in the upright subject) may have alveolar pressures higher than the pulmonary arterial pressures at that level. This would result in the virtual absence of blood flow to these areas. It should be noted that the total absence of pulmonary blood flow to these areas does *not* exist to any significant extent in the normally perfused lung.[63] However, if pulmonary artery pressure is significantly decreased (e.g., shock) or alveolar pressures significantly increased (e.g., intermittent

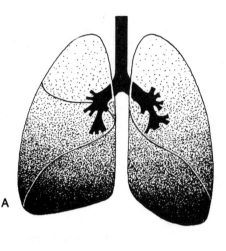

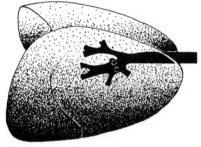

Fig 4–1.—The preponderance of pulmonary blood flow will normally occur in the gravity-dependent areas of the lung. Thus, body position has a significant effect on the distribution of pulmonary blood flow, as shown in the erect **(A),** supine (lying on the back) **(B),** and lateral (lying on the side) **(C)** positions. (From Shapiro, B. A., Harrison, R. A., and Walton, J. R.: *Clinical Application of Blood Gases* [2d ed.; Chicago: Year Book Medical Publishers, 1977].)

positive-pressure breathing or positive end-expiratory pressure), the absence of perfusion to the least gravity-dependent areas of the lung may become significant.

THE THREE-ZONE MODEL. — It has become well accepted to refer to the gravity effects of pulmonary perfusion in terms of the three-zone model (Fig 4–2).[62] Zone 3 is the gravity-dependent area of constant blood flow (arterial pressure greater than alveolar pressure); zone 1 is the least gravity-dependent area of potentially no blood flow (alveolar pressure greater than arterial pressure). The interceding area is zone 2, an area of complex and varying intermittent blood flow. The presence or absence of blood flow in zone 2 depends primarily on the relationship of pulmonary artery pressure to alveolar pressure. Under normal circumstances this is determined far more by the cardiac cycle (systole and diastole) than by the ventilatory cycle (inspiration and expiration).

Cardiac Output

The amount of blood ejected by the right ventricle per unit time (cardiac output) is a major determinant of blood flow through the pul-

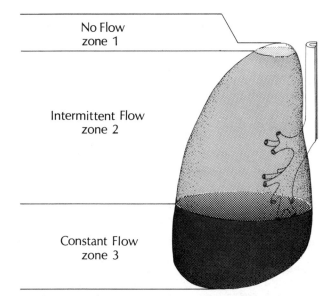

No Flow
zone 1

Intermittent Flow
zone 2

Constant Flow
zone 3

Fig 4–2. — The three-zone model illustrating the effects of gravity on pulmonary perfusion (see text). (From Shapiro, B. A., Harrison, R. A., and Walton, J. R.: *Clinical Application of Blood Gases* [2d ed.: Chicago: Year Book Medical Publishers, Inc., 1977].)

monary vasculature. In general, *the greater the cardiac output, the greater the pulmonary artery pressure.* Thus, in the normal lung, as the cardiac output increases, zone 3 extends upward (see Fig 4–2); conversely, as the cardiac output decreases, zone 3 descends. Since the pulmonary vascular system tends to react *passively* to changes in arterial pressure, the gravity effect on the distribution of blood flow secondary to cardiac output changes is greater in the pulmonary system than in the systemic circulation.[62]

Regional Differences in Ventilation

In normal man standing erect, *intrapleural pressure is more subatmospheric at the apex than at the base* (Fig 4–3). The most probable reason for this is that the lung is "suspended" from the hilus, and the weight of the lung requires a larger pressure for support below the

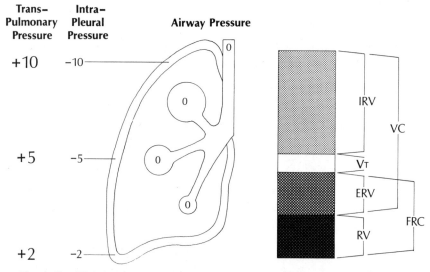

Fig 4–3.—The bar graph depicts normal total lung capacity and normal lung volumes. *RV* = residual volume; *ERV* = expiratory reserve volume; *Vt* = tidal volume; *IRV* = inspiratory reserve volume; *VC* = vital capacity; *FRC* = functional residual capacity. The lung diagram represents the erect lung and pleural space at *FRC*. Airway pressure and all alveolar pressures are zero (atmospheric). Interpleural pressures are negative—to a greater degree at the apex than at the base (see text). The numbers are for illustrative purposes and do not necessarily represent actual physiologic measurement. Note that transpulmonary pressure (airway opening pressure minus intrapleural pressure) is greater at the apex than at the base. This is the primary reason why the alveoli are larger at the apex and smaller at the base of the lung.

hilus than above.[62] Thus, pressure near the base is greater, and thereby the intrapleural negativity is less. This phenomenon is completely gravity dependent.

Approximately one half of the total lung capacity remains in the lung at the end of expiration; i.e., normal FRC is approximately one-half the normal TLC. The distribution of this lung volume will be primarily a function of the transpulmonary pressure (TPP), which is greater at the apex than at the base (see Fig 4–3).

Alveolar volumes are greater at the apex due to the greater TPP; in fact, they are so large that they lie on a part of the compliance curve whose slope represents a lesser compliance than do the basilar alveoli (see Fig 24–3). Thus, during inspiration *the inspired gas will tend to go toward the bases* because the basilar alveoli are easier to inflate than the apical alveoli.

Regional differences in ventilation refer to volume changes in relation to resting volume. Compared to the apex, the base of the lung has a smaller resting volume and undergoes a larger volume change per unit of lung; therefore, basilar ventilation is greater. This will hold true for dependent lung in any body position.

In general, as end-expiratory volume (FRC) increases, apical ventilation decreases; as FRC decreases, apical ventilation increases.

Shunting and Deadspace

The basic pulmonary gas-exchange unit is composed of a single alveolus with its associated pulmonary capillary. This theoretical respiratory unit can exist in one of four relationships (Fig 4–4): (1) the *normal unit* is one in which both ventilation and perfusion are relatively equal; (2) a *deadspace unit* is one in which the alveolus is normally ventilated but there is no blood flow through the capillary—the alveolar gas cannot participate in molecular blood-gas exchange; (3) a *shunt unit* is one in which the alveolus is completely unventilated while the adjacent capillary has blood flow—the blood goes from the right to the left heart without undergoing gas exchange; (4) a *silent unit* is one in which both the alveolus and capillary are completely collapsed.

Any one of these absolute conditions may exist in the lungs at any time. It takes little imagination to appreciate that an infinite number of ventilation-perfusion relationships may exist between the deadspace unit, the normal unit, and the shunt unit. This spectrum is illustrated in Figure 4–5. The complexities of the ventilation-perfusion ratio are primarily due to the spectrum between the two extremes of deadspace and shunt.

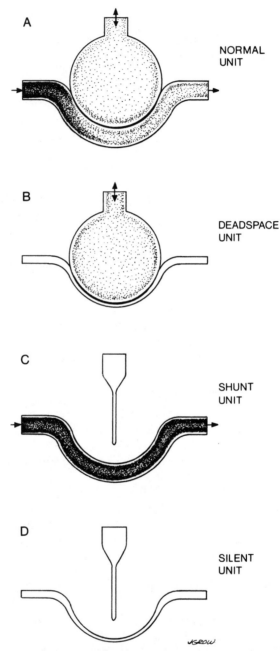

Fig 4–4. — The theoretic respiratory unit. **A,** normal ventilation, normal perfusion; **B,** normal ventilation, no perfusion; **C,** no ventilation, normal perfusion; **D,** no ventilation, no perfusion. (From Shapiro, B. A., Harrison, R. A., and Walton, J. R.: *Clinical Application of Blood Gases* [2d ed.; Chicago: Year Book Medical Publishers, 1977].)

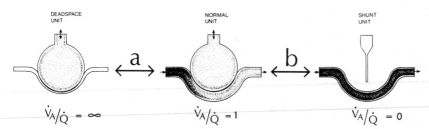

Fig 4–5.—The spectrum of ventilation-to-perfusion relationships. As shown, *a* represents the spectrum of ventilation in excess of perfusion; *b* represents the spectrum of perfusion in excess of ventilation. The true deadspace unit is represented as infinite $\dot{V}_A/\dot{Q}$; the normal unit is represented as $\dot{V}_A/\dot{Q}$, equalling 1; the shunt unit is represented as zero $\dot{V}_A/\dot{Q}$.

The Concept of Physiologic Deadspace

Further clarification of the deadspace concept is necessary to appreciate its clinical importance. The *physiologic deadspace* is defined as that portion of the total ventilation that does not exchange with pulmonary capillary blood. This has been previously described as "wasted ventilation." Physiologic deadspace can be divided into anatomic and alveolar components.

Anatomic deadspace is that portion of the total ventilation that occupies the space within the tracheobronchial tree; alveolar capillary gas exchange is impossible since the gas never reaches alveolar epithelium. As a general rule, the anatomic deadspace is equal to 1 ml per pound of ideal body weight.

Alveolar deadspace is that portion of the total ventilation that contacts alveolar epithelium without blood flow. This portion of the deadspace ventilation has the *potential* for exchange, but is not exchanging because of some physiologic or pathophysiologic condition curtailing pulmonary blood flow. The gas moving in and out of these alveolar areas is as "wasted" as gas occupying the tracheobronchial tree.

Using our previously developed concept of ventilation-to-perfusion inequity, some alveoli can be shown to have gas exchange significantly in excess of the blood flow through the respective capillaries. Some of this gas may not exchange with blood and will be deadspace ventilation.

The total ventilation must be composed of two portions: (1) *deadspace ventilation*—that portion which does not exchange with pulmonary blood; and (2) *alveolar ventilation*—that portion which physiologically exchanges with pulmonary blood. Since alveolar ventilation is "effective" ventilation, it is the only portion of the total ventilation essential to the life-support of the organism.

The Concept of Physiologic Shunt

A common cause of hypoxemia is a disease that produces intrapulmonary shunting. The physiologic (or total) shunt is that portion of the cardiac output that does not exchange with alveolar air. The physiologic shunt has been subdivided into three components: (1) anatomic shunt, (2) capillary shunt, and (3) shunt effect (perfusion in excess of ventilation or V/Q inequality).

Anatomic Shunt

In the normal person approximately 2–5% of the cardiac output is returned to the left heart without entering the pulmonary vasculature. This blood flow is via the bronchial, pleural, and thebesian* veins.[64] In addition to this normal anatomic shunt, pathologic anatomic shunts can exist, e.g., vascular lung tumors and right-to-left intracardiac shunts.

Capillary Shunt

Blood entering a pulmonary capillary that is coupled with an unventilated alveolus returns to the left heart without gaining oxygen. In other words, *capillary shunting is a result of pulmonary capillary blood in contact with totally unventilated alveoli.*

The sum of the anatomic and capillary shunts is frequently called the true or *absolute shunt*. This absolute shunt may be "refractory" to manipulation of oxygen therapy (see Chapter 7).

Shunt Effect

This physiologic defect is often referred to as *V/Q inequality* or *perfusion in excess of ventilation*. It occurs in an alveolar-capillary unit that has either a poorly ventilated alveolus or an excessive rate of blood flow.[65] Blood leaving this unit has a lower oxygen content than blood leaving a normal alveolar-capillary unit.[66]

This shunting secondary to ventilation/perfusion inequity is an extremely complex and variable component of the physiologic shunt. Its clinical importance is that it is responsive to oxygen therapy; that is, small increases in inspired oxygen concentration frequently result in dramatic increases in the amount of oxygen carried by the blood (see Chapter 7).[6]

A change in the characteristic of the alveolar-capillary membrane

*The minor or lesser venous drainage of the myocardium. The major veins empty into the coronary sinus and thus the right atrium. The minor system empties directly into the ventricles.

may act as an impedance to oxygen transfer from the alveolus to the pulmonary capillary. This defect in oxygen diffusion responds to oxygen therapy in a manner similar to ventilation-perfusion inequities.[555] Therefore, it is extremely difficult in the clinical setting of acutely ill patients to differentiate primary diffusion defects from inequities in ventilation-perfusion ratios. However, it should be remembered that the pathophysiology of each is distinctly different and should not be confused.

5 • CLINICAL EVALUATION OF THE PULMONARY SYSTEM

KNOWLEDGE OF appropriate anatomy, physiology, physics, and biochemistry is essential for the clinical application of respiratory care. The previous chapters have reviewed this broad span of information. It would be remiss to exclude the clinical and laboratory information necessary for the respiratory care practitioner to assess the pulmonary system. It is unfortunate that these areas have traditionally been considered the exclusive province of the physician. Modern critical care medicine places with the nurse and therapist responsibilities that may involve immediate clinical decisions of life or death.[67] For this reason, we feel it essential to include the basis of clinical evaluation of the pulmonary system in this text. The respiratory care practitioner must "master" four clinical areas to accomplish more than superficial clinical expertise: (1) physical examination of the chest; (2) interpretation of portable chest x-rays; (3) application and interpretation of bedside pulmonary function testing; and (4) interpretation of arterial blood gases.

Physical Examination of the Chest

Respiratory care is multidisciplinary, involving several medical specialities and allied health fields. The respiratory care practitioner holds great responsibility in the application of therapeutic and supportive techniques. To accomplish this responsibility the respiratory therapist, respiratory nurse specialist, and chest physical therapist must be capable of assessing the pulmonary system by observation, palpation, and auscultation of the chest.

The respiratory care practitioner is not responsible for initial or finite diagnostic evaluation. However, he must be able to assess (1) the quality of breath sounds; (2) the existence of bilateral air entry; (3) the significance of abnormal breath sounds; and (4) areas of the pulmonary tree that have decreased, or absent, breath sounds. The respiratory therapist must be able to evaluate the effects of his therapeutic modalities, and the respiratory nurse specialist must be able to constantly and accurately assess the acutely ill patient with a major respiratory problem. It is dangerous to become so involved with monitoring and machinery that the patient is forgotten. *Always look at the patient!* All individuals involved in acute care must use their sensory organs (eyes, ears, and tactile senses) to determine the status of the pulmonary system. The four primary techniques of chest physical examination are (1) observation, (2) palpation (feel), (3) percussion, and (4) auscultation.

Observation

Taking the time necessary to observe the patient is the first cardinal rule of physical examination. It takes no more than several seconds to observe the patient grossly in relation to sex, age, size, posture, skin color, state of sensorium, speech, and degree of ventilatory efforts. Immediate life-threatening abnormalities usually are apparent from this gross observation, and immediate supportive maneuvers can be initiated.

Following the initial, gross evaluation, an orderly observation of the anatomy and mechanics of the ventilatory system is carried out. The general appearance of the face, neck, chest, and abdominal structures in relation to the use of the muscles of ventilation is evaluated — specifically, the use of accessory muscles of ventilation in the neck and the position of the trachea in the neck. The chest is observed for bilateral chest expansion, and deformities of the rib cage are noted — especially paradoxical movement of the rib cage or surgical scars. The base of the rib cage is observed in relation to the degree of diaphragmatic movement and movement of the lateral rib cage. The tone of the abdominal musculature and its role, if any, in the ventilatory pattern are assessed.

Inspiration is observed for the use of rib cage and accessory muscles. The normal sequence of inspiration is (1) descension of the diaphragm; (2) slight lateral "flaring" of the lower ribs; and then (3) slight expansion of the upper chest.

The rate and depth of ventilation are noted along with such factors as the accessory muscles used and the position the patient assumes. A patient that assumes a reclining or relaxed position is probably having little or no difficulty breathing. The patient who is sitting, leaning forward, or attempting to support the chest wall in some manner must be assumed to be having difficulty breathing.

Expiration should be longer than inspiration and have some evidence of a pause prior to the next inspiration. Such factors as pursed lips, active abdominal muscular involvement, and ability to speak must be evaluated.

The terms "respiratory distress" or "shortness of breath" are clinical states that are evaluated by the observer. The term "dyspnea" refers to the patient's subjective complaint of difficulty in breathing — you cannot *observe* dyspnea.

Palpation

In certain circumstances, information that is not obtainable from observation can be gained from feeling the thorax. Palpation is usually accomplished by placing the palms on the chest and assessing the degree of chest movement. The presence of secretions can often be detected during palpation, especially fluid secretions that will cause turbulence and vibrations on deep breathing. The symmetry of chest expansion is best evaluated by palpation.

Percussion Technique (Fig 5–1)

The percussion technique takes advantage of the fact that tissue vibrations will produce different sounds with varying tissue density. A sound produced by the examiner's fingers travels through the underlying thorax and is reflected back to be evaluated by the examiner's fingers and ears. This process permits evaluation of disease states within the thorax.

The hand is lightly rested on the portion of the patient's chest to be examined. The middle finger is fitted between the ribs with slight but uniform pressure; the pressure must be uniform because the percussion note will vary as the pressure varies. The striking hand is used to create the percussion note. The middle finger is "crooked" or bent in a

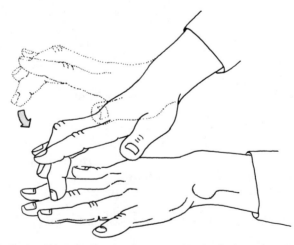

Fig 5–1. — Diagnostic chest percussion technique (see text).

semicircle from the wrist to fingertip—all the motion is accomplished by flexion of the wrist. The speed, force, and depth of the percussion note should be uniform for each blow.

With proper technique, the variations in resonance (echoing) can be assumed secondary to changes within the thorax. Percussion of the thorax is primarily used to compare one side with the other for: lung consolidation, pleural fluid, pleural air, and others.

Normally, the percussion note is the same over the entire thorax. Lung consolidation or fluid accumulation results in decreased resonance (dullness). Increased air in the lung results in increased resonance (tympany). In other words, a dull percussion note probably denotes consolidation or fluid. A tympanic percussion note probably denotes a hyperinflated area of lung. An extremely resonant note might mean air present in the pleural space.[68]

Auscultation

Chest auscultation is the technique employed to interpret the quality and quantity of breath sounds. The respiratory care practitioner must be familiar with the use of the stethoscope to determine and follow the progress of numerous disease states. Evaluation of sudden changes in chest pathology and effectiveness of various treatment modalities often depend entirely on auscultation.

The Stethoscope

The binaural stethoscope (Fig 5–2) has two heads: (1) a *diaphragm*, which is flat and is usually selected for the examination of high-pitched sounds; and (2) a *bell* portion used for auscultation of low-pitched sounds. Most often the diaphragm is used for auscultation of lung sounds. To understand what one is hearing through a stethoscope, there must be a basic understanding of the qualities and properties of sound.

Sound is the brain's interpretation of tympanic membrane vibrations. The tympanic membrane (eardrum) moves in sympathy with sound waves of various frequencies and intensities. *Pitch* is the frequency of vibrations—the lower the frequency, the lower the pitch. *Quality* of sound refers to the addition of certain matched frequencies, which gives the impression of a tone. *Intensity* is the amplitude of the vibration. Loudness depends not only on the intensity of the waves, but also on the sensitivity of the ear to the pitch or frequency. In chest auscultation, pitch, quality, and intensity are references; i.e., they are compared with the examiner's concepts of normal and with the various areas of that patient's chest.[69]

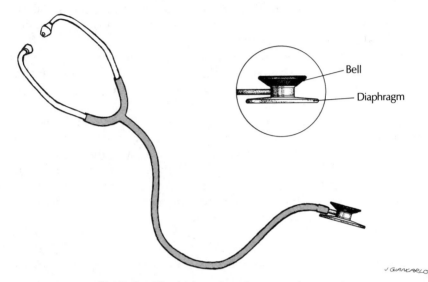

Fig 5–2. — The binaural stethoscope (see text).

Technique

Successful use of the stethoscope depends upon the ability of the examiner to know which sounds to disregard and which to give special attention. This can be learned only by listening with supervision and instruction. Mastering auscultation takes a great deal of experience. Unfortunately, in respiratory care the ideal conditions for auscultation of the chest are often impossible. For instance, it would be ideal to perform the examination in a very quiet area with the examiner free from all distractions and the patient completely relaxed in a standing or sitting position. Obviously, in the emergency room, intensive care unit, or hospital room, this is seldom possible.

If possible, the patient should be instructed to breathe deeply with his mouth open. The stethoscope is placed over the chest in a systematic manner so that all of the areas of the thorax are examined and compared. At least one full breath sound should be heard at each position and comparisons made between the left and right hemithoraces. If abnormal findings are heard, they should be compared with the opposite side and with normal areas on the same side.

Breath Sounds

Vesicular breath sounds are composed of normal inspiratory parenchymal sounds with little sound throughout the largest portion of expiration. This sound is heard in the normal lung because the distribution of air throughout the lung is unimpeded and the harsh quality of air rushing through tubes is not heard.

Bronchial breath sounds are those of air rushing through tubes; these are similar to the sounds heard by placing the stethoscope over the trachea. If bronchial breath sounds are heard over the thorax, it usually denotes parenchymal consolidation with transmission of the bronchial sounds through the consolidated tissue. Combinations of vesicular and bronchial sounds are often referred to as bronchovesicular sounds.

Rales are the most common abnormal sounds heard on auscultation of the chest. They are the sound of air entry into small airways or alveoli containing fluid. The sound is similar to the crinkling of cellophane or the sound heard by wetting the thumb and forefinger and opening and closing them next to the ear. Rales denote the movement of air into the alveoli or small airways containing fluid, i.e., the existence of pulmonary edema, heart failure, or pneumonia. Rales are usually heard during inspiration.

Rhonchi are sounds produced within airways where accumulation of fluid or secretions has occurred. The increased air turbulence produces a "rumbling" sound. Rhonchi are usually more pronounced during expiration. The presence of rhonchi suggests accumulated and/or retained secretions. Efforts should be made to mobilize the secretions and evaluate whether the rhonchi have disappeared or changed. A common diagnostic maneuver to distinguish rhonchi from rales is to ask the individual to cough. Rales will seldom clear on coughing; rhonchi will often clear with coughing.

Wheezes are often considered a type of rhonchi. The distinguishing feature of a wheeze is a *musical quality*. The noise is produced by high-velocity airflow through restricted air passages. Wheezes are most commonly associated with the clinical disease of asthma, a combination of bronchoconstriction and retained secretions. Wheezes may be heard both on inspiration and expiration when caused by bronchoconstriction. However, end-expiratory wheezes are often heard in patients with long-standing obstructive lung disease and are not bronchospastic in nature. *All that wheezes is not bronchospasm!*[70]

Abnormal Findings

Physical examination of the thorax allows the respiratory care practitioner to elicit the four pulmonary abnormalities most commonly found in acute respiratory care: (1) lung consolidation, (2) lung atelectasis, (3) pleural fluid, and (4) pneumothorax.

LUNG CONSOLIDATION. — Disease may transform normal, spongy lung parenchyma into a solid or semisolid structure. Breath sounds will be transmitted through this consolidated lung from centrally placed bronchi. Thus, we will hear *bronchial breath sounds* and have a *dull percussion note.* Consolidation may be produced by a process that fills alveoli with exudate (pneumonia), in which case fine rales may be heard over the involved lung portion.

ATELECTASIS. — When an air passage is occluded, the lung tissue distal to that occlusion will undergo resorption of gases and collapse. This collapse of lung parenchyma is termed *atelectasis.* Collapsed lung is consolidated lung and, therefore, will reveal a *dull percussion note.* There will be absent or decreased breath sounds over that area. The sounds present will be bronchial in nature. Other confirming signs of atelectasis are a shift of the trachea and mediastinum toward the side of the collapsed lung.

PLEURAL FLUID. — The accumulation of any fluid within the pleural space will separate lung parenchyma from the chest wall. Because the fluid layer does not transmit vibrations well, there will be distant or absent breath sounds. There will be a flat percussion note.

PNEUMOTHORAX. — Pneumothorax is defined as the presence of free air within the thoracic cavity and it is usually found in the pleural space. This will produce a *hyperresonant percussion note* with absent or distant breath sounds. Any shift in the mediastinum or trachea will be away from the side of the increased resonance.

With positive pressure ventilation, a *tension pneumothorax* may occur. A tension pneumothorax is defined as free air in the thoracic cavity with pressures in excess of atmospheric pressure. Tension pneumothorax with positive pressure ventilation is immediately life threatening. Because of the excessive pressure the lung tissue collapses and, more important, the great vessels in the mediastinum become compressed and occluded, resulting in circulatory collapse. Common physical findings include change in vital signs, tympany and hyperresonance, absent breath sounds, subcutaneous emphysema, and shift of the trachea away from the affected side.

The Infant Chest

Size and lack of cooperation make the physical examination of the infant chest difficult. Observation becomes the most useful technique of physical examination.

The frequency of breathing in the newborn may vary from 30 to 60 per minute in the first few days of life. Premature infants often manifest Cheyne-Stokes breathing—periods of apnea of 10 to 15 seconds between rapid ventilation. This Cheyne-Stokes ventilatory pattern must be recognized as an expected physiologic phenomenon in premature infants. However, it must be remembered that apnea lasting longer than approximately 15 seconds cannot be considered physiologic and may be associated with bradycardia.

The infant has a large protuberant abdomen and very high diaphragm; this makes the ventilatory efforts of a distressed baby extremely obvious. Since the infant's chest wall is very compliant, it is far easier to see retractions of intercostal and accessory muscles and the production of greater subatmospheric pressures in the pleural space. "Flaring" of the ala nasi is an extremely common sign of respiratory distress in the infant, and the *expiratory grunt* is a typical sign of severe respiratory distress.

Percussion and auscultation are extremely difficult to evaluate in the infant and small child, and for all intents and purposes should be left to the physician. The important fact for the respiratory care practitioner to understand is that abnormal findings are often easily overlooked in the infant chest. One must never assume that an absence of abnormal findings on physical examination of the chest of the infant means that there is no pathology existing.[71]

Assessment of the Portable Chest X-Ray

Numerous texts are available to describe the radiologic interpretation of the thorax. These texts are concerned with the finite points of diagnosis and are complete in description. The following material is presented to provide the respiratory care practitioner with some general, helpful points of portable chest film interpretation in the critically ill patient. The respiratory care clinician is usually forced to use *portable* chest x-rays which are rarely of optimal quality and usually available only in the anteroposterior (AP) view. These x-rays are used primarily to establish the existence of such entities as atelectasis, pneumonia, pneumothorax, and mediastinal shifts.

Principles of X-Rays

When a photographic film is exposed to x-rays it turns black. Thus, in a chest x-ray, the black portions represent areas where the x-rays went through the thorax essentially unimpeded. White areas represent tissue which has allowed very few x-rays to penetrate.

As illustrated in Figure 5–3, the source of x-ray emits a fan-shaped wave. The greater the distance between the x-ray source and the pho-

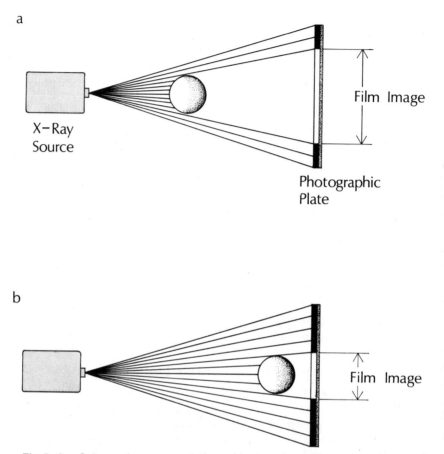

Fig 5–3. – Schematic representation of image size with x-ray exposure. **A** shows that the greater the distance between the x-ray source and the film, the larger will be the image because of "fanning" of the x-rays. The closer the object to the film (as in **B**), the smaller will be the x-ray image.

tographic plate, the more spread out the x-rays. The further an object is away from the photographic plate, the larger the object will appear on the film.[72]

The routine chest x-ray is taken with the patient facing and touching the photographic plate. The front of the chest is directly adjacent to the photographic film, and the x-rays penetrate the chest from the posterior to the anterior (PA view). This gives the sharpest and smallest cardiac shadow, since the heart lies close to the anterior wall of the chest.

Most portable chest x-rays are taken with the patient's posterior chest lying on the photographic plate. Therefore, this anteroposterior (AP) exposure will give a larger cardiac shadow. It is important to remember this fact in the interpretation of portable chest films. Lateral views are seldom obtainable in portable films.

Assessing the Chest Film

The thorax is an ideal region for radiologic examination since the aerated lung parenchyma offers little resistance to the passage of x-

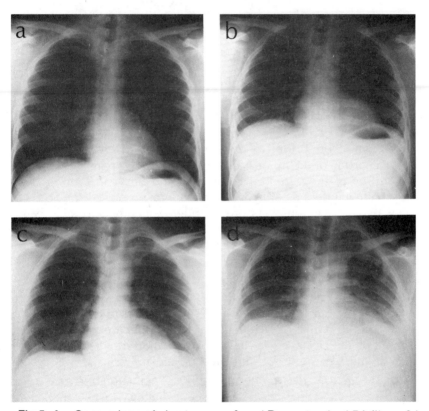

Fig 5–4. – Comparison of chest x-rays. **A** and **B** are standard PA films; **A** is inspiration and **B** is expiration. **C** and **D** are *portable* AP films (**C** is inspiration and **D** is expiration) in which the distance from x-ray source to film is significantly less than the standard films. Note that the chest image is larger in **A** than **C** because of distance from source to film; **A** has a smaller cardiac shadow in relation to the chest size because the heart is closer to the film in **A** than in **C**.

Portable films are more likely to be of less than full inspiration. Comparing the expiratory films (**B** and **D**) with full inspiration, it becomes obvious that interpretation is much more difficult when the lungs are poorly inflated.

rays. On the other hand, the soft tissues of the thorax (mediastinum, heart, great vessels, and diaphragm) do not permit x-rays to pass through as readily. They appear as white areas on the x-ray film. The bony structures (ribs, vertebrae, and sternum) are even less capable of allowing x-rays to penetrate and, therefore, their shadows are the whitest of all.

The normal appearance of the heart and lungs must be clearly understood before attempts are made to determine the existence of abnormalities or disease processes. Normal x-ray findings vary considerably with age, sex, and habitus. Different degrees of inspiration affect the appearance of the chest film (Fig 5–4).

It is necessary to approach the interpreting of chest films so that one will be sure not to miss significant findings. Our recommendation is that the x-ray be approached in the following manner: (1) examination of bony structures and the diaphragm; (2) examination of the heart shadow; and (3) examination of the tracheobronchial tree and lung parenchyma.

BONY STRUCTURES AND THE DIAPHRAGM. — The ribs, clavicles, scapula, and a portion of the humeri are clearly outlined on most chest films. The outline of the vertebral column should be visible through the heart shadow unless the film has been underexposed.

The two hemidiaphragms are rounded, smooth, and sharply defined. The right hemidiaphragm is normally situated slightly higher than the left because of the liver. The costophrenic angles are the junction of the rib cage and the diaphragm. These angles should be clearly delineated.

THE HEART. — The cardiac shadow should be sharply defined. Figure 5–4 shows the normal configuration, size, and location of the heart in the erect adult. Gross deviations from the normal are easily seen and assessed by the casual observer, but subtle aberrations must be left to the radiologist, cardiologist, and chest physician.

ASSESSMENT OF THE TRACHEOBRONCHIAL TREE AND LUNG PARENCHYMA. — The trachea is a vertical, translucent shadow situated in the midline overlying the cervical and upper thoracic vertebrae. The *hili*, or lung roots, are poorly defined areas of increased density in the midportion of the central lung field. The hilus is composed primarily of pulmonary blood vessels, bronchi, and lymph nodes. At the level of the fourth thoracic vertebrae, the trachea divides into the right and left main stem bronchi.

Normal lung appears black with fine white "strings" fanning out from the hili. These are shadows of blood vessels and are referred to as *vascular markings.* These should be present throughout the lung but should not be anything but very thin and wispy. Increased vascular markings or "fuzzy" vascular markings are abnormal.

Atelectasis will appear on the chest film as a density. A mediastinal shift to the side of the density may be present. Even segmental or subsegmental areas of collapse can usually be seen on a chest film.

The location of the atelectasis is extremely important for appropriate postural drainage and re-expansion. A helpful technique for locating atelectatic lung on the portable chest film is the use of the *silhouette sign.* The silhouette sign takes advantage of the fact that a density located next to or in front of the heart will obscure the border of the heart. Lung tissue that is collapsed and is located behind the heart will not obscure the heart border. If the heart border is obscured by the density, the collapsed lung must be adjacent to or in front of the heart; if the heart silhouette is intact, the atelectatic area of lung must lie behind the heart. This means that collapse of the posterior basilar segment, the lateral basilar segment, the superior segment of the lower lobe, and the posterior segment of the upper lobe will not obscure the heart silhouette. On the other hand, collapse of the middle lobe, lingula, and the anterior basilar segment of the lower lobe will obscure the heart border.

Miliary atelectasis is defined as physiologically significant atelectasis that is not detectable on chest x-ray because it is diffusely distributed throughout the lung.

Inflammation of lung causes fluid and blood cells to collect in the area. This shows up as a density on x-ray and is termed *infiltrate.* Infiltrate, or consolidation of lung, will usually show up as density, but may be extremely difficult to see. The *air bronchogram* can aid in assessing this lung condition. This radiologic sign takes advantage of the fact that the comparison of air-filled bronchi surrounded by consolidated lung tissue will be visible, whereas bronchi surrounded by normally aerated parenchyma will not be visible because of the lack of difference in density between the air in the bronchus and the air in the surrounding tissue. The existence of clear outlines of bronchi or bronchioles must mean that there is consolidated lung tissue around them.

The Application of Bedside Pulmonary Function Studies

Documentation of ventilatory mechanics is extremely important for initial quantification and for an objective method of following the patient's ventilatory state. The casual observer may completely miss ventilatory abnormalities because the patient is not obviously distressed; i.e., many observers do not delineate dyspnea from respiratory distress. When a patient is in respiratory distress he is experiencing a phenomenon which can be observed and measured. Dyspnea is the *subjective* perception of difficult breathing and cannot be observed or measured.[73]

There have been numerous theories to explain the perception of dyspnea. A popular theory is that the perception of respiratory distress is processed initially in the subcortical portion of the central nervous system (C.N.S.) and then perceived by higher cortical levels and interpreted.[74] Other experts believe the neurons in the lung and tracheobronchial tree affect the subjective perception of respiratory distress. Some believe that the sensation is mediated via the vagus nerve,[75] while still others suggest that chemical interaction and the relationship of the length of the respiratory muscle fibers to their tension contributes to the perception of dyspnea. *The complaint of dyspnea must always receive careful attention—it is a most sensitive and reliable indicator that the work of breathing has acutely changed.*

To further emphasize the difference between dyspnea and respiratory distress, let us take the example of the chronic obstructive pulmonary disease patient whose base-line state is one of obvious shortness of breath. He has existed this way for a long period of time and will deny dyspnea. In spite of shortness of breath and obvious objective signs of difficult breathing, the patient's subjective perception of his work of breathing is unchanged and, therefore, he is subjectively unstressed. At the opposite extreme, a patient may be experiencing a paralyzing disease and complain of difficult breathing far in advance of objective signs.

Pulmonary function studies are means of *objectively* documenting and quantifying the mechanics of breathing. They do not necessarily have any correlation with the subjective complaint of dyspnea.

Visual estimation of the tidal volume is notoriously inaccurate. Most observers are sensitive to increased ventilatory work and distress rather than the quantification of tidal volume. Clinical experience teaches that measurement of minute ventilation and tidal volume are often beneficial in exposing ventilatory pattern abnormalities not obvious to most observers. In addition, the gas exchange is documented so there can be serial comparisons throughout the clinical course.

A meter for measuring tidal volume and minute volume must add little or no resistance to breathing and be accurate over the expected range of flows. The spirometer (ventilometer) is the most commonly used bedside method of measuring tidal volume and minute volume. There are numerous types of spirometers that are portable, simple to use, and accessible. Many are hand-sized, and most have a one-way measuring system combined with a two-way flow system. In other words, the patient can breathe in and out through the apparatus but only the exhaled air will be measured.[44] The spirometer can be attached to a standard anesthesia mask and applied firmly but comfortably. The procedure must be explained to the conscious patient. If the patient is breathing through an endotracheal tube or tracheostomy, the spirometer can be connected through a universal 15 mm adapter. For accurate measurements, the cuff of the endotracheal or tracheostomy tube must be inflated.

The simple spirometer may be used to make three bedside measurements of value: tidal volume, minute volume, and forced vital capacity.

Tidal Volume

With a regular breathing pattern, 10 breaths are measured and the measurement divided by 10. The measurement must be made for one full minute and then divided by the ventilatory rate if the pattern is irregular. The measurement can be made easily in the comatose patient.

Minute Volume

Minute volume can be readily obtained by measuring the tidal volume and multiplying by the ventilatory rate.

FVC

Forced vital capacity (FVC) is an important measurement in the estimation of ventilatory reserve. The measurement depends on the cooperation of the patient and, therefore, is not obtainable in a semicomatose, comatose, or uncooperative patient. The patient is instructed to take the deepest inspiration possible and then, with the spirometer attached, exhale the air as quickly, forcefully, and completely as possible. *Success in obtaining an adequate forced vital capacity at the bedside can be achieved if you fully explain what you want the patient to do and how important it is that he make a maximum effort.* The maneuver should be done at least three times and the best effort recorded.

Since we are concerned with the patient's ability to meet stress by increasing his ventilatory work, the *forced* vital capacity is a far better reflection of ventilatory reserve than the slow vital capacity. Meeting stress means that the ventilatory system must work at a greater energy cost and, therefore, must be working under forced conditions.

Negative Inspiratory Force (NIF)

Estimation of ventilatory reserve is necessary in most patients when forced vital capacity measurement is not obtainable. A reasonable substitute measurement is the *negative inspiratory force* (NIF).[76] Experience has shown that the muscular power needed to provide a vital capacity of approximately 7 ml per pound (15 ml/kg) produces a negative inspiratory force of greater than −20 cm of water in 20 seconds. The normal NIF is in excess of −80 cm of water.

The equipment needed for this measurement is a manometer that will measure negative pressures and an adapter for connection to the anatomic mask or artificial airway. The manometer is attached and completely occluded for a period of 10 to 20 seconds while the inspiratory efforts of the patient are noted. Any degree of obvious distress or changes in vital signs calls for the immediate abandonment of the procedure and the reestablishment of a patent airway.

Clinical Interpretation

The clinical significance of such measurements depends primarily upon the experience and training of the practitioner and the patient. Clinical guidelines established over the last fifteen years have proven reliable as *aids* to clinical judgment—they must never be considered absolute.

1. Normal tidal volume is 6–7 ml/kg (3–4 ml per pound of normal body weight); 1 ml per pound is anatomic deadspace.

2. A decreased tidal volume usually means the presence of restrictive disease, central nervous system depression, or decreased ventilatory reserve.

3. The adult ventilatory rate is normally 12–18 per minute. Slow ventilatory rates (bradypnea) usually reflect severe central nervous system disease or narcotic overdose; increases in ventilatory rate usually indicate decreased ventilatory reserve, hypoxemia, acid-base imbalance, or C.N.S. disease.

4. Minute ventilation is normally between 5 and 10 liters per minute in the adult. This measurement gives us a general reflection of the individual's total mechanical ventilation and may be used in conjunction with blood gas measurements to indicate the efficiency of physiologic gas exchange (see Chapter 19).

5. The forced vital capacity is used primarily as a reflection of the patient's ability to breathe deeply and cough. Experience has shown that the previously non-diseased patient must have a vital capacity of

at least 15 ml/kg to assure that he can breathe deeply and cough effectively.

6. The forced vital capacity is the most readily accessible reflection of ventilatory reserve (see Chapter 3).

Arterial Blood Gases

Unquestionably, the most important single factor in the development of clinical respiratory care has been the clinical availability of blood gas and pH measurements. These are essential tools to the respiratory care practitioner and are as important to him as the electrocardiographic monitor to the coronary care nurse. One cannot be involved in respiratory care without an ability to evaluate and assess arterial blood gas measurements. The greatest confusion surrounding blood gas measurements stems from the fact that few people understand what is being measured and what the measurement reflects. Several textbooks and monographs are available concerning the use and interpretation of arterial blood gases. Respiratory care practitioners must establish a working relationship and familiarity with these measurements since it is impossible to clinically apply respiratory care without clinically applying blood gas measurements.

The partial pressures of arterial oxygen and carbon dioxide have no *direct quantitative* relationship with arterial *content* of carbon dioxide or oxygen; the arterial pH measurement is one of hydrogen ion activity.

Pco_2

The measurement of the partial pressure of carbon dioxide (Pco_2) in the arterial blood is a direct reflection of the adequacy of *alveolar ventilation*. The only nonmetabolic factor that affects the moment-to-moment level of arterial Pco_2 is the efficiency with which the lung exchanges air with blood. This efficiency of exchange, balanced against the metabolic rate that is producing carbon dioxide, will determine the arterial Pco_2. In other words, adequate physiologic ventilation may be defined as an arterial Pco_2 in the normal range. Inadequate physiologic ventilation would be an arterial Pco_2 above normal—a condition referred to as *ventilatory failure* or *respiratory acidosis*. On the other hand, if the arterial Pco_2 were significantly below normal it would signify physiologic hyperventilation—a situation referred to as *alveolar hyperventilation* or *respiratory alkalosis*. The major significance of the arterial Pco_2 measurement to the respiratory care practitioner is that it is an immediate measurement of the adequacy or inadequacy of physiologic ventilation.

pH

The arterial pH is a measurement of the free hydrogen ion concentration in the arterial blood. This measurement has a twofold clinical application: (1) the pH is a reflection of the total acid-base balance of the body and an excellent indicator of tissue milieu; and (2) a sudden significant change in the arterial carbon dioxide tension must chemically affect pH. Over a period of hours or days the kidneys will compensate for acid-base change. Therefore, a PCO_2 change that is accompanied by a normal pH signifies that the ventilatory event is not acute. *Whenever a PCO_2 change is accompanied by a concomitant pH change, it must be assumed that the ventilatory change was of recent onset since it is uncompensated.*

It is important to recognize the suddenness or acuteness of a ventilatory change because the direct threat to life is not only the degree of abnormality of ventilation, but also the rapidity of change in ventilatory status. *The arterial PCO_2 and pH measurements give the respiratory care practitioner a physiologic reflection of the ventilatory and acid-base status.*[35]

PO_2

The arterial PO_2 is a measurement of the dissolved oxygen gas tension in the arterial blood. This is closely related to the saturation of the hemoglobin with oxygen and therefore, the oxygen content of arterial blood. The arterial PO_2 is an extremely important measurement; however, it must be remembered that the measurement does *not* reflect the *tissue* oxygen state (see Chapter 6).

Blood gas measurements reflect the status of cardiopulmonary homeostasis and are, therefore, most useful in the critically ill or pulmonary diseased patient. The sicker the patient, the more frequently blood gas measurements are needed. A complete discussion of blood gases is outside the scope of this text; however, the reader is encouraged to study the subject in depth. No other single factor is more important in respiratory care!

SECTION II
OXYGEN THERAPY

6 • OXYGENATION

THE TRANSPORT and delivery of oxygen to body tissues is the essence of respiratory care. However, unlike modern "miracle" drugs, oxygen has been either taken for granted or ignored as a therapeutic agent. Oxygen therapy can be instituted with relative ease and, unfortunately, with little thought or rationale. Advances in respiratory care have made it obvious that our concepts of oxygen administration must be reviewed and revised. The foundation for the rational use of oxygen is knowledge of its pharmacokinetics and appreciation of the biomedical changes induced by too much tissue oxygen (hyperoxia) and too little tissue oxygen (hypoxia).

Oxygen is the third most abundant atom in the universe, the second most abundant atom in the biosphere, and the most abundant atom on the earth's crust. As the earth's atmosphere developed from one containing primarily hydrogen (a reducing atmosphere) to one containing primarily oxygen (an oxidizing atmosphere), oxygen became available as an energy source for the development of cellular life because it was abundant, accessible, and possessed a high potential. Thus, life forms developed utilizing oxygen as the primary biomedical storage type of energy; in fact, complex forms of life evolved only after mechanisms for maintaining the cellular oxygen environment were developed.

The transition to an oxygen atmosphere forced complex biologic systems to develop defenses against the toxic effects of oxygen. These toxic effects of oxygen were first alluded to by the discoverers of oxygen. In 1785 Lavoisier noted that oxygen must be considered a biomedical double-edged sword—it not only promotes life, but also destroys life.[77] He observed that when there is an excess of oxygen an animal undergoes a severe illness; when oxygen is lacking, death is almost instantaneous.

We now understand that increasing the oxygen tension in tissues will increase the available energy for biologic processes. However, more of the cellular constituents will be destroyed as oxygen tension increases. These two effects occur at all concentrations of oxygen— and, thus, *there must be an oxygen pressure at which biologic activity is optimal.*[78, 79] If the oxygen tension is significantly above or below this optimal pressure, biologic consequences will be dire.

Our biologic systems have evolved complex and varied forms of cellular anti-oxygen defenses.[80] The most universal defense in complex animal forms is the barriers placed in oxygen's path from the external environment to the intracellular environment. An inspired oxygen tension of 60 mm Hg results in an intracellular oxygen pressure in the rat cortex of only 0.6 mm Hg[81] – an oxygen tension reduction of 100-fold. Another major defense against cellular oxygen toxicity is that our atmosphere is composed mainly of nitrogen, an inert gas that suppresses oxidation. Oxygen, in the absence of inert gases like nitrogen, tends to make homeostatic systems decrease oxygen transport to tissues; e.g., atelectasis is more prevalent in pure oxygen environments.[82, 83]

Despite the dangers of cellular oxygen toxicity, there can be no serious objection to the administration of oxygen for the clinical support of the cardiopulmonary system. As is true with the administration of any drug, oxygen must never be administered without good reason and must always be administered properly and safely.

The process of oxygenation is complex and can be related to cardiopulmonary homeostasis in three stages: (1) external respiration, (2) blood oxygen transport, and (3) internal respiration.

External Respiration

External respiration is the transfer of oxygen molecules from atmosphere to blood (see Chapter 4). Oxygen molecules are constantly leaving the alveolus and entering the pulmonary blood. All alveolar oxygen exists as a free gas and, therefore, each molecule exerts a pressure. A decrease in alveolar oxygen content will result in a linear decrease in alveolar oxygen tension. On the other hand, most oxygen molecules entering the blood attach to desaturated hemoglobin and, therefore, do not directly exert a pressure (Fig 6–1). This means the blood will *not* show a linear oxygen tension increase for a linear gain in oxygen volume. At normal atmospheres, *a given volume of oxygen leaving the alveolus and entering the blood will result in alveolar oxygen tensions decreasing at a much faster rate than blood oxygen tensions will increase.*

Pulmonary capillary blood is ideally in equilibrium with alveolar air and, therefore, it is impossible for the left heart blood to have a higher oxygen tension than exists in the alveoli. *Alveolar oxygen tension is the major limiting factor in the oxygenation of desaturated blood.* Therefore, it is essential for us to review the major factors involved in determining the alveolar oxygen tension: (1) fraction of inspired oxygen, (2) alveolar gas exchange, (3) mixed venous oxygen content, and (4) distribution of ventilation.

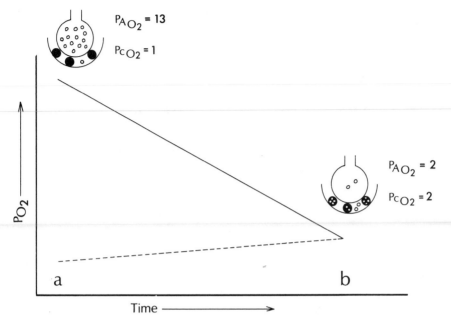

Fig 6–1. — Theoretic representation of alveolar-capillary oxygen equilibration. Solid line represents alveolar oxygen tension; dotted line represents capillary oxygen tension.

At point *a* the alveolus is enriched with fresh oxygen molecules, whereas the capillary blood is desaturated and has a low Po_2. If ventilation and perfusion were to instantaneously stop, oxygen equilibration would be achieved at point *b*. Alveolar oxygen pressure would decrease faster than capillary oxygen pressure would increase. Of course, numerous other factors are significant in the actual dynamic process of respiratory function.

Fraction of Inspired Oxygen (FI_{O_2})

At sea level, the normal individual breathing room air (20.9% oxygen) shows a drop in oxygen tension from 159 mm Hg just outside the mouth to 101 mm Hg in the alveolus. Table 6–1 shows the partial pressures of nitrogen, oxygen, carbon dioxide, and water vapor under normal circumstances. The decrease in oxygen tension from the atmosphere to the alveolus is due to several factors: (1) the addition of water vapor pressure; (2) the addition of a volume of carbon dioxide as well as the removal of a volume of oxygen from the alveolus; and (3) the incomplete pulmonary gas exchange with every breath.

Increasing the percentage of oxygen in the inspired atmosphere will obviously cause an increased alveolar oxygen tension. For practical clinical purposes, we must be able to calculate an approximate "ideal"

TABLE 6-1.—COMPOSITION OF AIR AT SEA LEVEL

AIR		TRACHEA (mm Hg)	ALVEOLUS (mm Hg)
Nitrogen	79.0% (601 mm Hg)	564	572
Oxygen	20.9% (159 mm Hg)	149	101
Carbon dioxide	0.04% (0.3 mm Hg)	0.3	40
Water vapor	Variable	47	47

alveolar oxygen tension. Table 6-2 delineates the universally accepted manner of clinically calculating ideal alveolar oxygen tension.

Alveolar Gas Exchange

It is essential for an alveolus to contain gas during inspiration and expiration so that respiration may occur throughout the entire cycle (see Chapter 4). This means that some gas volume must be maintained within the alveolus during expiration. The degree of replenishment of alveolar gas on inspiration will depend upon the resistance to gas flow in and out of the alveolus and the elastic properties of that alveolus (see Chapter 3). It should be obvious that the greater the alveolar gas exchange, the greater the delivery of oxygen molecules to the alveolus per unit time. Therefore, *a major factor in determining the alveolar oxygen tension would be the degree of alveolar gas exchange.*

Mixed Venous Oxygen Content

Normal transit time for blood through a pulmonary capillary is 0.3 to 0.7 second—more than ample time for complete equilibration with alveolar oxygen tensions as long as diffusion is normal and the alveolar oxygen tension is greater than 80 mm Hg.[41] The hemoglobin saturation curve (Fig 6-2) dictates that the less saturated the hemoglobin, the greater the volume of oxygen necessary to accomplish a predicted increase in oxygen tension. As venous blood becomes more desaturated, the demand for greater oxygen volumes is increased for any predicted rise in blood oxygen tension.

TABLE 6-2.—CALCULATION OF IDEAL ALVEOLAR OXYGEN TENSION

$$P_{A_{O_2}} = (P_B - P_{H_2O}) F_{I_{O_2}} - Pa_{CO_2} (1.25)$$

$P_{A_{O_2}}$ = Alveolar O_2 tension
P_B = Barometric pressure (760 mm Hg at sea level)
P_{H_2O} = Water vapor tension (47 mm Hg)
$F_{I_{O_2}}$ = Fraction of inspired oxygen
Pa_{CO_2} = Arterial carbon dioxide tension

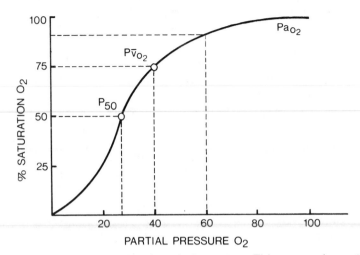

Fig 6–2.—The hemoglobin dissociation curve. This curve shows the relationship of plasma oxygen partial pressure to the degree to which potential
oxygen-carrying hemoglobin sites have oxygen attached (% saturation oxygen). This nonlinear relationship accounts for most of the oxygen reserves
in blood. Normally, hemoglobin is 50% saturated at a plasma Po_2 of approximately 27 mm Hg; this is designated P_{50}. Normal venous blood has an oxygen
partial pressure ($P\bar{v}_{O_2}$) of 40 mm Hg and an oxyhemoglobin saturation of
75%. A Po_2 of 60 mm Hg normally results in approximately 90% saturation.
Normal arterial blood has an oxygen partial pressure (Pa_{O_2}) of 97 mm Hg
and an oxyhemoglobin saturation of 97%. (From Shapiro, B. A., Harrison,
R. A., and Walton, J. R.: *Clinical Application of Blood Gases* [2d ed.; Chicago:
Year Book Medical Publishers, Inc., 1977].)

With a constant inspired oxygen concentration, a constant volume of
alveolar gas exchange, and a constant pulmonary blood flow, a drop in
venous oxygen content must result in a drop in alveolar oxygen tension. A corollary is that if alveolar oxygen tensions are to be maintained in spite of a drop in mixed venous oxygen content, either (1)
alveolar gas exchange must increase; (2) inspired oxygen concentrations must increase; or (3) pulmonary blood flow must decrease.

Distribution of Ventilation

Chapter 4 discusses the factors normally affecting the distribution of
inhaled gases. Many disease states change these relationships. For
example, diseases causing pulmonary mucosal edema, inflammation,
plugging of bronchioles, retained secretions, or changes in the elastic
properties of the alveoli result in extremely uneven gas distribution
throughout the tracheobronchial tree and alveoli. Since *air follows the*

path of least resistance, it must be remembered that any decrease in the diameter of a conducting tube greatly increases the resistance to airflow through that tube. The resistance change is a function of the fourth power of the radius (Poiseuille's law). In addition, the resistance to airflow in partially plugged bronchi is increased by turbulent flow replacing laminar flow (see Chapter 3).

Uneven distribution of ventilation will result in some alveoli being underventilated in comparison with others. Figure 6–3 depicts what occurs when one alveolus, *A*, receives less air exchange than another alveolus, *B*. We will assume blood flow to both alveoli is the same. Alveolus *B* has normal air exchange and normal blood flow so that the alveolar oxygen tension is maintained at 100 mm Hg. Remember, the *alveolar oxygen tension is always the result of fresh gas exchange in the alveolus in relation to the removal of oxygen molecules from the alveolus to the blood.* Alveolar gas exchange and blood flow are nor-

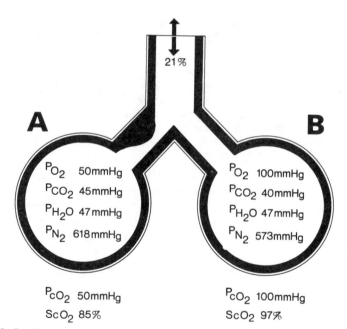

Fig 6–3.—Venous admixture. Alveolus *B* has normal ventilation and perfusion; therefore alveolar gas tensions and pulmonary gas tensions are normal. Alveolus *A* has a bronchiolar constriction, which results in decreased ventilation with normal perfusion. A decreased alveolar P_{O_2} results in a decreased capillary P_{O_2} and hemoglobin saturation. (From Shapiro, B. A., Harrison, R. A., and Walton, J. R.: *Clinical Application of Blood Gases* [2d ed.; Chicago: Year Book Medical Publishers, 1977].)

mal; therefore, alveolar ventilation (alveolar carbon dioxide tension) is 40 mm Hg. Water vapor pressure is 47 mm Hg, and nitrogen makes up the remaining gas pressure. The blood leaving this exchange unit has a carbon dioxide tension of 40 mm Hg and an oxygen tension of 100 mm Hg—the saturation of hemoglobin is 97%.

Alveolus A receives less alveolar gas exchange while blood flow and venous oxygen content remain normal. Therefore, the alveolar oxygen tension is somewhere between the inspired oxygen tension and venous oxygen tension. In this case, the alveolar gas exchange is poor enough to result in an alveolar oxygen tension of 50 mm Hg. The alveolar carbon dioxide tension is elevated (45 mm Hg) because alveolar air exchange is poor; i.e., physiologic alveolar ventilation is below normal. Alveolar P_{CO_2} can never be greater than the venous P_{CO_2}.

UNEVEN DISTRIBUTION OF VENTILATION WITH RESPECT TO THE PERFUSION IS THE MOST COMMON CLINICAL PHENOMENON RESPONSIBLE FOR HYPOXEMIA THAT IS RESPONSIVE TO OXYGEN THERAPY (SHUNT EFFECT). Blood leaving alveolus A has an oxygen tension of 50 mm Hg with a hemoglobin saturation of 85%. This phenomenon of "perfusion in excess of ventilation" is termed *shunt effect* or *ventilation-perfusion inequality* and results in left heart oxygen tensions below the calculated "ideal" alveolar oxygen tension (see Chapter 4). Note that the balance of alveolar gas tension is maintained by an increased nitrogen tension (P_{N_2}). Thus, nitrogen will go from alveolus to blood and cause an arterial P_{N_2} in excess of the theoretical "ideal" alveolar P_{N_2}. This is called *nitrogen shunting*.[84]

Blood Oxygen Transport

External respiration transfers oxygen from the atmosphere to the blood. Blood oxygen transport includes the processes which are responsible for the movement of oxygen from the blood in the left heart to the site of intracellular utilization. Blood oxygen transport is primarily a function of three variables: (1) cardiac output, (2) hemoglobin concentration, and (3) hemoglobin oxygen affinity.

Cardiac Output

Body tissues require a given amount of oxygen per unit time. It makes no difference whether the oxygen comes from a great quantity of blood or a small quantity of blood. Thus, when oxygen consumption remains constant, the amount of oxygen that must be extracted from a given quantity of blood is directly determined by the blood flow per unit time. In other words, if 25 ml of oxygen is required and utilized by an organ system every minute, this is the same as saying that the organ's oxygen consumption remains constant. Therefore, 25 ml of oxygen will be removed from the blood whether 1 L or 5 L is supplying the organ system. As blood flow per unit time increases, less oxygen will be extracted from any given quantity of blood. In this manner, *cardiac output has a significant effect on the venous oxygen content as well as on total oxygen availability.*

Hemoglobin Concentration

When a hemoglobin solution is exposed to a gas atmosphere containing oxygen, most of the oxygen entering the solution immediately attaches to hemoglobin. *Oxygen that is attached to hemoglobin is not dissolved and does not directly exert a gas pressure.* Exposing the hemoglobin to various oxygen tensions results in various degrees of oxyhemoglobin saturation. When the hemoglobin is exposed to oxygen tensions of 0 to 100 mm Hg, a sigmoid curve results. This is known as the *hemoglobin dissociation curve* (see Fig 6-2). Between oxygen tensions of 20 mm Hg and 80 mm Hg, the blood can exchange great amounts of oxygen with very small changes in oxygen tension. This means that the highest pressure of oxygen is maintained in the blood so that the greatest degree of driving pressure between blood and tissue is maintained for oxygen to be given to tissues.

The hemoglobin is the major determinant of the total amount of oxygen that is carried in the blood. When oxygen exchange with tissues takes place, the hemoglobin allows high blood oxygen tensions to be maintained while significant amounts of oxygen are given to the tissues. The oxygen content is the sum of the oxygen attached to he-

---

TABLE 6-3.—CALCULATING OXYGEN CONTENT

Grams percent (gm%) = grams of hemoglobin per 100 ml blood
Volumes percent (vol%) = milliliters of oxygen per 100 ml blood

STEPS

1. Hemoglobin content (gm%) $\times$ 1.34 $\times$ SO_2 = oxygen attached to hemoglobin (vol%)
2. PO_2 $\times$ 0.003 = oxygen dissolved in plasma (vol%)
3. Steps 1 + 2 = *oxygen content* (vol%)

Example 1: Hb 15 gm%, PO_2 100 mm Hg, SO_2 100%
    1. 15 $\times$ 1.34 $\times$ 1.00 = 20.10 vol%
    2. 100 $\times$ 0.003   =   0.30 vol%
    3.   20.40 vol%

Example 2: Hb 15 gm%, PO_2 50 mm Hg, SO_2 85%
    1. 15 $\times$ 1.34 $\times$ 0.85 = 17.09 vol%
    2. 50 $\times$ 0.003   =   0.15 vol%
    3.   17.24 vol%

moglobin plus that dissolved in plasma. Steps in the calculation of oxygen content are shown in Table 6-3. *Oxygen content* is a major factor in the process of tissue oxygenation. The role of hemoglobin concentration in maintaining adequate blood oxygen transport cannot be overemphasized.[35]

Hemoglobin Oxygen Affinity

Hemoglobin has a certain affinity for oxygen, allowing blood to readily oxygenate in the pulmonary capillary bed. Extreme changes in this affinity can make the hemoglobin less capable of releasing oxygen to the tissues. Various factors alter this affinity, and in so doing change the normal relationships between hemoglobin saturation and oxygen tension. In other words, *a change in the hemoglobin affinity for oxygen changes the position of the hemoglobin dissociation curve.* This is called "shifting the curve" (Fig 6-4).

1. Decreasing oxygen affinity results in a "shift to the right": for any given oxygen tension there is a lower percentage of oxyhemoglobin. *The oxygen transport capability of the blood is decreased because oxygen content is decreased.* It should be pointed out that a shift to the right aids oxygen movement from blood to tissue. However, it also results in a decreased oxygen content. This decreased oxygen content limits the *amount* of oxygen that can be given to tissue regardless of how easily it leaves the hemoglobin.

2. Increasing oxygen affinity results in a "shift to the left": for any given oxygen tension there is a higher percentage of saturated hemoglobin. This means that the oxygen content of the blood is increased. The significance of increased affinity on tissue oxygenation *may* be profound. Hemoglobin may be thought of as an "oxygen magnet" in the blood: the stronger the magnet, the less effective is a given oxygen blood-to-tissue pressure gradient in transferring oxygen to the tissues. *The greater the hemoglobin affinity for oxygen, the less effective any arterial oxygen tension may be in delivering oxygen to the tissues.*

It has been known for years that hydrogen ion concentration, carbon dioxide tension, temperature, and other factors affect hemoglobin affinity for oxygen. An increase in any of these factors produces a shift to the right. *Whenever there is a shift to the right, there is automatically a decreased oxygen content.* Within limits, acidemia, hypercarbia, and hyperthermia all tend to cause decreased blood oxygen content and, by inference, increased oxygen availability to the tissues. This decreased oxygen content may greatly enhance the possibility of tissue hypoxia because the oxygen transport capability of the blood is decreased.

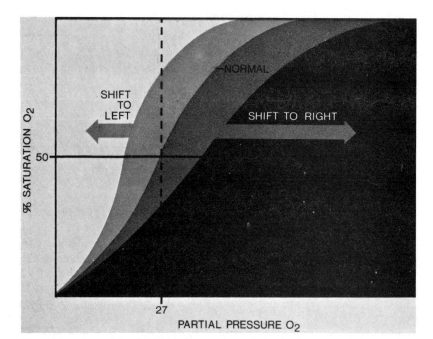

Fig 6–4. — Hemoglobin affinity for oxygen. Increased oxygen affinity *(shift to the left)* means there will be a higher oxygen content at any given Po_2. Conversely, decreased oxygen affinity *(shift to the right)* means there will be a lower oxygen content at any given Po_2. A shift to the left is the result of alkalemia (decreased H^+), hypothermia (cold), hypocarbia (decreased Pco_2), and decreased 2,3-diphosphoglycerate. A *shift to the right* is the result of acidemia (increased H^+), hyperthermia (fever), hypercarbia (increased Pco_2), and increased 2,3-DPG. (From Shapiro, B. A., Harrison, R. A., and Walton, J. R.: *Clinical Application of Blood Gases* [2d ed.; Chicago: Year Book Medical Publishers, 1977].)

Studies of red blood cells have revealed that certain enzyme systems are responsible for aiding the dissociation of oxygen from hemoglobin. Many phosphorylase enzyme systems seem to be involved, but the most completely studied at present is the enzyme producing the substrate 2,3-diphosphoglycerate (2,3-DPG). This enzyme system enhances the dissociation of oxygen from hemoglobin by competing with oxygen for the iron-binding site.[85] Thus, lowered levels of the enzyme will produce an increased hemoglobin affinity for oxygen, which has the same effect as shifting the curve to the left. The laboratory ability to measure such changes led to the development of the P_{50} measurement.

The P_{50} is defined as the oxygen tension at which 50% of the hemo-

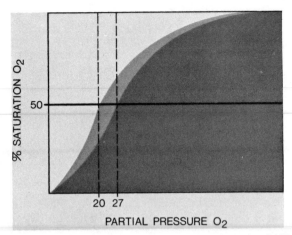

Fig 6–5. — P_{50}, a measurement of oxygen affinity. At normal pH and temperature the hemoglobin curve will be such that 50% of the hemoglobin will be saturated at a Po_2 of 27–28 mm Hg. If hemoglobin affinity for oxygen is increased for some reason other than alkalemia, cold, or hypocapnia, hemoglobin will be 50% saturated at a lower Po_2. Thus, a P_{50} of 20 mm Hg means the oxygen affinity is increased. (From Shapiro, B. A., Harrison, R. A., and Walton, J. R.: *Clinical Application of Blood Gases* [2d ed.; Chicago: Year Book Medical Publishers, 1977].)

globin is saturated under very specific conditions of laboratory measurement: 37°C, Pco_2 40 mm Hg, and pH 7.40.[86, 87] Figure 6–5 illustrates the concept of the P_{50} measurement. Whatever the laboratory method for determining P_{50}, the conditions of a pH of 7.40, a Pco_2 of 40 mm Hg, and a body temperature of 37°C must be included. In most laboratories Pco_2 and pH are calculated in the final determination.[88] It must be emphasized that pH, Pco_2, and temperature changes in the patient will affect the hemoglobin affinity for oxygen (see Fig 6–4) but will not affect the P_{50} measurement.

The normal adult P_{50} is approximately 27 mm Hg; in other words, normal adult hemoglobin is 50% saturated at a Po_2 of 27 mm Hg when the temperature is 37°C, the Pco_2 is 40 mm Hg, and the pH is 7.40.[89] The clinical significance of P_{50} measurement is not clear—in fact, some doubt its usefulness completely.[90, 91] The *concept*, however, is essential in understanding blood oxygen transport.

Hypoxemia

Hypoxemia is traditionally defined as "a relative deficiency of oxygen in the blood." Since arterial Po_2 measurement has become the standard means for clinical evaluation of blood oxygenation, we shall define hypoxemia as *a relative deficiency of oxygen tension in the arterial blood.*[35] Such a definition is completely compatible with current medical literature and lends itself most readily to the clinical care of acutely ill patients.

In the absence of a significantly increased hemoglobin concentration, hypoxemia is synonymous with a decreased oxygen content. It must be emphasized that hypoxemia is *not* always synonymous with tissue hypoxia. An arterial oxygen tension of less than normal is a *potential* threat to adequate tissue oxygenation but is *not* a direct reflection of tissue oxygenation.

Physiologic Causes of Hypoxemia

A simplistic statement that serves as a clinical generality is: *All arterial hypoxemia is due either to a decreased alveolar oxygen tension or intrapulmonary shunting.*

1. *Decreased alveolar oxygen tensions* must result in decreased pulmonary capillary oxygen tensions. We have seen previously that numerous factors can cause alveoli to have decreased oxygen tensions: (1) alveolar underventilation in relation to perfusion (shunt effect), (2) decreased venous hemoglobin saturation, and (3) alveolar hypoventilation when breathing room air.

2. *Intrapulmonary shunting* is blood from the right heart entering the left heart without exchange with alveolar gas (see Chapter 4). When the adequately oxygenated blood returning from the lungs mixes with this desaturated blood, a decreased oxygen content results. Since the shunted blood contains poorly saturated hemoglobin, even small amounts (10–20%) may result in significant decreases in arterial PO_2. Intrapulmonary shunting is a common manifestation of pulmonary disease and is often responsible for arterial hypoxemia. It must be remembered that the degree to which a shunt will manifest hypoxemia is dependent upon the hemoglobin saturation of the blood that is being shunted. Thus, *the hypoxemic effect of a shunt is as much dependent upon mixed venous hemoglobin saturation as it is upon the size of the shunt.*

The Pulmonary Response to Hypoxemia

A significant decrease in oxygen supply (e.g., decreased oxygen content; decreased arterial oxygen tension; or decreased blood flow) may result in *peripheral chemoreceptor hypoxia* (see Chapter 1). This initiates afferent signals to the midbrain where efferent signals are then sent to the ventilatory muscles. Theoretically, the increased ventilation should produce an increased alveolar oxygen tension, which in turn should produce more blood oxygen and, thereby, relieve the chemoreceptor hypoxia. This mechanism for compensating for hypoxemia is inefficient for two reasons: (1) It has little effect on hypoxemia secondary to true physiologic shunting, since the blood that is exchanging with alveolar air is already adequately oxygenated. The increased alveolar tensions add little oxygen to the exchanging capillary blood and have no effect on the shunted blood. (2) A point may be reached at which the oxygen consumed for the increased work of breathing cancels any oxygen gained from increased ventilation (see Chapter 3).

The pulmonary response to hypoxemia is quite efficient in circumstances where the hypoxemia is secondary to decreased alveolar oxygen tensions. Of course, increasing inspired oxygen concentration is a far more efficient method of raising alveolar oxygen tensions since it does not demand increased ventilatory work.

The Cardiovascular Response to Hypoxemia

The most effective mechanism by which the body responds to hypoxemia is that of increasing cardiac output. It is important to understand that tissue demand for oxygen is constant over a given period of time. Thus, if the cardiac output increases while metabolic rate stays stable, the amount of oxygen extracted from any 100 ml of blood decreases. *The effect of this is to increase the venous oxygen tension and its corresponding hemoglobin saturation.* Of course, systemic A-V shunting will produce the same result but at the *expense* of tissue oxygenation.

Hypoxemia and Oxygen Therapy

Only hypoxemia caused by a decreased alveolar oxygen tension will respond dramatically to oxygen therapy! This should be obvious since the prime purpose of breathing an increased oxygen concentration is to increase the alveolar oxygen tension. It is essential to remember that ventilation-perfusion mismatch will result in regional areas of decreased alveolar PO_2's. This type of V/Q inequality (or perfusion in excess of ventilation) is responsive to oxygen therapy.

The primary compensatory mechanisms for hypoxemia caused by true physiologic shunting are either (1) an increase in cardiac output; (2) a decrease in the oxygen utilization (A-V systemic shunting); or (3) a direct decrease in the amount of shunting by a change in the pulmonary distribution of perfusion.

Internal Respiration

The volume of oxygen consumed by the body in one minute is defined as *oxygen consumption* (V_{O_2}). Many factors determine the amount of oxygen to be consumed, such as temperature, stress, thyroid function, adverse biochemical effects of disease, and physical activity. At complete rest, the body is considered in a *basal metabolic state,* and the oxygen consumption per minute is known as the *basal metabolic rate.* The respiratory care practitioner must appreciate that there are numerous factors affecting oxygen consumption besides the demand of cells for oxygen. Obviously, the adequacy of transport of oxygen to the tissues is significant along with the existence of an adequate oxygen pressure gradient between blood and tissue. It must be remembered that the *microvascular system* (capillaries) plays a great role in determining oxygen consumption. There is no way for oxygen to be consumed if the blood does not flow through the systemic capillaries. Therefore, internal respiration involves diffusion of oxygen into the cell and appropriate utilization of the oxygen.

Tissue Hypoxia

Cellular energy is necessary to accomplish chemical reactions. Many essential biochemical reactions for sustaining life require a considerable amount of energy, in fact, such a high degree of energy that they have been referred to as "thermodynamically improbable."[92] This means that the energy required for many necessary biochemical cellular functions is so great that it is almost impossible to conceive that the cell can manufacture such energy. The cell obtains this great degree of energy from substances called *high-energy phosphate bonds.* In respiratory care we are primarily concerned with the high-energy phosphate bond that is contained in adenosine triphosphate (ATP). Most cellular energy is utilized, transported, and stored in the form of these high-energy phosphate bonds. Breakdown of these bonds is accompanied by a tremendous energy release.[93]

Oxidative metabolism is the normal mechanism by which energy is stored and released from high-energy phosphate bonds. The *mitochondria* are cellular constituents that contain all the components necessary to form and break down ATP. Molecular oxygen must be available in the cell in order for the biochemical process within the mitochondria (Krebs cycle) to produce high-energy phosphate bonds and allow the release of energy for biochemical processes.[93]

When the delivery of oxygen to the mitochondria becomes impaired, the energy contained within the Krebs cycle can no longer be made available. The cellular oxygen tension at which the mito-chondrial respiratory rate begins to decrease is called the *critical oxy-gen tension*.[93] Various studies show that as long as other factors are normal, the mitochondria can function adequately when cellular oxy-gen tension is less than 5 mm Hg.[93] At the present time, however, it is not possible to delineate critical oxygen tensions for various vital or-gan systems under various conditions.

We make the clinical statement that tissue hypoxia exists when the cellular critical oxygen tensions are inadequate. This seems clinically appropriate since the importance of the presence of tissue hypoxia is that mechanisms other than oxidative ones must be utilized to provide metabolic energy. These *anaerobic* mechanisms are homeostatically undesirable because (1) they are far less efficient than aerobic path-ways, and (2) they produce metabolites other than carbon dioxide.

Dysoxia

Dysoxia has been suggested as a term to characterize abnormal utili-zation of oxygen in the tissues.[94] It appears to be a useful term because it encompasses not only tissue hypoxia (a reflection of altered oxygen transport) but also alterations in cellular oxygen utilization. Such ab-normal tissue oxygen utilization in the presence of adequate cellular oxygen tension may be due to two factors: (1) intrinsic mitochondrial malfunction or (2) hyperoxia. Discussion of the former is beyond the scope of this text and has no clinical application at present. The second factor (hyperoxia) is of critical importance to the respiratory care practitioner.

Dysoxia related to hyperoxia is associated with four disorders sec-ondary to erroneous application of techniques: (1) depression of ven-tilatory stimulus in chronic hypercarbic patients who depend on peripheral chemoreceptor hypoxia; (2) use of capillary P_{O_2} measure-ments as a guide for oxygen therapy in neonates; (3) adult blood ex-change transfusion in neonates;[94] and (4) direct cellular toxicity. The lung appears more susceptible to direct cellular toxicity than other tissue — this pulmonary oxygen toxicity is discussed in the following chapter.

Summary

Appropriate oxygenation depends upon adequate external respira-tion, oxygen blood transport, and internal respiration. Hypoxemia is the primary means by which we clinically assess oxygenation status. Various pathophysiologic causes of hypoxemia are responsive to different supportive techniques. True intrapulmonary shunting disease is supported by increasing cardiovascular function and reversing pulmonary pathology (e.g., bronchial hygiene therapy, PEEP therapy). However, a major therapeutic technique for supporting hypoxemia is oxygen therapy, which is discussed in the next chapter.

7 • OXYGEN THERAPY

THE APPLICATION OF OXYGEN to ill patients was first attempted over a century and a half ago, and since then it has been shrouded in uncertainty. As late as 1945 there was serious debate in the medical literature as to whether oxygen should have a therapeutic place in medicine. Although blood gas measurements give us the means of properly monitoring oxygen therapy and advances in respiratory therapy have made it possible to administer oxygen properly, few physicians or allied health personnel understand oxygen therapy. Thus, before considering how oxygen therapy affects ventilation and the oxygenation state, it is necessary to clearly state the objectives of oxygen therapy and explain oxygen administration.

Goals of Oxygen Therapy

Before hospitals were air conditioned it was common practice to place a patient in an oxygen tent primarily to cool him on a warm day. Unfortunately, many physicians felt this was the *only* purpose of oxygen administration. Another common practice was to place an oxygen apparatus on the critically ill patient to alleviate his emotional stress. Undoubtedly there is some psychologic value in this, but it is by no means the basic advantage of proper oxygen therapy, which is its physiologic value.

The only direct effect of breathing fractions of inspired oxygen ($F_{I_{O_2}}$) above 21% is one of the following:

1. The alveolar oxygen tensions may be increased.
2. The ventilatory work necessary to maintain a given alveolar oxygen tension may be decreased.
3. The myocardial work necessary to maintain a given arterial oxygen tension may be decreased.

Through a sound understanding of cardiopulmonary physiology it becomes obvious that there are three clinical goals that can be accomplished with proper oxygen therapy.

Treat hypoxemia. — When arterial hypoxemia is a result of decreased alveolar oxygen tensions, that hypoxemia may be dramatically improved by increasing the inspired oxygen fractions.

Decrease the work of breathing. — Increased ventilatory work is a common response to hypoxemia and/or hypoxia. Enriched inspired oxygen atmospheres may allow a more normal alveolar gas exchange to maintain adequate alveolar oxygen levels. The result is a decreased need for total ventilation, which means a decreased work of breathing at no expense to the oxygenation status.

Decrease myocardial work. — The cardiovascular system is a primary mechanism for compensation of hypoxemia and/or hypoxia. Oxygen therapy can effectively support many disease states by decreasing or preventing the demand for increased myocardial work.

Administration of Oxygen

Fraction of Inspired Oxygen

Having established clear clinical goals, the evaluation of the adequacy and effectiveness of oxygen therapy is a matter of clinical examination and blood gas measurement—as long as the administration of oxygen is consistent and predictable! This necessitates a knowledge of oxygen devices, techniques, and inspired oxygen fractions.

Normal variances in the distribution of ventilation and pulmonary blood flow make the measurement of alveolar oxygen concentrations impractical and complex. Significant variation in oxygen concentration may occur throughout the inspiratory cycle; where and when to make the measurement is not universally agreed upon. Attempts at sampling tracheal air have been limited because of the slow electrode response time of available equipment.[95, 96] Recent technical advances have made this measurement more practical, but the clinical application of an "invasive" technique remains difficult to justify for routine use. The necessity exists for having a measurement that can be easily, practically, and consistently used in the clinical setting to reflect inspired oxygen concentrations. Such a measurement might be the percent (fraction) of inspired gas that is oxygen ($F_{I_{O_2}}$).

Clinical definition of $F_{I_{O_2}}$. — Since the final judgment of the adequacy of oxygen therapy is made by blood gas analysis and clinical examination, the major requisites of oxygen administration are *consistency* and *control*. Logic dictates that the most reasonable approach is to define the $F_{I_{O_2}}$ as the *measurable* or *calculable* concentration of oxygen delivered to the patient; i.e., if a tidal volume of 500 ml is composed of 250 ml oxygen, the $F_{I_{O_2}}$ will be considered 50%. In other words, we will not be concerned with how the gases are distributed throughout the tracheobronchial tree and the lung parenchyma; the concern will be solely with the fact that 50% of the entire inspired atmosphere is oxygen. This provides us with a consistent, practical, and understandable terminology that is easily applied to any method of oxygen therapy. With this arbitrary definition accepted, reliable oxygen therapy becomes a matter of methodology and thorough understanding of oxygen delivery systems.

Gas Delivery Systems

The advent of anesthetic gases and their clinical administration necessitated the development of gas delivery systems to meet various needs. The past century has seen a myriad of techniques developed for delivering controlled gas concentrations.[97] All these techniques fall into one of two categories: non-rebreathing and rebreathing systems.

NON-REBREATHING SYSTEMS (FIG 7–1).—A non-rebreathing system is designed so that exhaled gases have minimal contact with inspiratory gases. In most cases, this is simply a matter of venting the exhaled gases to the atmosphere via one-way valves. A primary advantage to non-rebreathing systems is that exhaled carbon dioxide does not have to be dealt with in the inspiratory gas system. However, a gas flow sufficient to meet the requirements of the minute volume and peak flow rate must be supplied. This is usually accomplished by an inspiratory reservoir which allows an additional amount of gas to be available during the transient times when inspiratory demands are beyond the capabilities of the uniform flow rates delivered by the apparatus.

To better meet this problem of sufficient gas delivery, non-rebreath-

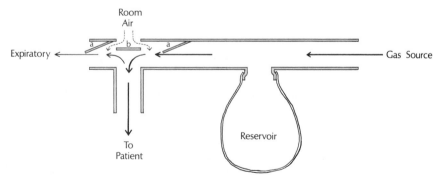

Fig 7–1.—A model non-rebreathing system. The gas source must supply a volume at least equal to the patient's minute ventilation. A reservoir bag serves to make gas available to meet peak flow requirements. A one-way valve system (at points a) assures the patient will inhale only fresh gas and exhale only to the room atmosphere. A one-way valve (b) will allow room air to supply a portion of the inspiratory volume if the gas source and reservoir prove inadequate.

ing systems have been developed in which a one-way valve allows room air to enter if the system itself is not adequate to meet the ventilatory demands. In this way, adequate minute volume and peak inspiratory flow volume are assured. This is accomplished at the expense of diluting the initially delivered gas concentrations with room air.

A non-rebreathing system in which the minute volume, flow rates, and reservoir system are adequate to meet the total ventilatory needs of the patient is called a *high-flow system*. Whenever room air must enter the system to meet total gas requirements, the system is considered a *low-flow system*. In other words, *low-flow non-rebreathing systems do not allow inspired gas mixtures to be determined precisely*.

REBREATHING SYSTEMS. — A rebreathing system is one in which a reservoir exists on the expiratory line and a carbon dioxide absorber is present so that the exhaled air minus the CO_2 can re-enter the inspiratory system. Rebreathing systems gained popularity in anesthesia because of their potential for conserving expensive anesthetic gases and because many anesthetic gases are explosive.

During induction of anesthesia, the rebreathing system is often used as a high-flow, non-rebreathing system. By preventing exhaled gases from diluting fresh inspired gas, the concentration of anesthetic gases delivered to the patient is kept constant. In other words, anesthesiology has long recognized that high-flow, non-rebreathing systems are most desirable for precise control of inspired gas mixtures.[98]

Oxygen Delivery Systems

Modern oxygen therapy is properly administered by *non-rebreathing systems* because (1) oxygen is a nonexplosive agent, (2) the expense is not prohibitive, and (3) rebreathing CO_2 is easily avoided. Since we are dealing with oxygen delivery and non-rebreathing systems, we may think in terms of high-flow and low-flow systems.

The *high-flow system* is defined as one in which the gas flow of the apparatus is sufficient to meet all inspiratory requirements. A *low-flow system* is one in which the gas flow of the apparatus is *in*sufficient to meet all inspiratory requirements. Thus, room air must be used to provide part of the inspired atmosphere.

Most of the confusion surrounding oxygen therapy results from referring to the *technique* rather than to the *device*. Low-*concentration* oxygen techniques were unfortunately described in terms of oxygen *flow rate* through a nasal cannula. This "low-flow oxygen administration" has led much of the medical world to believe that low flow is synonymous with low concentration. *Since it is the fraction of inspired oxygen that is important, oxygen flow should be considered only in relation to the total gas flow.* The concentration of oxygen delivered by any oxygen flow rate is determined solely by the apparatus and patient.

HIGH-FLOW OXYGEN SYSTEMS. — A high-flow oxygen system is one in which the flow rate and reservoir capacity are adequate to provide the total inspired atmosphere. In other words, the patient is breathing only the gas that is supplied by the apparatus. The characteristics of a high-flow oxygen delivery system are distinct from the *concentration* of oxygen provided; both high and low oxygen concentrations may be administered by high-flow systems.

Most high-flow oxygen delivery systems use a *Venturi device* (Fig 7-2), i.e., a system using the Bernoulli principle to "entrain" room air in static proportion to oxygen flows (Table 7-1). Such a device provides high total gas flows of fixed FI_{O_2}. The Bernoulli principle states that the lateral pressure of a gas decreases as its velocity of flow increases. Therefore, an oxygen flow through a constricted orifice, be-

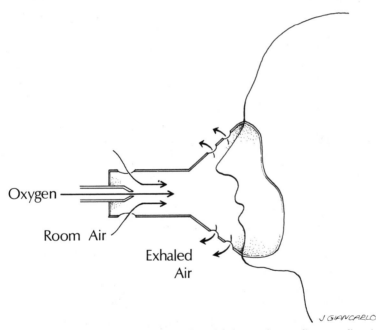

Oxygen

Room Air

Exhaled
Air

J. GIANCARLO

Fig 7-2. — A Venturi device providing high total gas flow at fixed FI_{O_2}. Pressurized oxygen is forced through a narrowed orifice; Bernoulli's principle determines the amount of room air "entrained" (see text). A Venturi mask is depicted; however, the Venturi mechanism is found in almost all high-flow oxygen delivery systems.

TABLE 7-1.—APPROXIMATE AIR
ENTRAINMENT RATIO

OXYGEN CONCENTRATION (%)	AIR°/100% O_2
24	25/1
28	10/1
34	5/1
40	3/1
60	1/1
70	0.6/1

Examples:
    a. 40% Venturi device—10 L/min O_2 flow will produce a total gas flow of approximately 40 L/min.
    b. 28% Venturi device—4 L/min O_2 flow will produce a total gas flow of approximately 44 L/min.
    ° Room air is assumed to be 20.9% oxygen.

cause of its great increase in velocity of flow, can create a "subatmospheric" pressure just after leaving the orifice. This subatmospheric pressure "entrains" room air. By varying the orifice size and oxygen flow, the $F_{I_{O_2}}$ may be varied.

High-flow systems can provide concentrations of 24–100% oxygen. There are *Venturi masks* available that provide 24–40% oxygen in addition to nebulizers utilizing the Venturi principle that can provide 30–100% oxygen concentrations. Numerous valves and appliances are available to provide varying $F_{I_{O_2}}$'s through high-flow systems.

High-flow systems have two major advantages: (1) because consistent $F_{I_{O_2}}$'s are provided as long as the system is properly applied, changes in the patient's ventilatory pattern do not affect the $F_{I_{O_2}}$; and (2) since the entire inspired atmosphere is provided, the temperature and humidity of the gas may be controlled.

$F_{I_{O_2}}$ can be directly measured in a high-flow system with an oxygen analyzer. Numerous analyzers are commercially available and most are reliable and accurate when properly used and maintained. The fact that oxygen concentration can be *measured* in a high-flow system is a significant advantage for critically ill patients. If not for the disadvantages of economics and patient comfort, high-flow systems would certainly be the method of choice for all oxygen therapy.

LOW-FLOW OXYGEN SYSTEMS.—The low-flow system does not provide sufficient gas to supply the entire inspired atmosphere; therefore, part of the tidal volume must be supplied by breathing room air. Any concentration of oxygen from 21% to 90+% can be provided by such a system. The variables controlling $F_{I_{O_2}}$ are (1) the capacity of the available oxygen reservoir; (2) the oxygen flow (L/min); and (3) the patient's ventilatory pattern. These systems are used because of tradition, familiarity, patient comfort, economics, and availability—*not* because of accuracy or dependability.

In principle, low-flow systems depend primarily upon the existence of a *reservoir* of oxygen and its dilution with room air. To demonstrate the use of low-flow systems, let us consider a "normal" person with a "normal" ventilatory pattern:

Tidal volume (V_T)	500 ml
Ventilatory rate (RR)	20/min
Inspiratory time	1 sec
Expiratory time	2 sec
Anatomic reservoir	50 ml

The anatomic reservoir is composed of the nose, the nasopharynx, and the oropharynx (Fig 7–3). We will assume that the volume of the anatomic reservoir is one third of the anatomic deadspace; therefore, $1/3 \times 150$ ml $= 50$ ml.

A nasal cannula with an oxygen flow of 6 L/min (100 ml/sec) is placed on this patient. We can safely assume that most of the expired flow occurs during the first 1.5 sec (75%) of the expiratory time; i.e., the last 0.5 sec of expiration has negligible expired gas flow. This allows the anatomic reservoir to fill completely with 100% oxygen because the flow rate is 50 ml/0.5 sec (100 ml/sec).

Assuming all oxygen supplied by the cannula and contained in the anatomic reservoir is inspired by the patient, the next 500 ml tidal volume, which takes 1 sec, is composed of:

50 ml of 100% oxygen from the anatomic reservoir.

100 ml of 100% oxygen supplied by the cannula flow rate.

350 ml of 20% oxygen (room air); thus, 0.20×350 ml $= 70$ ml oxygen.

The 500 ml of inspired gas contains 220 ml of 100% oxygen: 50 ml + 100 ml + 70 ml = 220 ml. We calculate:

$$\frac{220 \text{ ml oxygen}}{500 \text{ ml}} = 44\% \text{ oxygen}$$

This means that a patient with an "ideal ventilatory pattern" who receives 6 L/min of oxygen flow by nasal cannula is receiving an FI_{O_2} of 44%.

If we compute for this person all flows from 1 L to 6 L by nasal cannula or catheter, we see that for every liter-per-minute change in flow rate there is approximately a 4% change in the inspired oxygen fraction (Table 7–2, A).

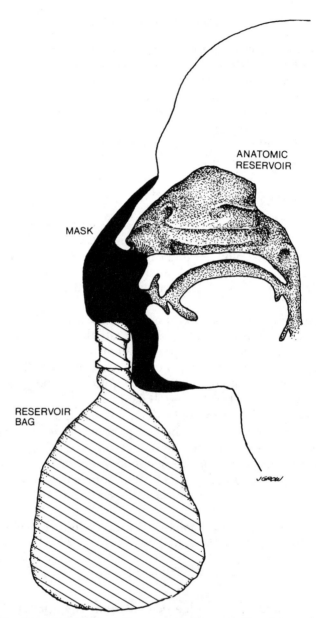

Fig 7–3.—Reservoirs in low-flow oxygen therapy. The *anatomic reservoir* consists of the nose, the nasopharynx, and the oropharynx. This reservoir is estimated to be approximately one third of the anatomic deadspace. The *appliance reservoir* consists of (1) the mask—100–200 ml volume, depending on the appliance; and (2) the reservoir bag—600–1,000 ml of added volume. (From Shapiro, B. A., Harrison, R. A., and Walton, J. R.: *Clinical Application of Blood Gases* [2d ed.; Chicago: Year Book Medical Publishers, Inc., 1977].)

TABLE 7-2.—GUIDELINES FOR
ESTIMATING $F_{I_{O_2}}$ WITH LOW-FLOW
OXYGEN DEVICES

100% O_2 FLOW RATE (L)	$F_{I_{O_2}}$ (%)
A. Nasal cannula or catheter:	
1	24
2	28
3	32
4	36
5	40
6	44
B. Oxygen mask:	
5-6	40
6-7	50
7-8	60
C. Mask with reservoir bag:	
6	60
7	70
8	80
9	90
10	99+

Note: Normal ventilatory pattern is assumed.

For practical application, we must have some guidelines for "estimating" the $F_{I_{O_2}}$ that a given low-flow apparatus with a given oxygen flow will deliver to a patient. It is essential to understand that *the $F_{I_{O_2}}$ in a low-flow system varies tremendously with changes in tidal volume and ventilatory pattern.*

Let us consider the same patient with his tidal volume reduced by half: 250 ml instead of 500 ml. The quantities now are

50 ml of 100% oxygen from the anatomic reservoir.

100 ml of 100% oxygen determined by the cannula flow rate.

100 ml of 20% oxygen (room air).

Thus, the 250 ml of inspired gas contains 170 ml of 100% oxygen: 50 ml + 100 ml + 20 ml = 170 ml. We calculate:

$$\frac{170 \text{ ml oxygen}}{250 \text{ ml}} = 68\% \text{ oxygen}$$

In a low-flow system, the larger the tidal volume, the lower the $F_{I_{O_2}}$; or the smaller the tidal volume, the higher the $F_{I_{O_2}}$.

A low-flow system delivers consistent oxygen concentrations as long as the ventilatory pattern is unchanged. However, it is erroneous to assume *that a nasal cannula guarantees low-concentration oxygen.* Obviously, a 1 or 2 L oxygen flow in a patient breathing shallowly can deliver much higher oxygen concentrations than one would be led to believe.

A nasal cannula can be used as long as the nasal passages are patent, since mouth breathing does not affect $F_{I_{O_2}}$. The airflow in the oropharynx creates a Bernoulli effect in the nasopharynx and air is inspired through the nose. Remember, the *nasal passages must be patent*.

A nasal cannula or catheter with more than a 6 L flow does little to increase inspired oxygen concentrations, primarily because the anatomic reservoir is filled. Thus, in order to provide a higher $F_{I_{O_2}}$ with a low-flow system, one has to increase the size of the oxygen reservoir. This is accomplished by placing a mask over the nose and mouth, thus increasing the volume of the potential oxygen reservoir (see Fig 7-3). This type of apparatus gives the inspired oxygen concentration shown in Table 7-2, *B*, as long as the ventilatory pattern is normal.

An oxygen mask should never be run at less than a 5 L flow; otherwise, exhaled air accumulating in the mask reservoir might be rebreathed. Above 5 L/min, most of the exhaled air will be flushed from the mask. Above an 8 L flow there is little increase in the inspired oxygen concentration because the reservoir is filled. Of course, changes in ventilatory pattern are as important in affecting the inspired oxygen concentrations as they are with the cannula and the catheter.

To deliver more than 60% oxygen by a low-flow system, one must again increase the oxygen reservoir (see Fig 7-3). This is accomplished by attaching a reservoir bag to the mask (see Table 7-2, *C*). Without a one-way valve between the bag and mask, this apparatus is called a *partial rebreathing mask*. This bag is neither a carbon dioxide reservoir nor a rebreathing bag. It is meant to be an *oxygen reservoir;* therefore, the bag must never be totally collapsed during inspiration. The very early exhaled air (the first one third of exhalation) will go back into the bag. This is deadspace air from the mouth and the trachea and contains little carbon dioxide. Again, it must be remembered that this is a low-flow system, in which the inspired oxygen concentrations vary according to the ventilatory pattern. At flow rates from 6-10 L/min, a close-fitting mask with reservoir bag gives approximately 60-90+% oxygen.

Summary

With these basic guidelines for oxygen administration in mind, one can readily provide a patient with a consistent and predictable oxygen concentration. Increasing or decreasing the inspired oxygen concentrations within reasonably predictable limits is possible and, most important, we can deliver a *consistent* oxygen concentration. A patient with a shallow, deep, or irregular ventilatory pattern should receive oxygen therapy from a high-flow system rather than from a low-flow system. It must be clearly understood that even though the term *low-flow oxygen* is generally considered to mean low-concentration oxygen, this may not be the case. The ventilatory pattern must be assessed! *As long as oxygen administration is consistent and predictable, clinical observation plus blood gas measurement will assure proper oxygen therapy.*

Clinical Guidelines for Administration of Oxygen Therapy

Following the decision that a patient needs oxygen therapy, the approach for determining the appropriate system depends primarily upon answering the following two questions: (1) is a low-flow system adequate or must a high-flow system be employed; and (2) will the needs be primarily for low concentration or high concentration oxygen? Low concentration oxygen is an $F_{I_{O_2}}$ below 35%; high concentrations of oxygen are those above 50%; 35-50% are considered moderate concentrations.

Low-flow delivery systems are better tolerated by the patient and more convenient for the therapist to set up and deliver. Therefore, it follows that whenever a low-flow system is adequate it should be employed. Adequacy is determined by whether or not the system will provide *consistent* and *predictable* inspired atmospheres of oxygen. Table 7–3 outlines the general criteria for evaluating whether a low-flow system will be adequate. In general, one may say that a low-flow system is adequate when a patient is stabilized clinically and has a reasonably normal ventilatory pattern and minute volume. It has been our experience that the adult patient whose tidal volume is between 300 ml and 700 ml, whose ventilatory rate is below 25 times per minute, and whose ventilatory pattern is regular will receive consistent and predictable $F_{I_{O_2}}$'s on a low-flow oxygen system. A high-flow sys-

TABLE 7–3.—CRITERIA FOR USE
OF LOW-FLOW SYSTEM

Low-flow system is adequate if:
A. Tidal volume
   300 ml-700 ml
B. Ventilatory rate
   Below 25/min
C. Ventilatory pattern
   Regular   Consistent

tem should be used if any one of these three criteria are not met. If it is anticipated that the oxygen therapy will have an effect on the ventilatory pattern, a high-flow system should be utilized so that the change in ventilatory pattern will not change the inspired oxygen concentration. In our experience, over 75% of patients requiring oxygen therapy are appropriately treated with low-flow systems.

Following the guidelines, we can choose an appropriate appliance that can deliver a consistent oxygen concentration in the *range* of desired FI_{O_2}. More important, we will be capable of increasing or decreasing the inspired oxygen concentration within reasonably predictable limits! It must be clearly understood that even though the term "low-flow oxygen" is considered to mean low-concentration oxygen delivered via low oxygen flow rates through a nasal cannula, this may not be as low an oxygen concentration as believed. If the patient has a very shallow tidal volume or an unusually slow ventilatory rate, the inspired oxygen concentrations may be much higher than anticipated.

This discussion has been purposely conceptual rather than technical — primarily because the field of respiratory therapy is advancing so quickly that any consideration of specific equipment would be quickly outmoded and unsatisfactory for many regions of the country. For specifics concerning various types of apparatus, the reader is referred to various technical respiratory therapy textbooks and to recent journal publications.

Evaluation of Oxygen Therapy

Evaluation of the adequacy and effectiveness of oxygen therapy is simple and direct when cardiopulmonary homeostasis is understood. This evaluation is primarily concerned with two factors: (1) physical examination of the cardiopulmonary system; and (2) the measurement of arterial blood gases.

Physical Examination of the Cardiopulmonary System

The goal of oxygen therapy is usually to provide adequate tissue oxygenation while minimizing cardiopulmonary work. Therefore, the evaluation of oxygen therapy must include a basic evaluation of the cardiovascular and the ventilatory status.

Cardiovascular vital signs are composed of *blood pressure, pulse,* and the *perfusion state.* It is always desirable to have a base line with which to compare, but this is not always possible. Certainly, these measurements and observation should be made each time an evaluation is undertaken. Systolic and diastolic blood pressure, pulse rate (counted for one full minute), and arrhythmias should be noted. The perfusion state is best approximated by noting the patient's skin color, texture, and capillary refill. Skin that is warm and dry is being adequately perfused. Urine output and the level of consciousness are good indications of over-all perfusion. A patient who has an intact sensorium is a patient who probably has adequate brain tissue perfusion. A patient who is confused and agitated should be assumed to have inadequate cerebral oxygenation until proven otherwise.

The ventilatory system is observed and evaluated by measurements of *tidal volume, ventilatory rate,* and an assessment of the *work of breathing.* Perhaps the most common mistake in clinical medicine is to assume that the tidal volume can be adequately evaluated by observation alone. Experience has taught that the clinician is far more aware of degrees of stress in breathing than the volume of breathing. *It is imperative to measure the tidal volume whenever oxygen therapy is critical.* The ventilatory rate should be counted for one full minute; irregularities in rate or tidal volumes must be noted. *There is no single factor that can affect oxygen therapy to a greater extent than the ventilatory pattern.* The work of breathing can be generally assessed by noting the muscular work involved with the ventilatory cycle, especially the use of accessory muscles. In the conscious patient, it is always helpful to investigate the degree of dyspnea. One should never discount or underestimate the meaning when the patient tells you that it is easier or harder to breath. The most sensitive indicator of a recent change in the state of a patient's work of breathing is his own subjective complaint of dyspnea.

Arterial Blood Gas Measurements

Arterial blood gas measurements are an essential part of the evaluation of oxygen therapy and must be accomplished as frequently as deemed necessary by the clinical situation. It is not only the PO_2 measurement that is significant in the assessment of oxygen therapy — the ventilatory state, hemoglobin content, and acid-base state must also be evaluated. Only in the perspective of these factors can a meaningful appraisal of arterial PO_2 be accomplished. Recent cardiopulmonary measurements and observations should accompany each blood gas sample.

To illustrate the principles of oxygen therapy evaluation, let us study an illustrative example: 35-year-old man with severe bilateral pneumonia. This shunting and venous admixture disease produces an arterial hypoxemia to which both the healthy cardiovascular system and the diseased pulmonary system respond. We would predict that the cardiopulmonary system would work hard enough to maintain an arterial oxygen tension at which the peripheral chemoreceptors would be minimally stimulated (approximately 60 mm Hg).

When an increased oxygen atmosphere is breathed, the alveolar oxygen tensions are increased. This means that the heart and the ventilatory muscles can do less work while the arterial oxygen tension is maintained so that tissues are adequately oxygenated. The organism will *not* preferentially increase the arterial oxygen tension if ventilatory work is great or if myocardial work is significantly increased. In essence, the patient who is alveolar hyperventilating (decreased P_{CO_2}) in response to hypoxemia will preferentially decrease ventilatory and myocardial work in response to oxygen therapy. This individual will *not* increase arterial oxygen tensions significantly until any increased cardiopulmonary work is relieved.

Here are the blood gas measurements and the vital signs of this 35-year-old male with bilateral pneumonia, breathing room air:

pH 7.52	BP 150/80
P_{CO_2} 28 mm Hg	P 130/min
P_{O_2} 60 mm Hg	RR 35/min

Hemoglobin content is 15 gm%. Physical examination shows the patient to be sweating, anxious, and complaining of difficulty in breathing. Note the elevated systolic blood pressure, tachycardia (rapid pulse), and tachypnea (rapid breathing). His arterial blood gases reveal an acute alveolar hyperventilation (acute respiratory alkalosis) with mild arterial hypoxemia.

The patient was given approximately 40–50% oxygen. Thirty minutes later the patient was comfortable and had no subjective complaints. No treatment was given other than oxygen therapy. The arterial blood gas measurements now are:

pH 7.45	BP 120/80
P_{CO_2} 35 mm Hg	P 100/min
P_{O_2} 70 mm Hg	RR 22/min

His blood pressure is normal, and the tachycardia and tachypnea are significantly decreased. There is a marked decrease in alveolar ventilation and a small increase in arterial oxygen tension. *It must be appreciated that the most striking changes caused by oxygen therapy are the decreases in ventilatory and myocardial work.*

The need for oxygen therapy cannot be appreciated if one judges the need solely by the arterial oxygen tension. The value of oxygen therapy is obvious when one understands that the original purpose of delivering oxygen to this patient was to support the cardiovascular and ventilatory systems primarily by decreasing their need to do increased work. In other words, the oxygen therapy was not only used to treat the hypoxemia; just as important, it was used to manipulate the cardiopulmonary compensatory status so that both the work of breathing and the myocardial work could be decreased while a satisfactory tissue oxygenation state was maintained.

Pulmonary Oxygen Toxicity

Although most of our concern in oxygen therapy is concentrated on preventing or reversing the hypoxemic state, the respiratory care practitioner must be knowledgeable and concerned about giving too much oxygen. This necessitates an unbiased and objective look at the subject referred to as "oxygen toxicity."

As early as 1897, the importance of pulmonary dysfunction in the critically ill patient was recognized and emphasized.[99] At the same time it was debated whether or not the inherent toxicity of oxygen for tissues might limit its clinical applicability. We have previously stated that shortly after the discovery of oxygen, it was appreciated that there was a *minimum* concentration of oxygen that was compatible with life. Shortly thereafter came the appreciation that there must also be a *maximum* concentration compatible with normal cellular function. Investigators in the field of oxygen toxicity recognized this circumstance and unequivocally demonstrated oxygen toxicity nearly eighty years ago.[100]

It was not until about 1920 that oxygen was *medically* employed as a therapeutic regimen on any noticeable scale. In fact, it has been only over the last three decades that oxygen therapy has been in widespread use. The major manifestations of oxygen toxicity have always been evident in the adult and were described as early as 1899. However, from the clinical viewpoint, there was little practical importance attached to oxygen toxicity until the advent of efficient mechanical ventilators that were capable of delivering continuous high oxygen concentrations and prolonging life in critically ill patients.[101]

It is well known that with chronic hypercarbic patients and premature infants, severe clinical tragedies have resulted from the improper administration of oxygen. Nevertheless, the basic interest and attention of excessive oxygen must be focused on the lung, since it is this vital organ that is most often affected, most easily affected, and that has been most intensely studied.

Pathology of Pulmonary Oxygen Toxicity

There are numerous factors that make the study of pulmonary oxygen toxicity difficult. Most information gathered about the pathology of pulmonary oxygen toxicity comes from animal studies. The identification of changes attributable directly to oxygen and not to other factors is tenuous. The role of intermittent positive-pressure ventilation in relation to pulmonary pathology and oxygen toxicity is debatable. It seems fair to conclude at our present state of knowledge that intermittent positive-pressure ventilation does *not* play an important role in the *advent* of pulmonary oxygen toxicity, as long as the positive pressure applied is not excessive.[101] However, IPPV may well play a significant role in the *course* of pulmonary oxygen toxicity.

There are two types of pulmonary changes that arise from excessive oxygen. The "chronic" type of oxygen toxicity is found in response to low concentrations over many months — this is associated with proliferative changes in lung endothelium and epithelium. In contrast to this type of toxicity are the changes produced by exposure to high concentrations of oxygen over short periods of time (several days to weeks). This *acute toxicity* is usually divided into two phases: an immediate "exudative" phase and a slightly delayed "proliferative" phase. Our discussion will be limited completely to the syndrome of "acute toxicity."

Knowledge concerning the structural changes in the lung because of oxygen has been considerably advanced by (1) the application of new techniques for quantifying lung damage, and (2) the widespread application of electron microscopy. These methods have been utilized in both hyperbaric (above-atmospheric pressure) and normobaric (atmospheric pressure) conditions, and have revealed interesting differences between rats and monkeys.[102, 103] One must question how this pertains to man. In general, the pathologic findings that have been found in acute pulmonary toxicity are consolidation, edema, alveolar cell hypertrophy, hyperplasia, degeneration, and desquamation. In addition, hyaline membranes have been reported surrounding or lining the alveolar cells and ducts. Recent studies show that hyaline membranes seem more likely to be found in oxygen toxicity of long standing. The electron microscope has made possible the study of the ultrastructural (sub-light microscope) changes in oxygen-poisoned lungs. The overwhelming evidence is that prolonged exposure (from 3 days to weeks) to high concentrations of oxygen leads to abnormal changes within the mitochondria of alveolar type II cells[104] (see Chapter 1). It must be emphasized that many of these pathologic changes are nonspecific and may be seen in pneumonia, postradiation lung, and postcytotoxic (anticancer) drug administration.

Not all studies have been limited to animals. There have been numerous attempts to study pathologic lung findings in humans who receive high concentrations of oxygen for prolonged periods. Most of these studies are inconclusive because (1) they are retrospective and, therefore, present obvious difficulties in interpretation; (2) many are dealing with hyperbaric conditions; and (3) many involve circumstances where pulmonary disease was present prior to oxygen administration. At the present time, these studies are far too inconclusive to be used as a basis for clinical application of oxygen therapy.

Human Tolerance to Oxygen

The preceding review makes it obvious that most of our information concerning acute pulmonary oxygen toxicity is based upon animal studies and human hyperbaric studies. *The respiratory care practitioner is concerned with the effects of oxygen in man at atmospheric pressure.* Reports that occasional patients have survived exposures to oxygen much greater than was thought possible has led some to question whether oxygen toxicity actually exists in man at normal atmospheric pressures. However, it is fair to state that sufficient data exist to demonstrate unequivocally that *acute pulmonary oxygen toxicity is a real entity in man!*

In healthy man there seems to be a threshold (50–70% oxygen) below which there is little evidence of acute oxygen damage. It also seems apparent that despite wide variations in human susceptibility, there is little identifiable risk in the administration of pure oxygen at 1 atmosphere for 24 hours to healthy man.[101] *It appears that the rate of the onset of the disease process (oxygen toxicity) is proportional both to the tension of oxygen and to the duration of exposure.*

Reasonable interpretation of data obtained from the manned space program indicates that no measurable changes in pulmonary function or gas exchange occur in man during exposures to less than 350 mm Hg (0.5 atmosphere) of oxygen. There seems to be little argument that it is primarily the *pressure* (tension) of oxygen, not the concentration of oxygen, which is the determinant of the development of toxicity.

Obviously, adequate arterial oxygen tensions are the endpoint of oxygen therapy. *Cellular toxicity due to blood hyperoxia should never occur.* However, clinical situations arise that *appear* to demand high $F_{I_{O_2}}$'s. The danger of such therapy is that it will eventually lead to pulmonary disease that will threaten tissue oxygenation. There appear to be two mechanisms that play a major role in creating pulmonary abnormality purely as a result of high $F_{I_{O_2}}$: (1) alveolar cell malfunction (pulmonary oxygen toxicity) and (2) absorption atelectasis.

Pulmonary Oxygen Toxicity

The entity of acute pulmonary oxygen toxicity is a biochemical process of great complexity.[105-107] Since lung parenchyma is exposed to higher oxygen tensions (alveolar P_{O_2}) than any other tissue, it is small wonder that under normobaric conditions the lung is the first and most common organ to manifest oxygen damage. Mitochondrial dysfunction (dysoxia) is related to the *inspired* oxygen level and the duration with which the epithelial cells are exposed to high alveolar tensions. Alveolar epithelial cells (see Chapter 1) are sensitive to hyperoxia. This is true for both types I and II; their dysfunction leads to a clinical entity known as adult respiratory distress syndrome (see Chapter 30).

Biochemical oxygen toxicity is not the same in normobaric and hyperbaric conditions.[108] Hyperbaric pressures seem to offer significant protection against central nervous system and pulmonary oxygen toxicity. However, there is no evidence to support the concept that the same protection exists in normobaric conditions.[102] Available evidence indicates that the neuroendocrine system plays a much greater role in the response of the lung to hyperbaric oxygen than to normobaric oxygen.[109] However, it is apparent that the neuroendocrine system plays a role in both situations. It has been suggested that the variation in individual susceptibility to acute pulmonary oxygen toxicity may be due to the variation in neuroendocrine activity.

Absorption Atelectasis

Nitrogen is an inert gas; i.e., it does not enter into chemical reactions within the body. It freely distributes throughout the total body water and therefore the nitrogen tension (PN_2) is equal in the alveolus, blood, and cellular water.

Under normal conditions, approximately 75% of the alveolar gas is nitrogen. When 100% oxygen is administered, the entire body will "denitrogenate" within 30 minutes.[110] It is believed that this denitrogenation may result in some alveoli collapsing due to absence of gas volume.[84, 111] However, this process appears to be of great import in diseased lungs where poorly ventilated alveoli have low P_{O_2} but adequate nitrogen gas volume. These "hypoxic" alveoli receive little blood flow because of the local hypoxic vasoconstriction. When the FI_{O_2} is increased, the alveolar hypoxia is relieved, resulting in increased perfusion. This redistribution of pulmonary blood flow may be responsible for these areas of lung collapsing.

When this process occurs, shunt effect is replaced with true shunt — a refractory hypoxemia. This may lead to the situation where higher and higher $F_{I_{O_2}}$ results in lower and lower arterial P_{O_2}.[112]

Summary

The fact that high concentrations (greater than 50–60%) of oxygen administered for long periods (3 days to weeks) may cause acute pulmonary toxicity is well documented.[113] *However, it is essential to keep in mind the relative danger of hypoxia and hyperoxia.* The pathophysiology of hypoxia in the critically ill patient has been aggressively treated for only two decades. In that time, numerous therapeutic manipulations, including oxygen therapy, have become normal practice. In the application of these treatment techniques, oxygen has often been abused and there is little room for disagreement that oxygen toxicity is a real iatrogenic (doctor-induced) disease. However, an overreaction to the dangers associated with oxygen supplementation has led to an extremely hazardous circumstance — poorly informed clinicians withholding essential oxygen therapy from hypoxic or hypoxemic patients. *To allow a patient to be exposed to dangerous levels of hypoxia for fear of developing oxygen toxicity is intolerable!* It is essential to remember that hypoxia is common and that the damage it causes is rapid and severe. On the other hand, pulmonary injury from oxygen is uncommon and its development is relatively slow.

Careful consideration of all the evidence, along with sound clinical principles, leads us to make three generalizations concerning oxygen therapy and oxygen toxicity.

1. Inspired oxygen tensions below 40% at 1 atmosphere rarely produce acute pulmonary oxygen toxicity — even with prolonged exposures. Under normobaric conditions there should be no hesitation in providing appropriate low-concentration oxygen (less than 40%) for supportive therapy of the cardiopulmonary system. Even in conjunction with appropriately administered intermittent positive-pressure ventilation, low-concentration oxygen rarely produces pulmonary toxicity.

2. Pulmonary oxygen toxicity in man has *not* been demonstrated from breathing 100% oxygen for 24 hours or less. Therefore, oxygen toxicity should not be a consideration intraoperatively, in resuscitation, or in transport situations. *Pure oxygen has no contraindication for brief periods in emergency situations!* However, absorption atelectasis must be kept in mind as a potential problem since this can occur within 30 minutes.[110] The lowest possible $F_{I_{O_2}}$ should be administered as early as feasible in the clinical course.

3. Patients with pre-existing pulmonary disease are no more prone to develop acute pulmonary oxygen toxicity than patients with normal lungs. However, pre-existing pulmonary disease is more susceptible to absorption atelectasis. Our clinical concern of acute pulmonary oxygen toxicity must not differ between the pre-existing nondiseased and diseased lung. *The general principle of minimal oxygen administration consistent with adequate cardiopulmonary homeostasis always holds true!*

High FI_{O_2}'s are most commonly administered to patients with primary cardiopulmonary disease. Therefore, although the pre-existing pulmonary diseased patient has no *inherent* increased risk of acute pulmonary oxygen toxicity, he is the patient who will most likely receive high oxygen concentrations. All measures possible must be instituted to allow minimal FI_{O_2}'s for maintenance of adequate oxygenation. Such measures include optimal ventilatory patterns, fluid restriction, maintenance of electrolyte and acid-base balance, and the institution of positive end-expiratory pressure (PEEP) where indicated. Of course, basic modalities of bronchial hygiene to improve distribution of ventilation and decreased work of breathing are essential.

The avoidance of excessively high inspired oxygen concentrations is a common issue in critical-care units. One must realize that appropriate tissue oxygenation is essential to the maintenance of life, especially in patients with multi-organ systems disease. There can be no dogmatic guidelines concerning appropriate degrees of arterial oxygenation to assure tissue oxygenation. This must always be a clinical decision based on thorough knowledge of cardiopulmonary homeostasis, careful monitoring, and physical examination.

Arterial blood gas measurement is essential for the appropriate administration of oxygen therapy!!

SECTION III
BRONCHIAL HYGIENE THERAPY

8 • RETAINED SECRETIONS

PULMONARY PHYSIOLOGY is traditionally taught almost exclusively in terms of pulmonary gas exchange. There can be no challenge to the statement that the prime function of the pulmonary system is to allow atmospheric gases to exchange with blood. A clean tracheobronchial tree must be maintained to adequately accomplish this function. Since atmospheric air is constantly moving in and out of the tracheobronchial tree, there must be mechanisms for keeping the conducting tubes free of foreign particles. In addition, there must be mechanisms for "preparing" the inspired gas for contact with lung parenchyma— the air must be warmed, humidified, and cleansed.

Prior to 1955, there was little concern for the *nonrespiratory* functions of the pulmonary system. Over the past twenty years there have been numerous investigative studies on this subject; however, clinical medicine has been slow to appreciate the importance of these nonrespiratory functions in health and disease. This slow acceptance stems in part from the fact that the pulmonary system is mechanical, and therefore many of the therapeutic modalities applicable to its care and maintenance are mechanical rather than pharmacologic. Internal medicine has paid great attention to the bronchospastic elements of pulmonary disease primarily because bronchospasm is readily reversible pharmacologically. Retained secretions occur with far greater frequency than bronchospasm in the critically ill, but there has been great hesitancy to accept the techniques and modalities for bronchial hygiene.

The progress of clinical respiratory care over the last decade has erased any legitimacy to the question: Is bronchial hygiene necessary? Today the question is: How should bronchial hygiene be applied and how do we evaluate its effectiveness?

Before addressing ourselves to the particular techniques and modalities of bronchial hygiene therapy, it is essential to discuss the normal bronchial hygiene mechanisms. Only if we understand these processes, and what occurs if they fail to function adequately, can we begin to understand the rationale for the application of respiratory therapy modalities of bronchial hygiene.

The Mucociliary Escalator

The scanning electron microscope has been applied ingeniously to document the existence and function of the *mucociliary escalator*. In the large airways, this is a continuous blanket of mucus covering the tracheobronchial tree epithelium that is mobilized by the forward motion of cilia (see Fig 1–5). The ciliary action causes the mucous blanket to be mobilized in a continuous motion toward the hilus of the lung, moving eventually to the larynx where the mucus is moved into the pharynx and swallowed.[114] How the mucus flows through the larynx and into the pharynx is unknown at the present time. Since the larynx does not have cilia, it is a mystery how this flow continues to the pharynx.

The process of moving mucus has been referred to as *mucokinesis*.[115] The mucous blanket moves at a reasonably rapid rate (1–2 cm/min) and can completely cleanse the normal adult lung in less than 20 minutes.[116] This normal bronchial hygiene mechanism depends primarily on two factors: (1) appropriate ciliary activity, and (2) appropriate mucus production.

Ciliary Activity

Ciliary activity appears to be affected by numerous pulmonary and nonpulmonary stresses. Numerous direct pulmonary insults, such as smoking, tracheal foreign bodies, positive-pressure ventilation, high inspired oxygen concentrations, tracheobronchial disease processes, and many others affect the action of the ciliary processes.[117-120] For our purposes, *normal ciliary action can be assumed only in the presence of a healthy and undiseased state.* Any physiologic stress may result in abnormal ciliary function.

Mucus Production

Mucus production is a complex and poorly understood process at the present time. We know that the prime sources of mucus are the *goblet cells* of the pulmonary epithelium and the *mucous glands* of the submucosal area; the mucus is constantly being produced and extruded onto the surface of the pulmonary epithelium.[121] The mucus must have very specific hydration, pH, electrolyte balance, and numerous other factors for proper mucokinesis to occur.[122]

Mucus rheology (the study of flow characteristics) is a very complex subject with many highly controversial factors. In general, the mucus has viscous and elastic properties that allow a continuous motion to result from the intermittent forward pulling of the cilia. The outer mucus layer (gel layer) is extremely viscous and normally flows continuously toward the larynx (see Fig 1–5). Any mucus abnormality can cause the mucous blanket to slow or stop. Obviously, any discontinuity in the mucous blanket in the large airways would cause poor forward motion and result in retained secretions. There are a multiplicity of factors that can cause abnormalities in mucus production: any pulmonary epithelial inflammation; any abnormality of the mucous and serous glands; or, in fact, almost any disease process that involves the tracheobronchial tree.

In summary, normal bronchial hygiene is dependent upon normal mucus production and ciliary function. Any disease process, but especially one involving the pulmonary system, may result in abnormal mucokinesis which will lead to retained secretions.[123] Although investigations into the details of mucus production and ciliary motion continue, there is more than enough evidence to substantiate these generalizations.

Parenchymal Hygiene

Alveolar Fluid Lining

The mucous blanket is not found beyond the terminal bronchioles. There are no mucus-secreting glands nor cilia in alveolar epithelium. However, alveolar epithelium is lined with a fluid, and it is believed that this fluid is mobilized into the bronchiolar mucous blanket.[6] Although this is a controversial subject, it seems reasonable to assume that the alveolar fluid lining is constantly mobilized in some manner to become part of the mucous blanket.

Macrophages

An important defense mechanism of the lung parenchyma is the *alveolar macrophages* (see Fig 1–4). These are large cells that are mobile and ingest foreign material (phagocytes). Their origin is believed to be in the bone marrow. These macrophages play an important role in pulmonary disease; their role in normal parenchymal hygiene is controversial.[7]

The "Sigh"

The normal breathing pattern involves varying tidal volumes in conjunction with intermittent deep breaths (sighs) 6 to 10 times an hour. This variability of inspiratory volumes plays a great role in preventing alveoli from collapsing (miliary or patchy atelectasis).[124, 125] Many believe this is a normal bronchial hygiene function.

The Cough Mechanism

When malfunction of the mucociliary escalator occurs, a very basic defense mechanism comes into play—*the cough*—a pulmonary defense mechanism which attempts to maintain adequate bronchial hygiene in spite of inadequate normal mechanisms.[126] There is no evidence that the cough is necessary in normal pulmonary hygiene; rather, it functions in the presence of abnormalities such as copious, dry, or thick mucus; poor ciliary activity; and diseased pulmonary epithelium. *The cough is the major defense against retained secretions* and is often obtunded or destroyed in pulmonary disease.[4, 23]

Much of respiratory therapy is involved with the maintenance of bronchial hygiene and, therefore, it is aimed at augmenting or replacing the function of a deficient cough mechanism. It is essential to completely understand the factors involved in the cough mechanism.

Anatomy of the Cough Mechanism

The initiation of the cough mechanism is provided by vagus nerve (X cranial nerve) reflexes, either from the trachea or the carina. Any foreign body or irritation in the tracheobronchial tree will elicit an afferent vagal impulse to the midbrain which will result in efferent vagal impulses to the appropriate muscles. Assuming appropriate sensory and motor reflexes, we may consider the cough mechanism as having five separate mechanical components: (1) a deep breath; (2) an inspiratory pause; (3) glottic closure; (4) increased intrathoracic pressure; and (5) glottic opening.

ADEQUATE INSPIRATORY VOLUME.—One can exhale no more than what has been inhaled, and an effective cough must be preceded by an adequate inspiration. *Coughing without adequate inspiration is ineffective;* e.g., multiple coughs in a row without intermittent inspirations are called "paroxysmal coughing" and are noneffective coughs.[127] Various investigators have attempted to quantitate the minimum adequate inspiratory volume for an effective cough, and most agree that an inspiratory capacity of at least 75% of normal is necessary. Others have found that a vital capacity below 15 ml/kg (6 ml/lb) will result in an inspiratory capacity that is inadequate to provide an effective cough. Regardless of the rules of thumb applied, the principle that an individual must have the mechanical capacity to breathe deeply for an effective cough cannot be ignored.

INSPIRATORY PAUSE.—Common sense dictates that if the cough is to be effective, as much of the inspiratory volume as possible must find its way distal to mucus that is to be mobilized. Following a deep inspiration, a breath-holding maneuver is accomplished for a period of time to allow maximal peripheral distribution of air. In essence, a tracheal-to-alveolar driving pressure is maintained for as long as possible so that a maximum volume of gas can overcome resistance to flow. The inspiratory pause is a significant part of an effective cough. An individual who is breathing rapidly and shallowly will not hold his breath for any length of time. Thus, he will not provide an adequate inspiratory pause and usually will have a poor or ineffective cough.

GLOTTIC CLOSURE. — After maximal peripheral distribution of air, the glottis must close tightly. This means that the laryngomusculature must be intact so that there will be no gas leaving the larynx in spite of greatly increased airway pressures. Adequate glottic function is as important a part of an effective cough mechanism as any other factor.

INCREASED INTRATHORACIC PRESSURE. — The basic purpose of the cough mechanism is to provide a high velocity airflow on expiration. This means that the greater the differential between intra-alveolar and atmospheric pressures, the greater will be the velocity of flow when expiration begins.

With the glottis closed, the prime mechanism for increasing intrathoracic (and, therefore, intra-alveolar) pressures is to increase *intra-abdominal* pressure. Increased intra-abdominal pressure will push the diaphragm upward, thereby decreasing the volume of the thoracic cavity. At the same time, the intercostals are brought into play to resist the expansion of the chest wall as the diaphragm is forced up. According to Boyle's law, this must cause an increase in intrathoracic and intra-alveolar pressures since the gas cannot leave the lung. A normal cough produces intra-alveolar pressures in excess of 100 cm of water, sometimes exceeding 200 cm of water.

The muscles of greatest importance in the cough mechanism are the *anterior abdominal wall muscles* (Chapter 1). These are the muscles that increase intra-abdominal pressure and thereby force the diaphragm up to increase intrathoracic pressure against the closed glottis. Much of bronchial hygiene therapy is involved in the evaluation and augmentation of abdominal musculature function.

GLOTTIC OPENING. — After intra-alveolar pressures are increased, the glottis suddenly opens and allows high-velocity airflow from the lungs. Peak flow rates may be as high as 300 L per minute.

Purpose of the Cough Mechanism

A high-velocity airflow out of the pulmonary tree will mobilize mucus. Obviously, the more fluid and continuous the mucous blanket, the greater will be the degree of mobilization. It must be appreciated *that no matter how effective the cough may be mechanically, it must have an intact mucous blanket to mobilize!* In other words, to mobilize retained secretions, an effective cough is essential – but without an intact mucous blanket the cough will be raspy, painful, and relatively nonproductive.

Pathophysiology of Retained Secretions (Table 8–1)

Retained secretions are so common in diseased patients that etiologic classification is useless. Any insult to the pulmonary system may interrupt normal bronchial hygiene mechanisms and create a potential for retained secretions. Thus, we see that retained secretions are the most common cause of pulmonary malfunction in sick patients.

1. Retained secretions lead to an inflammatory response of the pulmonary mucosa. The hyperemia (capillary congestion) and edema (swelling) resulting from this inflammatory reaction cause increased resistance to airflow. The narrowing of bronchial lumens caused by partial plugging of retained secretions also causes increased resistance to airflow. This increased resistance to airflow leads to an increased work of breathing, since it will take more energy to move an adequate amount of air in and out of the lungs.

The plugging and inflammation secondary to retained secretions are seldom evenly distributed throughout the lung. Thus, uneven areas of airflow resistance cause uneven distribution of ventilation, which leads to ventilation-perfusion mismatch (shunt effect) which leads to

TABLE 8-1.—POTENTIAL RESULTS OF
RETAINED SECRETIONS

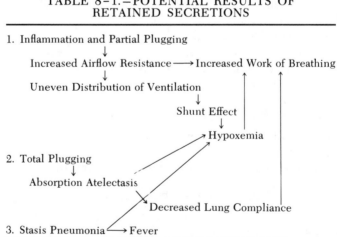

hypoxemia. Even minor degrees of retained secretions may lead to an increased work of the heart and lungs because of the subsequent hypoxemia.

2. Greater degrees of retained secretions will cause total plugging of bronchioles and absorption atelectasis of the distal lung parenchyma. Such atelectasis will result in a decreased lung compliance and increased true shunting. The decreased compliance will cause an increased work of breathing. The shunting will cause hypoxemia.

Thus, either minor or major degrees of retained secretions may lead to increased work of breathing and hypoxemia. *These processes are reversible by mobilizing the retained secretions!*

3. When areas of lung become atelectatic because of plugging of bronchioles, glandular and cellular activity continue. This leads to *stasis* of secretions, which is a perfect culture medium for bacteria. Such "stasis pneumonia" is a common result of retained secretions.

In summary, retained secretions are a potentially hazardous condition. Any patient with cardiopulmonary disease or a disease limiting the effectiveness of bronchial hygiene may retain secretions if the disease is severe enough. The respiratory care practitioner must maintain a high index of suspicion. It seems reasonable to suspect that any patient with pulmonary disease who manifests hypoxemia and/or increased work of breathing has retained secretions until proved otherwise.

Clinical Manifestations

It would "boggle the mind" to look back over the years and think of how many patients were afflicted with "retained secretions" that went undetected or were mistaken for some other pathology. With a reasonably high index of suspicion, it is not difficult to spot patients who may have retained secretions. Observation and clinical examination should be aimed at uncovering the symptoms caused by the pathophysiology: (1) increased work of breathing, (2) hypoxemia, (3) an inadequate cough, and (4) infection.

INCREASED WORK OF BREATHING. — A patient who has a sudden increase in the work of breathing will complain of *dyspnea* — the subjective complaint of difficult breathing. Dyspnea is the result of acute change in ventilatory work. It is not observed; it is *related* by the patient. Objective signs are (1) the use of accessory muscles of ventilation, (2) tachypnea (rapid respiratory rate), and (3) preference for sitting positions. In general, the individual who has an increased work of breathing will tolerate positional changes poorly.

HYPOXEMIA. — Hypoxemia (decreased arterial oxygen tensions) will initially be suspected by changes in the cardiovascular system: (1) tachycardia (rapid heart rate), (2) arrhythmia (irregular heart rate), and (3) elevated systolic blood pressure.

INADEQUATE COUGH. — A patient who makes frequent, feeble, nonproductive attempts to cough probably has retained secretions. He may be lethargic, sweaty, and anxious. These patients are often taking cough suppressants to find relief from the annoying, nonproductive, and, sometimes painful, coughing episodes. Chest auscultation may reveal rhonchi and distant breath sounds.

Common Etiologies of Retained Secretions

DEHYDRATION. — Whenever an individual has inadequate body water, the mucous glands have less water available and, therefore, produce thick and tenacious mucus.

ACUTE PULMONARY DISEASE. — Whether obstructive or restrictive, an acute pulmonary disease will often lead to retained secretions. The existence of acute pulmonary disease must be accompanied by the clinical anticipation of retained secretions.

TRACHEAL FOREIGN BODY. — The placement of endotracheal and tracheostomy tubes will cause a decrease in ciliary action and contaminate the trachea with bacteria. Both factors may lead to retained secretions.

GENERALIZED MUSCULAR WEAKNESS. — Generalized muscular weakness is most commonly caused by either neuromuscular disease, electrolyte imbalance, or exhaustion. Numerous neuromuscular diseases can cause generalized muscular weakness and an ineffective cough mechanism resulting in retained secretions. Acute illness is often accompanied by electrolyte imbalance — severe potassium depletion and/or chloride depletion can cause muscular weakness. Physiologic stress may lead to a lack of sleep over a prolonged period of time. Patients who experience such exhaustion are impaired in their ability to clear secretions from the airway.

BULBAR MALFUNCTION. — Bulbar malfunction may be caused either by nervous system disease or anatomic malformation. Certain central nervous system and neural diseases, such as multiple sclerosis and polio, can cause selective bulbar malfunction. The recurrent laryngeal nerve may be involved in neck disease or surgery and cause malfunction of the vocal cords. Central nervous system vascular accidents (strokes) can cause malfunction of the glottis. Prolonged intubation of the larynx causes malformation of the vocal cords on a temporary basis and, therefore, an inability to appose the cords completely for a period of time. In addition, such vocal cord problems as granuloma and other benign or malignant growths can cause malfunction of the glottis.

ABDOMINAL MUSCULATURE LIMITATION. — Abdominal musculature limitations are commonly the result of postabdominal surgery, or peritonitis (inflammation of the abdominal cavity lining), or paraplegia (paralysis of the lower part of the body). Abdominal surgery involves pain and stress to abdominal musculature that is often a significant limitation to adequate coughing and deep breathing. The pain caused by peritonitis is also responsible for limiting the ability of increasing intra-abdominal pressure. The paraplegic has lost neural control of his abdominal musculature and, therefore, is unable to increase intra-abdominal pressure. The paraplegic patient usually has few problems with retained secretions as long as the cough is not needed. When stressed by even a mild "cold," he may have severe retained secretions because of his inability to cough.

9 • HUMIDITY AND AEROSOL THERAPY

THE UPPER AIRWAY humidifies inspired air and thus maintains hydration of the mucous blanket. Disease processes interrupt this water balance and necessitate supportive measures to either prevent airway water loss or add water to the airway. The relationship of humidity to nonrespiratory pulmonary function must be fully comprehended prior to discussing the clinical application of aerosol therapy.

Humidity

Vaporization is the process of converting a liquid to a gas. *Humidity* can be defined as (1) water in the gaseous state, (2) water vapor in a gas, or (3) molecular water in a gas. The amount of water vapor a volume of gas can *potentially* contain is dependent upon the temperature. The higher the temperature, the greater the amount of water vapor that volume of gas can contain. The greater the surface area of water in a gas, the greater the rate of vaporization.

When a volume of gas at a given temperature contains all the water vapor it can possibly hold, it is said to be *saturated*. When saturated gas is cooled, a portion of the water vapor will condense (turn to liquid water); when saturated gas is heated, it becomes capable of increasing its water vapor content.

Absolute humidity is the weight of water vapor in the gas volume. Traditionally, this is measured as mg of water vapor per liter of gas (mg/L). The *maximum absolute humidity* is defined as the weight of water vapor in a *saturated* gas.

Table 9–1 illustrates that 37°C. (body temperature) air has a maximum absolute humidity of approximately 44 mg/L; 21°C. (room temperature) air has a maximum absolute humidity of approximately 18 mg/L. If *saturated* air at 21°C. was heated to 37°C., it would have an absolute humidity only 40% of the gas' potential (maximum absolute humidity). This ratio of absolute humidity to maximum absolute humidity is termed *relative humidity*. Fifty percent humidified air at 37°C. has a higher absolute humidity (22 mg/L) than 100% humidified air at 21°C. It is well to remember that when humidity is a concern, temperature must always be kept in mind.

TABLE 9-1.—RELATIONSHIPS OF HUMIDITY AND TEMPERATURE

TEMPERATURE	ABSOLUTE HUMIDITY (mg H_2O/L GAS)	RELATIVE HUMIDITY
37° C.	44 mg/L	100%
37° C.	22 mg/L	50%
37° C.	18 mg/L	40%
21° C.	18 mg/L	100%
21° C.	9 mg/L	50%

Airway Humidification

Alveolar air is 100% humidified at 37°C. and, therefore, contains 44 mg of water vapor per liter of gas. This water vapor exerts a partial pressure (P_{H_2O}) of 47 mm Hg. Under most climatic conditions on earth, the water vapor content of inspired air is something less than 44 mg of water per liter; in fact, average U.S. "room air" conditions (21°C., 50% humidified) have water vapor contents of less than 10 mg. The difference between water vapor content in alveolar air and inspired air is termed the *humidity deficit*.[23]

Ambient air inspired through the nose is warmed to 34°C. and is 80–90% humidified in the oropharynx. It is 37°C. and 100% humidified at the carina. If the same air is breathed through the mouth, it is 21°C. and 60% humidified in the oropharynx—but still 100% humidified and 37°C. at the carina.[128] Thus, *if the water and heat are not supplied by the nose, they must come from the mucosa and mucous blanket of the tracheobronchial tree.*

The "insensible water loss" (water lost primarily by the skin and the pulmonary tree) in the resting normal adult is approximately 1 L in 24 hours; the pulmonary tree is responsible for approximately 250 ml. Even more than 250 ml is lost from the nasopharyngeal mucosa when (1) hyperventilation occurs, (2) the inspired air is extremely dry (as it ordinarily is when oxygen is breathed), or (3) when fever develops.

In the normal resting adult the nasopharyngeal mucosa gives up approximately 0.35 ml of water per minute in changing ambient air (21°C., 50% humidified) to alveolar air (37°C., 100% humidified). If this rate of water loss were not counteracted by opposite forces, it would amount to over 500 ml per 24 hours. Since the actual loss is only 250 ml per 24 hours, it is evident that the nasopharyngeal mucosa must recapture about 250 ml of water per 24 hours from the exhaled air. Fluid exchange in the nose is best considered in terms of the dehydration and rehydration of the mucous secretions. These secretions are produced in response to stimuli which are not completely understood. In cold weather, the mechanisms allow condensation of exhaled vapor to be reabsorbed by the mucous lining and re-used for humidification of inspired air.[129]

Inadequate humidification of inspired gases via the upper airway will lead to an adverse chain of events in the lower airways. When the upper airway is not functioning properly, the humidity deficit must be provided by the mucous blanket. This results in drying of the tracheo-bronchial tree which leads to (1) impairment of ciliary activity; (2) impairment of mucus movement; (3) inflammatory change and necrosis of ciliated pulmonary epithelium; (4) retention of viscid, tenacious secretions with secondary incrustation; (5) bacterial infiltration of mucosa; (6) atelectasis; and (7) pneumonia.[130, 131]

It stands to reason that great concern must be given to patients whose upper airways are not functioning properly or in whom the upper airways have been bypassed completely with an endotracheal tube or tracheostomy. It is also obvious that mouth breathing in the presence of very dry inspired air can be detrimental to the pulmonary tree.

Humidifiers

Humidifiers are designed to deliver a maximum amount of water vapor without producing particulate water. The water may be at room temperature or heated. Water will transfer heat to the gas that passes through and allow for a greater water vapor content. The gas must cool to body temperature before reaching the patient; this cooling process causes water vapor to condense ("rain out") in the delivery tubing.

There are two major types of humidifiers in common use: the pass-over humidifier and the bubble diffusion humidifier.

Pass-Over Humidifier

The pass-over humidifier is the simplest of all humidifiers and operates on the principle that water will evaporate as air is passed across its surface. Heated or not, this type of humidifier is not in exceptionally common use today except for some volume ventilators. It has been replaced by far more efficient humidifiers and nebulizers.

Bubble Diffusion Humidifier

A method of increasing efficiency is to break up the gas into small bubbles and allow it to come into intimate contact with the liquid. This provides a great gas-to-liquid surface contact (interface) and enhances evaporation. Figure 9–1 illustrates a basic model of a bubble diffusion humidifier. Although the actual techniques vary from one appliance to another, essentially it is a method of breaking up the gas

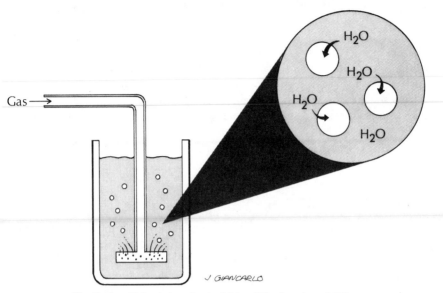

Fig 9–1.—Principle of a bubble diffusion humidifier.

into small bubbles and allowing intimate contact between the bubbles and the liquid. The liquid can be easily heated to provide for higher water vapor content. At room temperature and low-flow rates these appliances produce gas that is maximally saturated. However, when heated to body temperature the relative humidity is seldom over 40%. The past decade has seen the jet aerosol gain great popularity as a means of better humidification; however, the bubble diffusion principle is still widely used for low-flow oxygen systems and some newer designs have proved very efficient.

Of special interest is a type of bubble diffusion humidifier made for mechanical ventilators that is known as a "cascade humidifier." This appliance effectively breaks inspired gas into minute bubbles by a cascading process and passes these bubbles through water heated by an adjustable immersion heater. The temperature of the humidifier can be raised to such a level that the gas will be 100% saturated when it reaches the patient.

Clinical Application of Humidifiers

Oxygen Therapy

All medical oxygen is stored in cylinders or liquid tanks. The oxygen delivered from these sources is anhydrous (dry) and must be humidified prior to patient contact. Totally dry gas delivered to a patient will have a rapid drying effect on the nasal and pulmonary mucosa. The bubble diffusion humidifier is a popular means for routine humidification of oxygen; enough humidity is added to mimic the humidity of room air. Thus, its purpose is simply to restore the dry oxygen to room air conditions. The advantages are the simplicity of the apparatus and its ease of maintaining sterility. Unheated humidifiers are used with small-caliber tubing since the gas temperature will not decrease in transit to the patient. This means water condensation in the tubing will be nonexistent.

Artificial Airways

Heated (37°C.) and humidified (100%) gas is essential when the upper airway is bypassed, but such air is poorly tolerated when breathed through the intact upper airway.[132] Anyone who has been in a steambath or sauna will attest to this fact. Remember, a humidifier can *prevent* airway water loss; it *cannot add* water to the airway. Heated humidifiers must be used with wide-bore tubing since "rain-out" is expected as a result of the cooling of gas in transit to the patient.

Sterility

Humidifiers will rarely transmit bacteria because there is no particulate water.[133] However, one must be careful since many jet aerosol appliances are used for humidity therapy; i.e., a nebulizer can be used for humidity purposes. Since this is a common practice in respiratory care, the respiratory care practitioner must be aware that such an apparatus can transmit bacteria.[134]

Aerosols

An aerosol may be defined as a suspension of very fine particles of liquid in a gas. *Of all the pharmacologically and physically active aerosols used in medical practice, water is the most important.* The use of water in the treatment of bronchopulmonary disease requires an understanding of the physical principles of aerosols.

The last ten years has produced a flurry of investigative techniques attempting to discern the complexities of medical aerosol therapy. The authors recognize the problems involved and realize that differences in technique account for much of the variance found in the medical literature, especially pertaining to effective particle sizes and to the degree of alveolar penetration by aerosols. We suggest that the interested reader delve further into the complexities involved in studying medical aerosol therapy.[135-137] The following discussion reviews the most widely accepted behavioral characteristics of medical aerosols *as they apply to clinical medicine.* We can only alert the reader to the fact that it is by no means a totally valid application of the physics of aerosols. In addition, new developments in this field may well change basic concepts.

Medical aerosols must deal with particle sizes of less than 3 microns in diameter because it is at this mass that gravity begins to lose its influence on particles and, as we shall see, it is at this size that deposition of particles in the pulmonary tree becomes feasible.

Aerosol Stability

The ability to remain in suspension for significant periods of time reflects the stability of an aerosol. Numerous characteristics affect this stability. Among the more important are (1) concentration of particles; (2) size and nature of the particulate matter; and (3) ambient humidity. Instability is the tendency for particles to be removed from suspension. The stability or instability of an aerosol will greatly affect its clinical usefulness.

Medical aerosols are believed to have optimal stability when the particle diameter is from 0.2 to 0.7 micron and the concentrations are from 100 to 1,000 particles per cubic centimeter of gas. We must accept the generalization that water particles (or saltwater particles) are reasonably stable in the 0.5- to 3-micron diameter range, and that these particles maintain a basically spherical state under normal conditions.[131]

A medical aerosol must traverse tubular structures in which turbulent flow is the rule. Water (or saltwater) solutions will not change basic chemical or physical properties when inhaled, and they have the tendency to coalesce when contact is made; i.e., when two particles of water collide, they tend to form one larger particle. Water particles have the physical tendency to form spheres, so that the least surface area is exposed to the gas. Since the volume of a droplet is proportional to the cube of its diameter, one thousand 4-micron particles must coalesce to form a single 40-micron diameter particle.[23]

We can make the generalization that as droplets are traveling down the pulmonary tree, turbulence will cause the particles to collide and form larger diameter particles. How far the aerosol will penetrate and how much will be deposited in the tracheobronchial tree is a subject to which we must devote some depth of study.

Penetration and Deposition

Penetration refers to the maximum depth that suspended particles can be carried into the pulmonary tree by inhaled tidal air. *Deposition* is the result of an aerosol's eventual instability, permitting the particles to "fall out" on a nearby surface. *Clearance* generally refers to the process of removal of particles once deposited in the pulmonary tree. In relation to therapeutic aerosols, there are four major factors that are known to influence penetration and deposition: (1) gravity, (2) kinetic activity, (3) inertial impaction, and (4) ventilatory pattern.

Gravity

Gravity will influence a suspended particle in direct relation to the particle mass. Suspended water particles between 0.1 and 70 microns follow the prediction of *Stokes' law of sedimentation.*[138] This is a complex law which deals with the rate at which small particles will fall to the earth, taking into account physical factors such as particle volume, density, acceleration of gravity, and viscous resistance of air.

Since we are dealing solely with water particles at the earth's surface, we may simplify Stokes' law into a proportionality which states that as the diameter doubles, the forces of gravity tending to make that particle "rain out" increase fourfold. Remember that it takes a very large number of small water particles to coalesce and form a particle with twice the diameter. We may generalize the effect of gravity on water aerosol by stating that as the diameters of the particles become larger, the gravitation forces that tend to make the particles remove themselves from suspension become greater.

Kinetic Activity of Gas Molecules

Small particles suspended in a liquid can be seen to have an erratic movement pattern seemingly independent of the direction of the liquid flow. This movement is due to molecules of water moving at random as a result of kinetic energy and hitting the suspended particles. The particle movement caused by this molecular phenomenon is known as brownian movement. This same phenomenon will occur with small water particles in gas suspension.

This phenomenon has little application in the tracheobronchial tree, but is an essential concept in the study of the efficiency of aerosol equipment.[139] The random lateral movement of particles may result in unwanted coalescence and deposition in the generator and tubing. As aerosol generators become more efficient in producing smaller particles and denser mists, this factor becomes more important.

Inertial Impaction (Fig 9-2)

Inertial impaction is an important theoretic concept in the penetration and deposition of medical aerosols. It is based upon the physical

——————— Water Particles

Gas Molecules

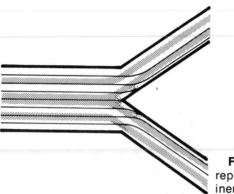

Fig 9–2. — Schematic representation of the principle of inertial impaction (see text).

fact that water particles have a greater mass than gas molecules.[140] The force moving water particles in a straight line is greater than the force on gas molecules. Thus, when an airstream containing liquid particles undergoes a sudden change in direction, the particles tend to continue on a straight course. This directional divergence of the water particles from the airstream will cause a great number of water particles to collide with the sides of the bronchi and bronchioles either at points of branching or in areas where there is retained mucus. Whether a particle will deposit in such a manner depends in part upon its location within the airstream. Therefore, *the probability of deposition caused by inertial impaction increases as the diameter of the conducting tube decreases.* This type of deposition is far more important in the bronchioles than in the bronchi.

In clinical practice the aerosolized solutions will vary, as will the method of administration. There are two additional factors that may affect particle deposition: tonicity of the liquid and temperature variation. Hypertonic fluid tends to absorb water, whereas hypotonic fluid tends to lose water. Therefore, hypertonic aerosols would theoretically gain water and increase droplet size; hypotonic aerosols may theoretically evaporate. Although it is an interesting theory, there is little to document its occurrence in clinical practice. A more realistic concern may be associated with injecting the aerosol into a heated and humidified gas stream that will cool on the way to the patient. The evaporated water that must "rain out" may well coalesce with the existing droplets and increase their size.[141]

Ventilatory Pattern

The previously mentioned factors that determine the penetration and deposition of aerosols are basically dependent upon the appliance and the state of the airway. This means the therapist has little control of these factors. However, the ventilatory pattern is potentially within the control of the therapist and, therefore, *becomes the most important clinical variable determining the penetration and deposition of medical aerosols.*

In general, *deposition and retention of aerosol particles are directly related to inhaled volume and inversely related to ventilatory rate.*[142] This generalization holds true with water particles of at least 1 micron in airways larger than the terminal bronchioles. Distal to terminal bronchioles it is believed that gas stream flow stops and mass gas movement in and out of the alveolar structures is by diffusion. Gas movement is in response to pressure gradients. Thus, depth and frequency of ventilation have little influence on the deposition of particles once they have reached the alveolar level.[23]

Deposition of water particles within the tracheobronchial tree is very definitely related to the ventilatory pattern. Since the nose will filter particles, the patient must inhale the aerosol through the mouth. Shallow breathing carries a reduced volume of aerosol per tidal volume, and a rapid breathing rate reduces the time available for the particles to settle. *If penetration and deposition are the objectives, the ideal ventilatory pattern consists of slow, deep breathing and holding the breath at the end of inspiration.* This pattern facilitates the introduction into the pulmonary tree of a significant volume of particles. This is a practical point that the respiratory care practitioner will have to keep in mind as he instructs and supervises patients in the proper technique of effective aerosol therapy.

Water Content

Penetration and deposition of aerosol are obviously dependent on the density of the aerosol mist. The total water content of aerosol gas (water vapor plus water particles) greatly affects the potential for depositing water within the tracheobronchial tree. Gas containing 50 mg of water per liter of gas at room temperature will guarantee 100% humidification of inspired gas, but will not be significant in depositing water in the airways. Water contents of greater than 50 mg of water per liter at room temperature have the *potential* for depositing water in the airway. When aerosol mists contain appropriate 1-micron droplet size and water contents in excess of 100 mg of water per liter, they are

TABLE 9-2.—NEBULIZER OUTPUT
VS. WATER CONTENT

OUTPUT	GAS FLOW (L/min)	WATER CONTENT (mg/L)
6 ml/min	5	1,200
	15	400
	25	240
3 ml/min	10	300
	20	150
	30	100
1 ml of H_2O = 1,000 mg of H_2O.		

extremely effective mists for deposition in the tracheobronchial tree when appropriately administered.

It is important to differentiate between water content of an aerosol and the output of an aerosol generator. The fact that an appliance has a liquid output of 6 ml per minute says little about the mist (Table 9-2). It is obvious that the medical efficiency of aerosols is dependent upon the water content—the appliance output is important only in relation to total gas flow.

Airway Resistance

Introduction of aerosol into the tracheobronchial tree will cause an increase in total airway resistance.[143] It is noted that this increase in resistance is greatest when the aerosolized material is distilled water. Aerosols of normal saline also cause an increase in total airway resistance, but to a lesser degree. The airway resistance caused by distilled water is partially reversible by bronchodilators, whereas the airway resistance in response to normal saline is not reversible by bronchodilators. There is great controversy about the causes for these reactions, and at the present time it is not clear what roles tonicity and salt content play.

A widely acceptable clinical observation is that the optimal solutions for aerosol therapy are 0.25% or 0.45% saline (0.9% NaCl is normal saline).[144] These solutions seem to produce less increase in airway resistance than either distilled water or normal saline, and the increased airway resistance is partly responsive to bronchodilator therapy.

Clearance of Aerosols

We shall discuss only the removal of particles from the pulmonary tract by means other than that of exhaled air. Much of the inhaled particulate water is removed from the pulmonary tree by exhalation.

These exhaled water particles are not deposited and, therefore, are not of therapeutic significance.

We must consider the mechanisms by which the pulmonary tree clears the deposited water in both the tracheobronchial tree and the parenchyma. The pulmonary mechanisms for clearing of aerosols is the same as the discussion of the lung defense mechanisms in Chapter 1. We are concerned primarily with the deposition of water particles in the tracheobronchial tree for the purpose of promoting mobilization of the mucous blanket. Thus, the very act of clearing the deposited aerosol is the desired effect of aerosol therapy — the mobilization of the mucous blanket.

In summary, a medical aerosol ideally (1) is a weak salt water solution; (2) contains particles of 1 micron in diameter; (3) has water contents in excess of 100 mg/L; (4) is delivered with the patient mouth breathing; and (5) is delivered with a deep and slow ventilatory pattern.

The study of aerosol penetration and deposition is so technically unsure that there is no dependable information from direct study at the present time. We must make our basic evaluation on the theoretic application of physics and clinical observation.

Aerosol Generators

An *atomizer* generates an aerosol. Instruments that generate aerosols of uniform particle size are called *nebulizers*. Medical nebulizers are designed to deliver a maximum number of uniform particles for penetration and distribution in the pulmonary tree.

Medical nebulizers can be subdivided into two general categories; pneumatic and electric. A pneumatic generator operates from a pressurized gas source; an electric generator derives its power from an electric source. We shall consider two types of pneumatic nebulizers: the jet nebulizer and the hydronamic nebulizer. We shall consider one electric generator: the ultrasonic nebulizer. These three are the significant types of generators in use at the present time.

Figure 9–3 illustrates the principle of *baffling*. A baffle is a device that deflects gas flow. When such a device is placed in the path of a gas flow that contains water particles, the particles will "smash" against the baffle and break up into smaller particles. The heavier (larger) particles will collide with the sides of the tube or container and "rain out"; the smaller particles will again join the gas flow distal to the baffle. The more baffles in a series, the smaller and more uniform the particle size. The water surface, sides of the container, and right-angle

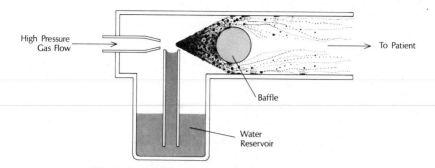

Fig 9–3.—The principle of baffling (see text).

bends in tubing may function as baffles. Most pneumatic nebulizers create uniform, small particle size by baffling systems. Atomizers do not contain baffles.

Jet Nebulizer

The jet nebulizer is a system in which a high-velocity gas flow is directed over a tube that is immersed in a water reservoir (Fig 9–4). The Bernoulli effect (see Chapter 7) causes the water to rise in the tube and be sprayed out into the high-velocity airflow. These gross particles are then baffled into uniform particle sizes. The pneumatic force comes directly from a gas cylinder, pipeline, or compressor. A

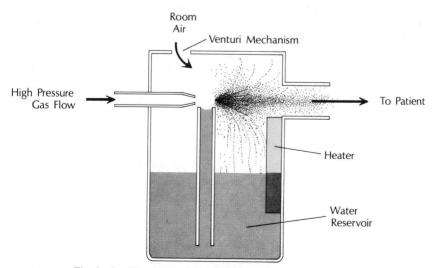

Fig 9–4.—The jet "all-purpose" nebulizer (see text).

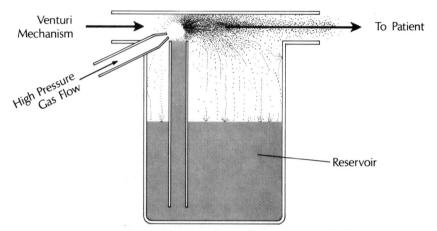

Venturi Mechanism

To Patient

High Pressure Gas Flow

Reservoir

Fig 9–5. — Model of a reservoir mainstream jet nebulizer.

Venturi mechanism (see Chapter 7) is incorporated to provide a high total gas flow. This makes a readily available oxygen dilution system for combining controlled oxygen therapy with the aerosol therapy. A water heater allows the temperature of the carrier gas to be controlled. The combination of (1) jet nebulizer action, (2) a Venturi oxygen device, and (3) a heater is called an "all-purpose" nebulizer. Such a device allows control of $F_{I_{O_2}}$, water content, and temperature — an ideal high-flow oxygen system (see Chapter 7).

Tradition has created a confusing nomenclature for categorizing types of nebulization units. The following discussion is compatible with traditional nomenclature, yet applicable to newly developed, disposable units. It is not our purpose to detail various commercially available nebulizers but, rather, to aid the therapist in evaluating and applying commercially available equipment. Before clinically classifying nebulizers, it is essential to define four types of nebulizing units:

1. *Reservoir jet nubulizers* have solution reservoirs in excess of 250 ml to provide long-term aerosol therapy.

2. *Standard jet nebulizers* have reservoir capacities less than 20 ml. The modern respiratory therapy prototype is the IPPB machine nebulizer whose power source may or may not be intermittent. The purpose of this nebulizing unit is twofold: (1) humidification of dry gases to approximately 50% humidity at room temperature, and (2) delivery of medication by aerosol.

3. *Mainstream nebulizers* create aerosol *within* the main gas flow chamber, allowing the outflow gas to be well humidified. Relative humidity may approach 100% if a heating element is included.

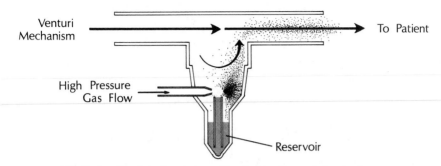

Fig 9–6. – Model of an intermittent sidestream jet nebulizer.

4. *Sidestream nebulizers* create aerosol *outside* the main therapeutic gas flow. As the aerosol enters the main gas flow, it partially evaporates and provides humidity while the remainder is carried in the gas flow to the patient. This is an effective means of humidifying dry gas and administering medication during IPPB therapy.

Clinical classification of jet nebulizers falls into two main categories: reservoir and intermittent. The reservoir jet nebulizer is almost always of the mainstream type (Fig 9–5) and is used for long-term aerosol and oxygen therapy. The intermittent jet nebulizer is usually of the sidestream type (Fig 9–6). These nebulizers are clinically applied almost exclusively for the purpose of delivery of pharmaceutical aerosol.

Hydronamic Nebulizer

Recently, another principle of pneumatic nebulization has been developed.[145] This hydronamic principle uses a system which prepares a film of water for aerosolization by flowing it over a hollow sphere (Fig 9–7). A small orifice in the sphere expels gas at supersonic velocity. This high-velocity gas ruptures the thin film of water and produces a continuous dispersion of fine, liquid particles. A baffle is used to assure uniform particles of small diameter.

The hydronamic nebulizer has proved to be extremely useful in the armamentarium of equipment available for clinical application of high volume aerosol therapy.

Ultrasonic Nebulizer

The electric nebulizer works on a completely different principle from pneumatically driven generators. It is a complex electronic instrument that has been described in much detail.[146] We shall review

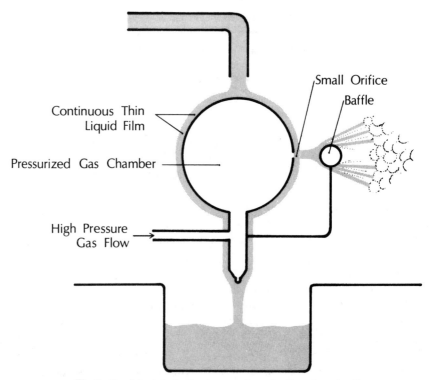

Fig 9–7. — Model of a hydronamic nebulizer (see text).

its major features (Fig 9–8) and applications. This nebulizer has two components: a *power unit* and a *nebulizing unit*.

The power unit receives standard alternating house current and converts it into an ultrahigh frequency of approximately 1.35 megacycles per second. This ultrahigh frequency electric current is conveyed to the nebulizing unit.

The nebulizing unit contains a small disk which will vibrate in sympathy with electric current. This *piezoelectric transducer* transforms the ultrahigh frequency electric current into ultrahigh frequency vibrations. In this way the disk vibrates in sympathy with the ultrahigh frequency of the electric current, and these ultrasonic vibrations are transmitted to a water bath in which the disk sits. This water bath is called the *couplant*.

A container is placed within the couplant fluid. This container has a bottom that is made of a very thin plastic material which will vibrate in sympathy with the couplant fluid, while not allowing water molecules to pass through it. Thus, the couplant vibrations are transmitted into

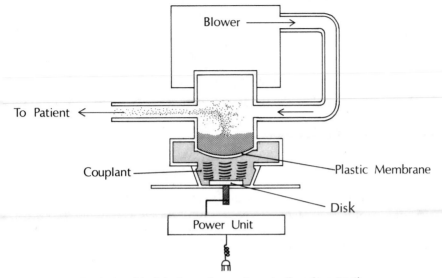

Fig 9–8. – Model of an ultrasonic nebulizer (see text).

the nebulizing cup where their intense energy physically breaks the surface water into small particles.

The precise mechanism by which the ultrasonic vibration forms the aerosol is not known. The mechanism has become a subject of controversy that is of no clinical significance. For our purposes we may conclude that the fine-particle nebulization occurs in the aerosol medicament chamber entirely by acoustic energy, i.e., without the use of air or gas. The aerosol particles are carried to the patient by a blower which provides a carrier gas.

The ultrasonic nebulizer is an extremely efficient instrument, nebulizing from 1 to 6 ml of water per minute. Because of the *high-volume* aerosol output, heating is not necessary and the therapy can be administered at room temperature.

It is a clinical error to assume that the efficiency of the ultrasonic nebulizer guarantees appropriate deposition of water in the pulmonary tree. The machine is undoubtedly an extremely efficient nebulizer, but does *not guarantee* the results of therapeutic aerosol – only the therapist can do that!

In summary, ultrasonic nebulizers produce very dense mists with water contents in excess of 100 mg/L. It is an extremely efficient appliance that is claimed to create better than 90% of its particles within the "effective" range of 0.5 to 3 microns. In contrast, most jet nebulizers produce approximately 55% of the particles in the effective range and seldom produce water contents of more than 50 mg/L. For this reason, ultrasonic nebulizers have gained great popularity in the administration of medical aerosol therapy.

Goals of Aerosol Therapy

The three clinical goals of aerosol therapy[141, 146] are as (1) an aid to bronchial hygiene, (2) a means to humidify inspired gases, and (3) a means to deliver medication.

Aid to Bronchial Hygiene

Desiccated and retained secretions are *hydrophilic;* i.e., they absorb water. Since dried, retained secretions cause significant pulmonary pathophysiology (see Chapter 8), it is appropriate to attempt to restore and maintain the mucous blanket. Although it is possible to increase the water content of secretions by systemic hydration (I.V. and oral fluids), this has little effect on dried, retained secretions present in the airways prior to systemic hydration.

The rationale for the administration of aerosol therapy as an aid to bronchial hygiene is to attempt to (1) hydrate dried, retained secretions; (2) restore and maintain the mucous blanket; (3) promote expectoration; and (4) improve the effectiveness of the cough. It is clinically apparent that where retained secretions exist, high-volume aerosol therapy may be effective in mobilization of those secretions, with improvement in pulmonary function and blood-gas exchange.

It is our opinion that intermittent, high-volume aerosol therapy is extremely effective in aiding bronchial hygiene and must always be accompanied by other appropriate techniques to promote expectoration, such as cough instruction and postural drainage. *The administration of high-volume aerosol therapy for 30 minutes every 4 hours will accomplish as adequate mobilization of dried, retained secretions as a continuous ultrasonic aerosol.* We believe little is to be gained from continuous administration of high-volume aerosol, but it does involve potential hazards, which will be discussed shortly.

Humidification of Inspired Gases

In circumstances where the upper airway is either bypassed or rendered inefficient, the application of aerosol therapy to assure proper humidification of inspired gases is indicated. Aerosol is preferred to humidifiers because artificial airways can better be kept moist and free from obstructive, dried secretions. We prefer pneumatic reservoir mainstream jet nebulizers that are heated, rather than continuous high-volume therapy.

Deliver Medication

The delivery of medication by aerosol will be discussed in Chapter 13. However, it must be mentioned here that aerosols are the method by which medications are delivered to the tracheobronchial tree and lung parenchyma. Studies have shown that most groups of drugs administered by aerosol therapy are not disrupted in their pharmacologic action by being delivered by aerosol route. We prefer sidestream intermittent jet nebulizers for this purpose.

Administration of Aerosol Therapy

Review of the medical literature concerning aerosol therapy presents conflicting and even diametrically opposed conclusions. The most likely explanation for this is the complexity of studying aerosols. It is our contention that aerosol therapy is an extremely effective modality when the clinical goals are kept clearly in mind and when properly administered. Therapy must be judged not only on its rationale, but also on the skill with which it is administered. If the prescription for aerosol therapy is rational and the therapy is applied skillfully, the results are both rewarding and dramatic.

The proper technique for the administration of aerosol therapy for purposes of bronchial hygiene comprises basically four steps: (1) the patient is placed in proper body alignment for maximal breathing efficiency and postural drainage when desired; (2) the patient *must* be instructed to breathe through his mouth, and to breathe slowly and deeply—a slight inspiratory pause is ideal; (3) the patient must be instructed in diaphragmatic breathing to assure that the maximum distribution and deposition of aerosol will occur in the basilar areas of the lung; and (4) proper cough instruction or cough assistance must be concomitant with the administration of aerosol.

Hazards of Aerosol Therapy

The hallmark of the efficient application of any treatment modality is the capability of recognizing and dealing with the potential hazards associated with its administration. We feel that there are four well-documented hazards of high-volume (ultrasonic, hydronamic) aerosol therapy that must be understood by the respiratory care practitioner.

Swelling of Dried, Retained Secretions

Dried, retained secretions result in partially obstructed airways, which can become completely obstructed with the addition of water. These secretions are hydrophilic (water-loving) and will swell when they absorb water. This results in acute lower airway obstruction and has caused death! Certainly, any individual who has had clinical contact with ultrasonic nebulization has experienced the circumstance where a patient manifests acute dyspnea and respiratory distress shortly after the initiation of therapy. A patient should never be left unattended while receiving ultrasonic therapy, especially during the early treatments. The water content should be carefully and gradually increased as tolerated. It is essential that efforts be made for mobilization of secretions immediately upon starting the aerosol therapy.

Precipitation of Bronchospasm

Aerosol droplets are foreign bodies that can precipitate bronchospasm. It is essential for the therapist to remain in attendance during ultrasonic therapy of any patient who has a tendency toward bronchospasm. This may be an indication for administering a bronchodilator before or with the ultrasonic treatment.

Fluid Overload

Fluid overload has been reported as a problem in infants receiving continuous ultrasonic aerosol therapy. However, an exhaustive search of the literature has failed to show documentation of fluid overload in the *adult* receiving *intermittent* therapy. Since intermittent ultrasonic therapy seems to be as effective in bronchial hygiene as continuous therapy, it seems reasonable to limit ultrasonic therapy to intermittent treatments, except in specific circumstances, such as patients with cystic fibrosis.

Cross-Contamination

Of great concern to all associated with respiratory therapy is the potential for infecting a patient through the respiratory therapy equipment. Hospital infections that are transmitted by particles are a type of *nosocomial* infection. Transmission of nosocomial infections via therapeutic aerosols has been extensively studied.[134] It is incumbent upon all in respiratory therapy to assure that equipment is properly sterilized. However, we must be aware that all aerosol generators utilize room air, and, despite excellent attempts to filter the air, the water reservoirs are inevitably contaminated with bacteria from the room. Since hospitals are notoriously associated with severe and dangerous airborne infections, it would stand to reason that therapeutic aerosols in the hospital would be a frequent source of contamination. An extensive culture program of respiratory therapy equipment should be devised by each department. Results of this can produce guidelines for routine changing of equipment.

It is incumbent upon all in respiratory therapy to do everything possible to assure that patients will not be *cross-contaminated!* It is impossible to protect the patient from his own organisms or from the organisms in room air—but he must be spared introduction of organisms from other patients in other locations. The inviolate rule of respiratory therapy must be that there is room for question about the efficacy of therapy, but we can never tolerate harming the patient with our therapy.

10 • IPPB THERAPY

IPPB THERAPY is defined as the therapeutic application of inspiratory positive pressure to the airway (usually via mask or mouthpiece) by a competent therapist or technician. It must not be confused with *IPPV* (mechanical support of ventilation)—inspiratory positive pressure which is administered to support cardiopulmonary homeostasis (see Chapter 22). This chapter is not intended to be a refutation of medical literature condemning IPPB therapy,[147-151] nor is it meant to be a justification for the lack of convincing studies. Rather, it is an attempt to place the clinical application of IPPB therapy on a basis upon which the respiratory care practitioner may judge its effectiveness and utilization. Only under these circumstances can we hope to provide the highest quality patient care at the least cost to the patient and society.

IPPB therapy has been controversial for more than three decades. Those who demand specific physiologic evidence attesting the qualitative and quantitative benefits of IPPB must be reminded that to appropriately study the efficacy of treatment regimens, their administration must be standardized. While relatively easy to accomplish in pharmacologic studies, it is very difficult with mechanical or manipulative regimens. On the other hand, those who believe that IPPB therapy is effective must be reminded that unsubstantiated clinical impression and dogma are far from irrefutable fact.[152]

The efficacy of any treatment modality must be judged by how well it accomplishes its goals. Most clinical studies of IPPB have failed to make clear delineation of methodology from equipment; positive-pressure breathing from bronchodilators; acute disease from chronic; pulmonary function improvement from clinical improvement; or clinical effectiveness from cost effectiveness. If objectivity is to exist in the support or nonsupport of IPPB therapy, reasonable and practical therapeutic goals must be clearly stated. Therefore, we shall begin the discussion by asking a very simple and straightforward question: What is IPPB therapy meant to accomplish?

Physiology

There are four documented physiologic effects of intermittent positive-pressure breathing. The physiologic effects of IPPB *alone*—not in conjunction with medication or aerosol—are (1) an increase in mean

184

airway pressure; (2) a decrease in the work of breathing; (3) manipulation of the inspiratory-expiratory ratio; and (4) an increase in tidal volume. The authors are unable to substantiate other purported physiologic effects of IPPB.

Increase in Mean Airway Pressure

Any method of breathing augmentation in which the inspiratory driving pressure is provided by applying a greater than atmospheric pressure to the upper airway will result in an increased mean airway pressure.[153-155] Thus, the *potential* for decreasing venous return results.

The Work of Breathing

Mechanical support of ventilation is, in part, the process of providing ventilatory power so the patient's ventilatory muscles can decrease their work (see Chapter 22). When an increased work of breathing exists, intermittent positive pressure may allow the same degree of physiologic ventilation with far less expenditure of muscular energy. This is true only while the therapy is being applied. There is no rationale for expecting the decreased work to continue after the therapy is ended.

Manipulation of the Inspiratory-Expiratory Pattern

Appropriate application of IPPB may result in a stressed patient accepting and being comfortable with ventilatory patterns not tolerated during spontaneous breathing. In the presence of disease that alters normal ventilatory patterns, the proper application of IPPB therapy may restore more efficient physiologic ventilatory patterns for the period of therapy.[156] This is true only in patients with appropriate disease entities — not healthy people.

Increasing Tidal Volume

An individual afflicted with a disease that limits the depth of breathing can be given an increased tidal volume with IPPB therapy. In some disease states the increase in tidal volume may be as great as three- or fourfold.[156-158] Although IPPB therapy may potentially increase tidal volume, *it is not guaranteed to do so!* Certainly, a given pressure limit does not assure volume delivery. Tidal volumes delivered by IPPB therapy should be measured.

Two additional physiologic effects are less well documented, but must be considered in this discussion: mechanical bronchodilation and collateral ventilation.

Mechanical Bronchodilation

The tracheobronchial tree possesses a potential of distensibility and collapsibility.[4] This characteristic increases as the lumen size decreases. There is a tendency for the tracheobronchial tree to dilate whenever intraluminal pressures exceed extraluminal pressures. The greater the intraluminal-to-extraluminal pressure difference, the greater will be the degree of dilation. When IPPB therapy is appropriately applied to a *diseased* lung, there is a greater degree of mechanical inspiratory bronchodilation than that which occurs with spontaneous inspiration.

Collateral Ventilation

Ventilation of alveoli via pores of Kohn (see Chapter 1) appears to take place in diseased lungs in which bronchiolar resistance is increased.[159, 382] It appears reasonable to assume that appropriate IPPB therapy may increase this collateral ventilation by increasing the tidal volume delivered and improving the ventilatory pattern.

Clinical Goals

IPPB therapy may provide a significantly deeper breath at physiologically advantageous inspiratory-to-expiratory patterns than the patient can produce with spontaneous ventilation. It is this statement and the facts contained therein that form the *rational clinical basis* for the application of intermittent positive-pressure breathing therapy.

Based upon available evidence and a preponderance of clinical experience, it is the authors' opinion that the goals of IPPB therapy should be (1) to improve and promote the coughing mechanism, (2) to improve the distribution of ventilation, and (3) to deliver medication. Each time IPPB therapy is applied to the patient, a concise thought process should be formed about which one (or combination) of these goals is desired. Only then can the therapist be guided in his approach to the patient and in his delivery of the therapy for maximum benefit. In addition, only after concise goals have been delineated can the respiratory care practitioner evaluate the benefit and effectiveness of therapy.

IMPROVE AND PROMOTE THE COUGH MECHANISM. — Bronchial hygiene is greatly dependent upon the effectiveness of the cough mechanism (see Chapter 8). Essential to an effective cough is the ability to take as deep a breath as possible and to accomplish the optimum peripheral distribution of that inspired air by providing a slow, inspiratory flow rate and inspiratory pause. A patient in whom these capabilities are significantly limited may receive significant benefit from IPPB therapy.[157, 158, 160, 161]

An acutely ill patient who will *not* produce a vital capacity of at least 15 ml/kg may benefit from IPPB therapy to improve the cough. However, if IPPB delivers less than 75% of the patient's vital capacity, the benefit of the treatment must be questioned, since theoretically the patient should be able to spontaneously inspire as much or more than is being delivered by IPPB.

IMPROVE DISTRIBUTION OF VENTILATION. — Appropriately applied IPPB therapy improves the distribution of ventilation in patients with ventilation-perfusion mismatch.[157, 158] Nitrogen washout studies, blood gas studies, and distribution of ventilation studies have concluded that IPPB therapy definitely improves the distribution of ventilation in the pulmonary-diseased patient.[162-165] A corollary to this is that *appropriately applied* IPPB therapy should have a great potential in decreasing the incidence of postoperative atelectasis and pneumonia, as well as re-expanding atelectatic alveoli.

Although clinical studies are contradictory and controversial, the authors have observed that when therapy is administered with expertise to the appropriate patient, the results are consistent and convincingly beneficial. An improved distribution of ventilation should be accomplished when a significantly diminished inspiratory capacity is present and/or a rapid ventilatory rate is present.

DELIVER MEDICATION. — Internal medicine depends primarily upon pharmacology for therapeutics. It is not surprising that the internist has come to view IPPB therapy primarily as a means of delivering medication. The unfortunate consequence has been that the *mechanical advantages* have been ignored while an inappropriate emphasis seems to have been placed upon the pharmacologic aspects. When an individual is limited in his ability to breathe deeply, there is a better distribution of drug if it is administered by IPPB as opposed to a hand nebulizer.[166, 167] However, in the individual who *can* breathe deeply, there is no advantage to IPPB administration over a hand nebulizer.[168, 169] *When medication can be safely and conveniently delivered by means other than IPPB therapy, it is an unjustifiable expense to use IPPB simply as a means of administering the drug!* It is the authors' opinion that IPPB therapy should seldom be administered *solely* as a means for delivering medication.

Much evaluation of IPPB therapy has been based upon its effect as a means of delivering bronchodilators.[157, 158, 165, 169-171] Controversy exists whether or not there is an advantage in delivering a bronchodilator by

IPPB vs. hand nebulizer vs. parenteral administration. The authors wish to emphasize that this is a question independent of the appropriateness of IPPB therapy. The need and desire for bronchodilator therapy must be considered separately from the use of IPPB therapy.

Administration

The efficacy of respiratory therapy is primarily dependent upon the *therapist*![156, 170] Ideal administration of *effective* IPPB therapy consists of (1) a knowledgeable and well-trained therapist completely familiar with the operation, maintenance, and clinical application of the machinery; (2) a relaxed, informed, and cooperative patient who meets the criteria for therapy and will respond to and work with the therapist and machine; (3) a concise concept of therapeutic goals by the physician, therapist, and patient; (4) a pressure-limited machine to accomplish maximal inspiration and a means of measuring tidal volumes; (5) appropriate coughing and breathing instruction; and (6) an *honest* appraisal by the therapist of whether or not the patient is benefiting.

Every patient treatment will not be successful. The therapist must not view the failure to adequately treat a patient as an embarrassment! The physician must not assume the failure to be due to incompetence or lack of skill! The therapist has a professional obligation to notify the physician of the inability to administer adequate therapy — both physician and therapist must work together to solve the dilemma!

Many clinicians believe the disparity in studies evaluating IPPB is due to variance in administration. It is the authors' opinion that this is the most significant factor causing the controversy surrounding *all* respiratory therapy. The essential fact governing the effectiveness and usefulness of respiratory therapy depends *not* upon the equipment, but upon the *therapist*!

"The" Criteria for IPPB

Therapy that is expensive must be judged on its cost effectiveness as well as clinical effectiveness. Whether administered to improve the cough, improve distribution of ventilation, or deliver medication, IPPB is only justified if the patient's ability to inspire adequately is limited. Therefore, for IPPB to be legitimately considered, the measured forced vital capacity must be below 15 ml/kg (ml/lb) and the IPPB tidal volume must exceed at least 75% of the limited vital capacity.

Effectiveness

Many attempts to study the effectiveness of IPPB therapy have been based on the *chronic* lung disease patient.[169, 171, 173] The negative results of these studies have been generalized to include *acutely* diseased patients. IPPB therapy does not reverse or improve *chronic* disease processes — this has never been stated as a clinical goal. The only logical basis for claiming benefit of IPPB therapy is in conjunction with its ability to provide deeper breaths and better physiologic ventilatory patterns.

Another common means of attempting to judge the effectiveness of IPPB therapy is to measure its effect on pulmonary function tests.[167, 172] No one would argue that pulmonary function testing will document many physiologic changes; to assume that these measurements can elucidate *all* of the potential benefits of therapy seems unjustifiable. IPPB therapy improves pulmonary function in some circumstances and causes deterioration in others. There is often subjective improvement even though pulmonary function studies do not improve.

To fairly judge the effectiveness and appropriateness of IPPB therapy, one must be willing to accept that there may be physiologic and psychologic factors involved that are not measurable or documentable at the present time. In the final analysis, one must judge and evaluate the effectiveness of IPPB therapy on how well it accomplishes the stated clinical goals.[156] Specific criteria upon which evaluation is based are discussed in Chapter 14.

Hazards

Effective therapy is accompanied by potential risks. Since a great deal of IPPB's efficacy depends upon the therapist, it stands to reason that the therapist must be sensitive to potential hazards that may be recognized early and prevented. The major hazards of significant frequency are (1) excessive ventilation, (2) excessive oxygenation, (3) decreased cardiac output, (4) increased intracranial pressure, (5) pneumothorax, and (6) hemoptysis.

Excessive Ventilation

When a patient is poorly informed or supervised in the use of the positive-pressure machine, it is common for the patient to rapidly cycle the machine and receive large tidal volumes. This rapid and deep ventilation results in an acute alveolar hyperventilation (decreased arterial P_{CO_2}) which may cause dizziness and/or loss of consciousness. In addition to the frightening experience of feeling faint, there is the possibility of the patient falling from his chair or bed and sustaining serious injury. The patient should be instructed to sit and rest for 5 to 10 minutes following a treatment to avoid dizziness on standing.

A well-trained therapist knows several maneuvers to avoid alveolar hyperventilation with the positive-pressure machine, e.g., manipulating the inspiratory sensitivity so the patient must exert a greater effort to start the inspiratory cycle, or slowing the inspiratory flow rate. The therapist must be knowledgeable about the clinical techniques as well as the machinery so the patient will take slow and deep breaths with the IPPB machine.

Excessive Oxygenation

Excessive oxygen administration can be extremely dangerous — especially in those chronic lung diseased patients who are "CO_2 retainers" and are dependent on a "hypoxic drive" for breathing. Oxygen is used in the hospital as the pneumatic power source because it is inexpensive and readily available in comparison with compressed air. IPPB therapy is not *designed* to deliver high oxygen concentrations; rather, the oxygen delivery is a result of using gas-driven machines in the hospital where oxygen is the primary pneumatic force available. For patients in whom excessive oxygen could be dangerous (even for a short period of time) care must be taken to give IPPB therapy with appropriate oxygen administration. This is readily accomplished by using machines powered by air compressors or using a compressed air pneumatic source.

Decreased Cardiac Output

It is possible to initiate a significant decrease in venous return with IPPB therapy, especially if the therapy is not properly applied. This venous return embarrassment may lead to a decrease in cardiac output, tachycardia, dyspnea, and a "feeling of impending doom." Needless to say, the patient will become anxious, frightened, and unwilling to continue with the therapy.

Proper inspiratory-to-expiratory ratios in conjunction with minimal airway pressures will usually prevent venous return embarrassment. More important, when the symptom complex occurs (1) it must be recognized immediately, (2) the therapy stopped, (3) the patient placed in a supine or head down position, (4) the patient reassured, and (5) the physician notified before continuing therapy.

Increased Intracranial Pressure

IPPB therapy creates an increased airway pressure which, in turn, may create an increase in the mean intrathoracic pressure. This means that venous drainage from the head is potentially impeded and may result in venous congestion inside the cranial cavity. This would result in an increased intracranial pressure since the volume of the cranial cavity is fixed. This pressure will compromise the capillary blood flow to brain tissue. This is of little consequence with appropriately administered IPPB therapy except in patients with pre-existent central nervous system disease. Care must be taken to administer IPPB while such patients are in a sitting position if at all possible. Care must be taken to allow long periods of expiration and periods of spontaneous breathing between positive-pressure breaths.

Pneumothorax

It is a common misconception that the IPPB machine itself causes a "bleb" to break and create a pneumothorax. Mouth pressures of 20 cm of water seldom create alveolar pressures above 10 cm H_2O — a pressure that will not rupture blebs. However, improvement in distribution of ventilation results in more gas entering poorly ventilated lung such as blebs. Under these conditions a good cough mechanism will result in high bleb pressures because of the increased gas volume. Thus, there is an increased incidence of pneumothorax secondary to bleb rupture when a good cough accompanies IPPB therapy. The therapist must be aware of any complaint of chest pain with or after coughing. This must be evaluated before giving further positive-pressure therapy. *Any complaint of chest pain must be evaluated before IPPB therapy is continued.* Pneumothorax plus IPPB results in tension pneumothorax unless chest decompression is accomplished.

Hemoptysis

The improvement of the cough mechanism with IPPB is occasionally associated with hemoptysis (blood in the sputum). Whenever this is seen by the therapist, the treatment must be stopped, the patient reassured, and the physician notified.

The bleeding is not due to the IPPB, but rather to the improved cough that results from IPPB therapy. Most hemoptysis is bronchial *venous* bleeding and readily stops; however, it may be secondary to tumor or left-sided heart failure and, therefore, the physician must be notified prior to continuing therapy.

Summary

The only absolute contraindication to IPPB therapy is pneumothorax without a functioning chest tube. The second most universally applied contraindication should be its use when not indicated or when it is replaceable by a less expensive technique.[200]

The overuse, misuse, and abuse of IPPB therapy are unquestioned. The clear delineation of its appropriate application must be the goal of every physician and respiratory care practitioner. Its use as a *prophylactic* bronchial hygiene technique is to be discouraged.

11 • SUSTAINED MAXIMAL INSPIRATORY (SMI) THERAPY (INCENTIVE SPIROMETRY)

SINCE THE INTRODUCTION of IPPB therapy in the 1950s as a therapeutic regimen for bronchial hygiene, few have questioned its effectiveness in the very ill or debilitated patient with acutely retained secretions or acute absorption atelectasis. However, as this technique became widely applied for "routine" prophylactic therapy, its dubious effectiveness in these patients, along with the considerable cost, led to seeking more *cost beneficial* methods for *prophylactic* bronchial hygiene.

Several techniques were attempted in the 1960s with little success. *Expiratory maneuvers* such as blow bottles, tracheal suctioning, and spontaneous coughing proved disappointing, probably because they did not improve lung inflation or improve the effectiveness of the cough.[174-176] *Carbon dioxide inhalation* via rebreathing techniques to induce hyperventilation enjoyed popularity for a period of time.[177, 178] This technique was not effective because patients with pain on inspiration tended to breathe faster rather than more deeply. The 1970s produced the *incentive spirometer,* a technique that appears effective and appropriate for *prophylactic* bronchial hygiene.

Defining SMI

Spontaneous inspiration is a result of the muscles of inspiration producing an increased transpulmonary pressure gradient (see Chapters 3 and 21). Inspiratory flow will continue as long as a transairway pressure gradient exists. Thus, if a patient is encouraged to *sustain* the inspiratory effort as long as possible, a *maximum inspiration* will result.

In normal man, a sustained maximal inspiration (SMI) can produce transpulmonary pressure gradients in excess of 40 cm H_2O for 5 to 15 seconds.[179] In the absence of significantly increased airway resistance or decreased lung compliance, this maneuver can result in tidal volumes in excess of 40 ml/kg.

193

Rationale for SMI Prophylaxis

Approximately 6–9 times per hour, the normal adult's tidal volumes of 6–7 ml/kg are interspersed with deep inflations ("sighs") that approach total lung capacity.[180, 181] Alteration of a normal breathing pattern to one of shallow tidal volumes without sighs results in gradual alveolar collapse within one hour.[182-184] Therefore, it seems logical to assume that the development of atelectasis, retained secretions, and pneumonitis in the acutely ill, obtunded, postoperative or bedridden patient may be due to a similar process.[185-187]

Studies in both dogs[182, 188] and patients[180, 182, 184, 187, 189] indicate that inflated alveoli remain open for at least one hour after the onset of hypoventilation. Thus, hourly sustained maximal inspiratory maneuvers should provide an ideal prophylactic measure for atelectasis and retained secretions.

The Incentive Spirometer

The *incentive spirometer* is a device that allows the patient to perform SMI without added resistance while presenting a visual quantitation of his effort. This provides an "incentive" or goal and hopefully encourages the patient to repeat the maximal effort frequently.

The original type of incentive spirometer has a variable preset inspiratory volume with a light that turns on when that volume is reached; the light stays on as long as an inspiratory flow rate is maintained.[190] The patient is encouraged to keep the light on as long as possible while increasing the preset inspiratory volume by increments. More recent devices utilize various mechanisms whereby flow through a tube lifts a colored ball up a column. The sustained inspiratory flow is rewarded by the ball's reaching its goal and being sustained. Each device has a simple method of increasing the flow required to reach the goal. The primary advantage of the newer generation of incentive spirometers is economic.

As with IPPB and aerosol therapy, the incentive spirometer itself does *not* assure effective therapy. Simply leaving the device in the patient's room without proper instruction, supervision, and follow up has little benefit. *The adequacy of SMI therapy is dependent upon the patient's physiologic and emotional limitations.*

The main advantages of the incentive spirometer over IPPB as a prophylactic regimen are that (1) it appears to be a more effective prophylactic technique,[191-193] (2) the patient potentially receives more frequent therapy, and (3) personnel time (and therefore cost) is minimized.

Another advantage of SMI therapy is that performance appears to dramatically decrease when acute pulmonary disease occurs. Our experience with quadriplegic patients clearly demonstrates that early acute pulmonary disease (pneumonia, atelectasis) is reflected in a sudden inability to perform previous levels of SMI therapy.[194] This most likely reflects an acute decrease in ventilatory reserve.

Clinical Goals for SMI Therapy

When appropriately applied and supervised, SMI therapy will (1) optimize lung inflation, (2) optimize the cough mechanism, and (3) allow early detection of acute pulmonary disease.

Optimize Lung Inflation

As often as each hour, the lungs are maximally inflated in a manner that assures optimal distribution of ventilation. This is believed to help prevent atelectasis and accumulation of bronchial secretions.

Optimize Cough Mechanism

Optimizing the inspiratory capacity should provide an optimal forced vital capacity for coughing.

Early Detection of Acute Pulmonary Disease

Frequent SMI efforts establish base lines for the patient, therapist, nurse, and physician. Sudden decreases in the ability to perform the maneuver demands careful pulmonary evaluation for acute disease. In our experience, this occurs 12–24 hours prior to obvious clinical evidence of pneumonia and atelectasis (fever, tachycardia, tachypnea).[194]

Criteria for SMI Therapy

Guidelines for appropriate administration of incentive spirometry (SMI) therapy for the acutely ill patient are as follows: (1) the patient must be cooperative and motivated; (2) the lungs should be without acute atelectasis, pneumonia, or obvious retained secretions; (3) an FVC greater than 15 ml/kg or inspiratory capacity greater than 12 ml/kg should be obtainable; (4) a respiratory rate of less than 25 per minute should be present. Under these circumstances the patient is potentially capable of effective SMI; it is then the responsibility of the therapist, nurse, or physician to properly instruct and supervise the patient.

Administration of Incentive Spirometry

1. The patient is appropriately evaluated and the procedure is carefully explained. Emphasis must be placed on *why* the therapy is prescribed and *what* it accomplishes.

2. Technical aspects of the device must be thoroughly explained — fear and embarrassment are founded in the unknown.

3. Proper breathing technique and positioning must be taught (see Chapter 12) in conjunction with the use of the device.

4. The initial inspiratory goal should be twice the patient's measured tidal volume, but this may have to be increased or decreased to find an appropriate initial goal. If the patient is unable to manifest twice his measured tidal volume after orientation of the technique, the appropriateness of (SMI) therapy should be re-evaluated.

5. The patient should be instructed to do the therapy every waking hour: one SMI maneuver each 60 seconds (by the clock), repeated four to five times. This routine will (a) avoid hypocarbia secondary to hyperventilation, (b) avoid exhausting the patient, and (c) limit the therapy to 5 minutes of each hour.

6. The patient's goals and performance should be evaluated at least twice daily.

Summary

Incentive spirometry appears to be the most cost effective technique for administering *prophylactic* bronchial hygiene therapy. The theoretic basis for effectiveness is valid, and it appears clinically to be *at least* as effective as (if not more effective than) other methods.

The appropriateness and effectiveness of incentive spirometry as a *therapeutic* bronchial hygiene technique are not clear since its rationale is based on prophylactic studies. It is hoped that future investigations will delineate its therapeutic value. *The incentive spirometer should not be considered the replacement for all IPPB, aerosol, and chest physical therapy!* However, SMI therapy as a *prophylactic* technique appears to be the much needed replacement for IPPB and CPT, which are so ubiquitously misused and abused.

12 • CHEST PHYSICAL THERAPY

AN INTEGRAL PART of respiratory therapy's recent advancement has been the adoption of chest physical therapy techniques. These techniques have enjoyed much earlier and wider acceptance in Europe than in the United States, where chest physical therapy remains a relatively unknown mode of treatment. There are numerous reasons for the slow acceptance in the United States, not the least of which is the sparsity of qualified individuals for teaching. The past five years has seen a great gain in the utilization of chest physical therapy in large teaching centers. Most of this has been due to the availability of skilled chest physical therapists in aggressive respiratory care programs. A deterrent to widespread acceptance is that physical therapy and respiratory therapy are separate allied health fields. There is great reluctance on the part of some physical therapists to view these modalities as an integral part of respiratory therapy. Experience demonstrates that a team approach between respiratory therapy and physical therapy results in maximum patient benefit.[195]

Physical therapists must have a basic knowledge of respiratory therapy to appreciate and understand the role that chest physical therapy plays in bronchial hygiene and ventilation. On the other hand, respiratory therapists must be familiar with chest physical therapy techniques and be qualified to deliver such therapy. It appears inevitable that the majority of hospital chest physical therapy treatments will be provided by respiratory therapists since the techniques are commonly used in conjunction with "inhalation therapy" modalities and are required in intensive care 24 hours a day. The role of the physical therapist is primarily one of supervision, teaching, and evaluation.

This chapter is limited to a superficial overview of chest physical therapy as it pertains to respiratory therapy. For more detailed and in-depth information, the reader is referred to other texts.[196]

Goals of Chest Physical Therapy

Chest physical therapy is a series of manipulative techniques designed to prevent pulmonary complications and improve function in acute and chronic pulmonary disease.[45] From the viewpoint of respiratory therapy it seems appropriate to classify the goals of chest physical

197

therapy: (1) to prevent the accumulation and improve the mobilization of bronchial secretions, (2) to improve the efficiency and distribution of ventilation, and (3) to improve cardiopulmonary reserve using exercise techniques to promote physical conditioning.

Chest physical therapy techniques may be classified in three categories: (1) techniques that promote bronchial hygiene, (2) techniques that improve breathing efficiency, and (3) techniques that promote physical reconditioning. Physical reconditioning is discussed in Chapter 32.

Techniques Promoting Bronchial Hygiene

Bronchial hygiene has been defined as the maintenance of clear airways and the removal of secretions from the tracheobronchial tree. The mucociliary complex and cough mechanism can be aided by techniques such as aerosol, IPPB, and (1) postural drainage, (2) percussion, and vibration, and (3) coughing assistance.

Postural Drainage

The diseased mucociliary escalator is greatly enhanced when aided by gravity; i.e., mucus drainage of a lung segment is facilitated by body positions that allow mucus to flow in the direction of gravity. Obviously, postural drainage must be based upon a firm knowledge of tracheobronchial anatomy. Since branching of the tracheobronchial tree is variable and complex, practical postural drainage positions are best limited to areas of lung that commonly retain secretions.

Lung Segments

As illustrated in Figure 12–1, the upper lobes are composed of an apical, anterior, and posterior segment plus a middle lobe. The lingula is considered a left middle lobe since the location and direction of the lingular segmental bronchus constitute a mirror image of the right middle lobe bronchus. Although there are more precise anatomic descriptions of segments and subsegments available, for all practical clinical purposes these four segments are the ones commonly involved in upper lobe disease.

The lower lobes have four segments: superior, anterior basilar, posterior basilar, and lateral basilar. The *posterior basilar* segment is the largest, encompassing at least half of the posterior chest wall and resting directly on the diaphragm. Figure 12–2 demonstrates that the superior and posterior basilar segmental bronchi do not have the advantage of gravity for drainage in the usual hospital bed positions.

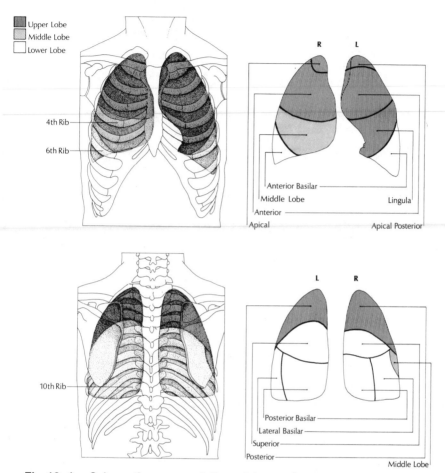

Fig 12–1.—Schematic representation of lung segments most commonly requiring bronchial hygiene therapy.

This is undoubtedly a major reason why these particular segments are most commonly involved in atelectasis and pneumonia. Topical landmarks for locating these lung segments are depicted in Figure 12–1. The *major fissure* or oblique fissure separates the upper and lower lobes. The right middle lobe is separated from the upper lobe by the minor fissure.

Figure 12–3 illustrates the basic positions for drainage of the most common segments demanding postural drainage. These positions are essential for respiratory care practitioners to know and implement.

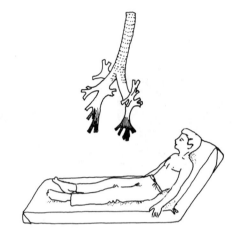

a

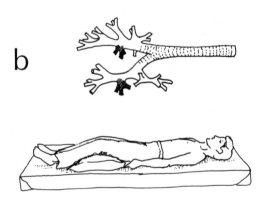

b

Fig 12–2. — Common body positions for ill or convalescent patients. **A** represents the common "hospital bed" position. Note that the shaded segmental and subsegmental bronchi of the posterior basilar segments of the lower lobes have no gravity drainage. These are the areas of lung most commonly involved with atelectasis and pneumonia in the acutely ill patient. **B** represents the absence of gravity drainage of the apical segments of the lower lobes in the supine position.

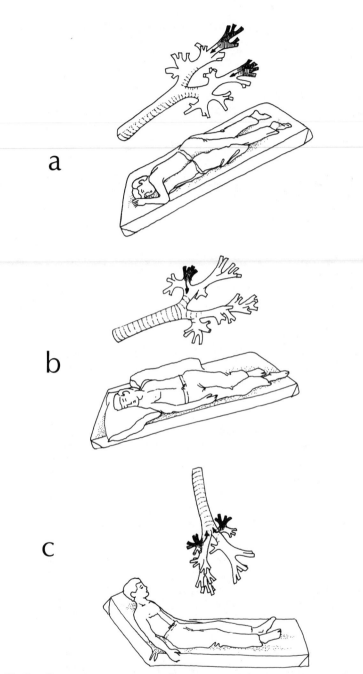

Fig 12–3. — Common postural drainage positions for **A,** posterior basilar segments; **B,** middle lobe and lingula; and **C,** apical segments of upper lobes.

Clinical Indications

When normal bronchial hygiene mechanisms malfunction and secretions are retained, the patient becomes a candidate for postural drainage therapy. Diseases often requiring postural drainage include, but are not limited to, bronchiectasis, cystic fibrosis, chronic obstructive pulmonary disease (COPD), acute atelectasis, lung abscess, ventilator care, and pneumonia. Postural drainage may also be required for postoperative patients and patients who have been on prolonged bed rest. There is always potential for contamination of the opposite lung when secretions are mobilized in unilateral disease. A general rule of postural drainage therapy is that care must be taken to assure prophylactic drainage of the opposite (contralateral) lung following therapeutic drainage of the diseased side.

Lung abscess is a collection of purulent material (pus) within lung parenchyma. *Empyema* is a collection of purulent material within the pleural space and may contain as much as 4–5 liters of pus. Postural drainage may result in the patient "drowning" in the pus or contaminating the opposite lung if bronchial drainage is established. *An empyema must be surgically drained prior to the application of chest physical therapy techniques.* On the other hand, lung abscess is usually drained best by appropriate chest physical therapy.

Precautions

There are several precautions which must be considered when applying postural drainage. Position change may be a significant physiologic stress to the cardiovascular system, especially in critically ill patients. Further, a head-down position may diminish venous return from the head and result in increased intracranial pressure. It is best to avoid head-down positions in postoperative neurosurgical patients and in patients with known intracranial disease.

Postural drainage positions must not place stress on "healing" tissue, e.g., patients with recent spinal fusion or skin grafts. Postural drainage techniques must be weighed in terms of the potential benefit versus potential risk. In the final analysis, the decision is based on the therapist's and physician's clinical evaluation!

Chest Percussion (Fig 12–4)

The technique of chest percussion is most often used in conjunction with postural drainage to loosen adherent bronchial secretions. The object is to have cupped-shaped hands "clap" the chest wall, trapping air between the hand and the chest wall. This sudden compression of

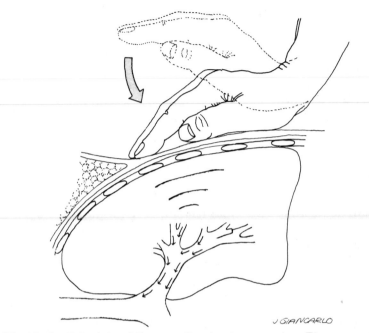

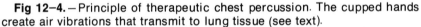

Fig 12–4. – Principle of therapeutic chest percussion. The cupped hands create air vibrations that transmit to lung tissue (see text).

air produces an energy wave that is transmitted through the chest wall tissues to the lung tissue. This energy wave will theoretically loosen adherent mucus plugs and allow better mobilization of secretions via gravity and coughing techniques.[197, 198]

The procedure is performed by rhythmically and alternately striking the chest wall with the cupped hands, producing a loud clapping noise without pain, discomfort, or bruising. Bony prominences (clavicle, spine of the scapula, spinal column) and female breast tissue should be avoided. Chest percussion is an excellent *adjunct* to bronchial hygiene therapy and is usually performed in conjunction with postural drainage.

Care and judgment must be exercised when a patient is fragile or "brittle." A skilled therapist can administer chest percussion to patients with brittle bones or fractured ribs; however, this takes great expertise and must not be done by the occasional therapist. In general, hemorrhagic conditions, "fragile" bones, bony metastases, and undrained empyema are contraindications to chest percussion. The procedure is usually avoided in patients with resectable tumors of the lung so that tumor spread is minimized prior to surgery.

Chest Vibration

The technique of chest vibration is accomplished by placing the hands on the chest wall and producing a very rapid vibratory motion in the arms while gently compressing the chest wall. A skilled therapist can develop a vibratory frequency in excess of 200 per minute. This becomes an extremely effective means of mobilizing secretions toward the gravity-dependent major airways in conjunction with postural drainage and following chest percussion. Chest vibration is performed during exhalation following a deep inspiration and is a very effective adjunct to IPPB therapy in the intubated patient.

Cough Instruction

Cough instruction is a simple technique requiring a thorough understanding of the normal cough mechanism (Chapter 8). The importance of a deep breath, the glottis, and the abdominal muscles must be appreciated. A patient receiving cough instruction must first be taught proper breathing techniques.

A simple technique is to have the patient take several deep breaths and then a maximum inspiration which he "holds" for a count of 3. After mastering this maneuver, he is taught to forcefully contract his abdominal muscles on the count of 2 and expel the air by opening his glottis on the count of 3. Two coughs in succession may also be tried as an aid to mobilization of secretions.[199]

Cough instruction is useful in conjunction with all respiratory therapy modalities and with postoperative abdominal and chest patients. A painful incision will limit the willingness of the patient to cough. It is helpful to have the patient "cuddle" a pillow to his abdomen in a sitting position or for the therapist to support the incisional area with slight hand pressure. These maneuvers decrease the need to tighten abdominal muscles, the procedure that produces most of the pain.

In patients with spinal cord injury or disease, the abdominal musculature may be severely weakened. It is often helpful to apply an abdominal binder or hand pressure to provide support. Compressing the abdomen at the end of inspiration will help to increase intra-abdominal pressure and, therefore, increase the cough effectiveness.

Knowledge of the cough mechanism and the muscles of ventilation makes cough instruction an extremely simple and effective method of improving bronchial hygiene.

Cough Simulation (Fig 12-5)

The respiratory care practitioner commonly encounters patients unable to cough effectively because of (1) the placement of an artificial airway (tracheostomy or endotracheal tube), (2) glottic disease, or (3) muscular inability. In these circumstances, it is effective to combine the bronchial hygiene techniques of chest physical therapy with IPPB therapy, thus *simulating* the cough mechanism.

The patient is provided a deep breath by positive pressure that is held for as long as reasonable. Chest vibration and compression is applied during this inspiratory pause. Exhalation is allowed to take place while the vibration and chest compression continue. This technique effectively produces a high-velocity airflow from the pulmonary tree, moving secretions to the trachea where they can be suctioned or coughed up. The positive pressure may be applied with a hand ventilator or an IPPB machine.

Techniques Improving Breathing Efficiency

Few nurses are trained in the application of breathing techniques, and those with training have too little time to spend carrying them out. All respiratory therapy treatments necessitate proper breathing patterns and, therefore, all respiratory therapy practitioners must have an understanding of the techniques of breathing instruction and breathing retraining. Thorough understanding of the normal ventilatory cycle and the ventilatory muscles is mandatory.

Normal inspiration is accomplished primarily by contraction of the diaphragm. This results in an increased thoracic volume and a greater subatmospheric intrapleural pressure. This transairway driving pressure (see Chapters 3 and 21) results in gas movement toward alveoli. Recall that normal expiration is entirely passive, depending upon the elasticity of the chest wall and lung itself (see Chapter 3). With unlabored inspiration one observes: (1) rise of the abdomen because of the descension of the diaphragm; (2) flaring out of the lower ribs; and then (3) a slight raising of the upper chest. During expiration, the abdomen moves in as the diaphragm rises and the lateral ribs return to the resting position.

A stressed inspiration includes use of the accessory muscles of ventilation, most commonly the scalenes, sternocleidomastoid, pectoralis major, and trapezius muscles. These muscles act to elongate the bony thorax and exaggerate the increase in thoracic volume resulting from contraction of the diaphragm. Forced expiration is primarily accomplished by using abdominal musculature to increase intra-abdominal pressure. This forces the diaphragm upward.[202]

These normal and forced ventilatory mechanisms are important to understand since it is the recognition of abnormal sequence or inefficient use of these mechanisms that allows the application of corrective

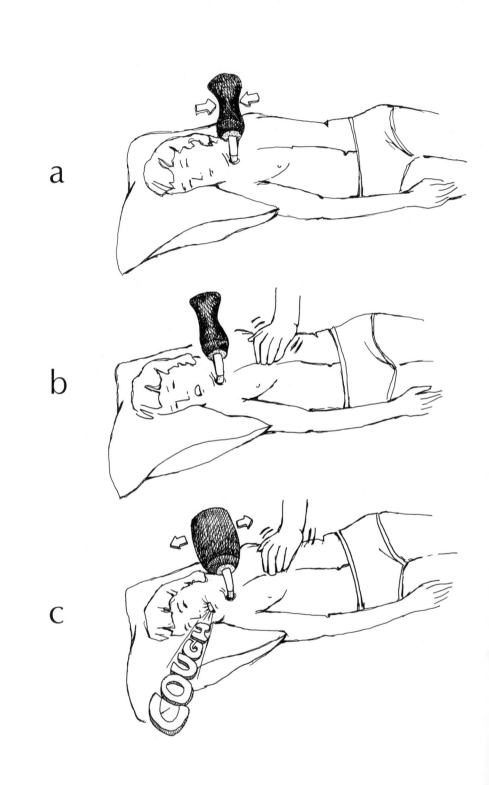

a

b

c

measures. Such measures may greatly improve the patient's breathing mechanics. Any circumstance in which there is an abnormal breathing pattern is a circumstance where breathing retraining may be of dramatic aid. The abnormal breathing may be due to pain, apprehension and nervousness, surgery, bronchospasm, airway obstruction, restriction of the lungs and/or chest wall, central nervous system disease, chronic lung disease, neuromuscular disorders, and countless others.

The tactile sense is most helpful in instructing a patient to assume a more appropriate breathing pattern.[203] The therapist's hands are placed over the areas where muscular movement is desired and the patient is encouraged to concentrate on expanding the part of the chest under the hands. Proper diaphragmatic breathing instruction may be aided by placing the hand on the abdomen just beneath the xiphoid process and asking the patient to "breathe in" against the hand. Proper diaphragm movement will cause the patient to feel his abdomen pushing away the hand. Relaxed shoulders and a slow, relaxed breathing pattern are essential to breathing instruction.

For segmental breathing instruction, the therapist's hand is placed on the chest area to be expanded. The patient is encouraged to breathe deeply and to preferentially "send air" to that area of the chest where tactile stimulation is being applied by the therapist.[204] On expiration, moderate compression is applied.

It is often helpful to have a patient with obstructive disease exhale through "pursed lips," a maneuver that increases resistance to exhalation at the mouth. This maneuver is believed to transmit an expiratory back pressure to the bronchial tree. This back pressure is believed to prevent early collapse of small bronchioles and improve exhalation from alveoli[205] (see Chapter 23).

The Pediatric Patient

The secret to the successful application of chest physical therapy techniques in the small child is patience and understanding. Children are usually inquisitive and require a great deal of assurance that you are not going to hurt them. Postural drainage is easy to accomplish because the child is small and can be held in the lap and easily manipulated. Percussion is accomplished by simply tapping several fingers

---

Fig 12–5.—Schematic representation of cough simulation by IPPB and chest physical therapy techniques. **A,** deep breath is provided and inspiration maintained while **(B)** chest compression and vibration are started. A sudden release of the positive pressure **(C)** allows expiration and may allow high-velocity airflow approaching that of a true cough.

against the chest wall. This can be extremely effective and should not be accompanied by a "slapping" sound which may frighten the child. Above all, the therapist must be able to play "a game" with the patient and to teach the family how to carry out the therapy in the chronically diseased child.

The most difficult modality of chest physical therapy to apply in pediatrics is coughing and breathing instruction. It is difficult to obtain the cooperation of a child who does not want to take a deep breath or is in respiratory distress. IPPB therapy is usually difficult and unrewarding in the small child because he is afraid of the mask and the machinery. Patience and understanding will often result in improved coughing technique and adequate bronchial hygiene.

In the infant and small child, laughing and crying may assure deep breaths and may occasionally induce coughing-like maneuvers.[206] Nasopharyngeal or oropharyngeal suctioning may be necessary if secretions cannot be mobilized by other means.

13 • PHARMACOLOGY IN BRONCHIAL HYGIENE THERAPY

THE INHALATION of medication has been a mode of therapy for centuries. Adding medical agents to boiling water and inhaling the vapors has been a "home remedy" since the beginning of recorded history; camphor, eucalyptus, and tincture of benzoin enjoy popularity to this day. Freon pressurized atomizers for administering bronchodilators are used by hundreds of thousands of asthma sufferers. When not abused they undoubtedly provide significant relief with little risk.

Medicine has adopted the unfortunate belief that IPPB and aerosol therapy are primarily sophisticated and efficient methods of delivering medication. If aerosol and IPPB therapy are being administered primarily for their pharmacologic effects, it is almost certain that those effects can be better and more economically accomplished by methods other than respiratory therapy techniques!

Pharmacology is the main therapeutic tool of the pulmonary medicine physician, but is merely a *supplement* to the respiratory therapist. With the exception of nurses, respiratory therapists are the only recognized non-physician practitioners administering drugs to patients. Therefore, they must understand the appropriate administration, indications, and contraindications of the various agents. Although the respiratory therapist is primarily concerned with the delivery of aerosolized medication, he must be familiar with the general field of pulmonary pharmacologic therapy since he treats patients who are commonly receiving multiple pharmacologic agents. This chapter is *not* meant to be a detailed discussion of medical pharmacologic therapy for pulmonary disease; it is meant to be a general exposure to the entire field of pulmonary pharmacology for the respiratory care practitioner.

Basic Principles of Pharmacology

A *drug* is a chemical compound that affects physiologic and biochemical processes. A *medication* is a drug applied for therapeutic purposes. *Pharmacology* is the scientific study of drugs and medications in all aspects.

Effects and Side-Effects

Few medications possess specific actions; most have varied effects on metabolic and physiologic processes. The administration of a medication carries the responsibility of comprehending all of the drug's effects. The physiologic actions of a medication other than those specifically desired are termed "side-effects." For example, if a medication is administered for purposes of affecting the heart—but also affects the lungs—the lung effects are considered side-effects. On the other hand, the same medication given for the lung would have its cardiac effects considered side-effects.

Mode of Action

A medication produces its effect by contacting cellular elements (e.g., receptors, cell membranes, mitochondria). This is accomplished either by direct application or by absorption into the bloodstream.

TOPICAL EFFECT. — Medication can be applied directly to epithelial or mucosal surfaces and have its effect by direct contact. The drug molecules pass through or among the cells to directly contact cellular elements. A topical mode of action is when there is *no* absorption of drug into the bloodstream; the drug has its effect by direct contact with the cells. This must be distinguished from topically applying a medication to an epithelial (mucosal) surface with absorption into the bloodstream occurring via the copious blood supply of the epithelium.

SYSTEMIC ABSORPTION. — Medications are usually absorbed into the bloodstream and distributed throughout the body tissues where contact is made with cellular elements. Whether the route of delivery is injection, G.I. tract, or inhalation, the drug is absorbed into the bloodstream and has its effects via that route.

Classic pharmacologic study pertains to drugs that have their effect via the bloodstream; most medications applicable to pulmonary disease act in this manner. Such drugs are traditionally studied in four phases: (1) absorption into the bloodstream; (2) distribution throughout the body tissues; (3) metabolic inactivation and destruction; and (4) excretion. We shall be concerned only with the first of these phases.

Routes of Administration

Figure 13–1 illustrates the generalizations that may be made pertaining to the rapidity and efficacy of systemic absorption by four routes of administration: (1) intravenous; (2) intramuscular; (3) gastrointestinal; and (4) inhalation.

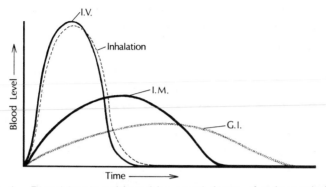

Fig 13–1.—Blood levels achieved by equal doses of a drug administered via different routes: I.V. = intravenous; I.M. = intramuscular; G.I. = gastrointestinal (pill or liquid). Only direct I.V. injection achieves a faster and higher blood level than the inhalation route.

INTRAVENOUS INJECTION.—The fastest and surest method of achieving a drug blood level is by injection directly into a vein. One is assured the total dose will enter the blood and it will do so rapidly. This is the preferred route of administration in critically ill patients.

INTRAMUSCULAR AND SUBCUTANEOUS INJECTION.—The deposition of a drug into a muscle will allow absorption via the copious blood flow. This is usually a dependable method of achieving a blood level as long as general circulation is good. Absorption occurs over a period of time—in comparison with an identical I.V. dose—and a lower blood level will be reached and maintained for a longer time.

Subcutaneous injection results in slower and less dependable absorption because of the less abundant blood supply to fatty tissues.

GASTROINTESTINAL ABSORPTION.—The small intestine is an excellent absorptive surface, the stomach and large intestine less so, but capable of significant absorption. The oral route (pill or liquid) is by far the most commonly used method of drug administration. Absorption is far slower and less reliable than with I.V. or I.M. injection. The convenience, toleration, and safety of the oral route, however, makes it the most widely used route for self-administration of medication.

Medications may also be given under the tongue (sublingual) or rectally. These routes have the advantage of bypassing the stomach where many drugs are inactivated or destroyed.

INHALATION ABSORPTION.—The lung has more potential surface area for molecular exchange with blood than any other organ. Only intravenous injection is more rapid than inhalation in achieving blood levels of a drug. The greatest absorptive area in the pulmonary system is the lung parenchyma; however, the medication must be delivered to the alveolar surfaces for absorption to take place across the alveolar-capillary (A-C) membrane. The tracheobronchial tree has a large mucosal surface area with copious capillary blood flow, so much so that some drugs are rapidly absorbed via this mucosa. Drugs administered via the pulmonary tree may act (1) topically; (2) by absorption through mucosa or A-C membrane; or (3) by both of these mechanisms.

With the exception of mucolytic and decongestant drugs, most medications delivered by aerosol may be as effective when administered by another route. Most inhalation drugs are administered because it is a convenient and safe method of self-administration. It is a common misunderstanding to assume that drugs administered by inhalation are working topically. The opposite is usually true – the lung and tracheobronchial tree are being used as a mechanism for rapid systemic absorption.

Dosages and Solutions

The calculation of dosages delivered by aerosol is unnecessarily confusing. Since the medication must be nebulized, concentrations are labeled either by the dilution factor of the drug or by the percent solution of the drug mixture. If several facts are committed to memory and several relationships understood, the use of these solutions is simple.

1. Solute = the drug dissolved.
2. Solvent = the fluid in which the drug is dissolved.
3. 1 ml of water = 1 gm (gm of water).
4. 1 gm = 1,000 mg.

Drug dilutions are expressed in terms of: GRAMS OF SOLUTE/ GRAMS OF SOLVENT. A 1:1,000 solution contains 1 gm of drug/ 1,000 gm of solvent. This is equal to 1,000 mg/1,000 ml; or 1 mg/ml.

Percent solutions are expressed in terms of: GRAMS OF SOLUTE/ 100 GRAMS OF SOLVENT. A 1% solution contains 1 gm/100 gm; or 1,000 mg/100 ml; or 10 mg/ml.

1:1,000 solution is a 0.1% solution.

1:200 equals 5 mg/ml, or a 0.5% solution.

Catecholamines

The catecholamines are widely used in cardiopulmonary disease and are among the most effective medications known to man. Over five thousand years ago, the Chinese discovered "ma huang," an herb

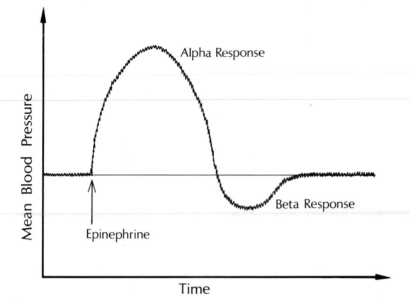

Fig 13-2.—Blood pressure response to appropriate dose of epinephrine (see text).

very successful in treating respiratory disease. The alkaloid "ephedrine" was isolated as the active ingredient in ma huang at the turn of the century. Shortly thereafter, the vasopressor action of adrenal gland extract was demonstrated. This adrenal gland activity was the basis for naming the sympathetic nervous system the "adrenergic" nervous system. In 1904, *epinephrine* was isolated and quickly became the prototype for all catecholamines.[207]

When epinephrine is injected into a dog in appropriate dosages, the blood pressure responds as illustrated in Figure 13-2. The initial vasopressor effect was named the "alpha" effect; the secondary vasodilating effect was named the "beta" effect. The receptor theory was soon put forth to explain these various effects. This theory is still universally accepted.

The Autonomic Receptor Theory

The autonomic nervous system does not come in anatomic contact with the target cells; rather, a chemical substance is released at the nerve ending that crosses a minute fluid gap and stimulates a receptor located on the cell membrane. This receptor activation is responsible for the reaction in the target cells.

The sympathetic nervous system has two categories of receptors: alpha and beta. *Alpha receptors* are located mainly in arteriolar vascular smooth muscle — when stimulated they cause constriction of that muscle. Beta receptors are also located in the vascular smooth muscle and have a weak dilating effect. *Beta receptors* are mainly located in the heart and lungs. Beta-1 receptors are on the heart cells and cause the myocardium to contract more rapidly and with more force; beta-2 receptors are located on the bronchial smooth muscle cells of the lung and cause active dilation of that musculature.

Alpha drugs will cause mucosal vasoconstriction and peripheral vasoconstriction (↑ BP). Beta drugs will cause tachycardia, arrhythmias, and bronchodilation. Although these are profound generalities, they will serve the respiratory care practitioner well.

Autonomics and the Lung

The tracheobronchial tree is supplied by both sympathetic and parasympathetic nerves. Stimulation of the sympathetic nerves primarily results in active relaxation of bronchial smooth muscle; stimulation of parasympathetic nerves primarily results in increased glandular activity and constriction of bronchial smooth muscle.

The sympathetic nervous system is believed to accomplish bronchodilation by stimulating the beta-2 receptors and causing relaxation of bronchial muscle. Therapeutically, epinephrine or related catecholamine drugs may be administered systemically or by inhalation to accomplish relaxation of airway musculature.

Bronchial smooth muscle can be made to contract by chemicals such as histamine or choline, or by stimulation of the parasympathetic nerves.[208] Historically, drugs that block the parasympathetics (such as atropine) have been used for bronchodilation.

Mechanisms of Bronchodilation

Although bronchodilating drugs have been successfully used for decades, the mechanisms through which they work have been discovered only within the last decade. The beta receptor on the smooth muscle cell is associated with an enzyme called adenylcyclase. When this enzyme combines with the beta-sympathetic drug, intracellular adenosine triphosphate (ATP) is rapidly converted to *cyclic AMP*. Intracellular levels of cAMP are responsible for relaxation of the muscle fiber.[209] Thus, increased levels of cAMP result in a series of biochemical reactions resulting in relaxation of muscle fibers; decreased levels of cAMP favor the reestablishment of bronchospasm in susceptible muscles.

Another intracellular enzyme, phosphodiesterase, is responsible for metabolizing cAMP. Thus, cAMP concentration may be increased by inhibiting phosphodiesterase. This is the pathway by which the methylxanthines (theophylline, aminophylline) achieve bronchodilation. In other words, all bronchodilating drugs cause an increase in cAMP levels, either by increased production or decreased breakdown. In general, catecholamines increase the production of cAMP; other bronchodilators decrease the breakdown of cAMP.[210]

Non-Inhalation Pulmonary Agents

Non-inhalation pulmonary pharmacologic therapy may be broadly categorized in seven areas: bronchospasmolytics, decongestants, mucokinetics, anti-inflammatories, antiallergics, anti-infectives, and antitussives.

Bronchospasmolytics

Bronchospasmolytics are drugs used in the management of bronchospasm. They may be categorized as active bronchodilators and preventatives. Active bronchodilators are either catecholamines or methylxanthines. The former increase production of cAMP; methylxanthines are phosphodiesterase inhibitors which decrease the rate of breakdown of cAMP.

EPINEPHRINE. — Epinephrine (Adrenalin) is the classic catecholamine. It has strong alpha and beta action and is both beta-1 and beta-2. Given subcutaneously, it is the standard therapy for acute asthma.

EPHEDRINE. — Ephedrine is similar to epinephrine and is the most common catecholamine oral bronchodilator. The dose of ephedrine needed to cause an optimal beta-2 effect would result in severe beta-1 effect and significant central nervous system stimulation. Therefore, it is usually given in suboptimal doses in combination with theophylline.

THEOPHYLLINE. — Theophylline is the most important of the methylxanthines for oral bronchodilation. In optimal beta-2 doses it is extremely irritating to the stomach and causes excessive central nervous system stimulation.

Suboptimal doses of both ephedrine and theophylline often are matched with a tranquilizer or sedative. Such combinations form the foundation of oral bronchodilators in the United States (e.g., Amesec, Bronkotab, Marax, Quadrinal, Tedral). Newer oral bronchodilators are effective and have fewer side-effects; these have been used extensively in Europe (metaproterenol, salbutamol, terbutaline). With their appearance on the American market, they will undoubtedly change present clinical regimens and concepts.

Aminophylline is theophylline dissolved in ethylenediamine for intravenous use; it may be given rectally or orally.[211]

CORTICOSTEROIDS. — Corticosteroids are clinically effective in relieving bronchospasm, especially in status asthmaticus. The specific actions affecting bronchodilation are unknown.[212]

CROMOLYN SODIUM. — Cromolyn sodium is a new agent whose main value is as a prophylactic bronchospasmolytic in allergic asthma.[213] It has been reported to allow steroid-dependent patients to significantly reduce steroid dosages or completely discontinue the drug.[214] The mechanism is believed to be the stabilization of the cellular membranes of mast cells. These cells are in abundance in allergic asthmatics and release histamine and other agents which induce bronchospasm. Cell wall stabilization is believed to decrease the release of these substances resulting from antigen-antibody reactions and thereby decreasing the bronchospasm of the allergic asthmatic.

This drug is of no use in the treatment of acute bronchospasm — it is a preventative. It is available as a powder and is inhaled with a special "spinhaler." The usual dose is 1 capsule four times a day; if the patient improves sufficiently, 1 capsule per day may eventually be adequate.

Decongestants

Nasal and pulmonary tree epithelium have a potential for copious capillary blood flow. When mucosal capillaries are dilated with maximal blood flow, they are said to be "congested." This mucosal congestion can lead to significant swelling of the mucosa, increasing airway resistance and causing nasal obstruction. A medicine that relieves this congestion is called a "decongestant."

True decongestants are alpha-adrenergic drugs that cause arterioles to constrict and thereby decrease blood flow to the area. This decreased blood flow diminishes capillary hydrostatic pressure and decreases fluid transudation to the tissues.

Allergic decongestants interfere with "histaminelike" irritation of tissues and thereby diminish the cause of the increased blood flow. Corticosteroids are commonly used as decongestants because of their anti-inflammatory action.

PHENYLEPHRINE (NEO-SYNEPHRINE). — Phenylephrine (Neo-Synephrine) is the most commonly used oral decongestant.[207] It is most often used in the liquid form in combination with antihistamines. *Pseudoephedrine* is a stereoisomer of ephedrine that is a reasonably good mucosal decongestant with little alpha side-effect. Although far more useful as a nasal decongestant, it is often used for therapy of the pulmonary tree.

ANTIHISTAMINES. — Antihistamines (e.g., Benadryl, Chlor-Trimeton) are very effective for nasal decongestion when the congestion is of an allergic origin. Antihistamines decrease glandular secretion and may have an effect of thickening the secretions.

Mucokinetic Agents (Expectorants)

Mucokinetic agents are used to help improve the removal of sputum. Most of these drugs are probably no better than water, which is an extremely effective agent for thinning mucus and decreasing its viscosity. Water may be administered by mouth, veins, rectum, or inhalation therapy. Nebulization is generally considered to be the most effective method for the administration of salt water solutions for the thinning of retained secretions. Aerosolized mucolytics will be discussed later; here we are concerned with the systemic mucokinetics. These agents fall into two general categories: vagal stimulants and direct bronchial gland stimulants.

VAGAL STIMULANTS. — Vagal stimulants work by stimulating the gastric mucosa, causing reflex vagal activation of the bronchial glands producing secretions. Glyceryl guaiacolate (Robitussin) and terpin hydrate are common expectorants that work via vagal stimulation.

DIRECT BRONCHIAL GLAND STIMULANTS. — Direct bronchial gland stimulants are exemplified by supersaturated potassium iodide solution (SSKI). When administered orally, this solution has a direct effect on the bronchial glands, causing increased secretions.

In terms of respiratory therapy, the use of oral expectorants appears self-defeating. A primary purpose of aerosol therapy is to *decrease* irritation to the pulmonary mucosa while improving and promoting mobilization of secretions. Although expectorants are widely used in general medicine, they are of no benefit in respiratory therapy.

Anti-Inflammatory Agents

Corticosteroids are used to decrease acute and chronic inflammatory processes of the pulmonary tree. The specific mechanisms are unknown, but there are many patients who obtain significant relief from no other regimen.

Antiallergic Agents

Allergic disease is responsible for a significant portion of pulmonary disease. Many patients are dramatically relieved by hyposensitization regimens ("allergy shots"). Antihistamines are useful in documented allergic disease, but must be accompanied by efforts to maintain fluid secretions since these drugs tend to dry mucus. Corticosteroids are also used as antiallergic agents.

Anti-Infectives (Antibiotics)

The application of antibiotic therapy for documented pulmonary infection is a well-tested mode of therapy. The greatest hazard is in the misuse and abuse of these excellent agents. Antibiotics are the most widely used category of drugs in pulmonary disease, with the exception of the bronchodilators.

Antitussives

Codeine is the most popular anti-cough agent. It is a potent central nervous system depressant of the cough center. This may be a very useful agent for the mildly ill, home therapy patient. However, in respiratory therapy the emphasis is placed on making the cough productive rather than suppressing the cough.

Inhalation Pulmonary Agents

The topical application of pharmacologic agents to the pulmonary tree is a well-accepted mode of therapy. In many circumstances the drugs are more effective by the inhalation route, and in other cases they are used only as an adjunct to systemic therapy. We shall discuss in detail the bronchodilators, decongestants, and mucokinetics. These major categories of aerosolized drugs must be completely understood by the respiratory care practitioner, both in their pharmacologic action and in their technical administration.

Catecholamines (Bronchodilators)

ISOPROTERENOL (ISUPREL). — Isoproterenol is the classic beta-adrenergic bronchodilator. A derivative of epinephrine, it was introduced into the medical arsenal in 1940. It is the most powerful bronchodilator marketed in the United States today and its use with IPPB has been extensively experienced over the past twenty years.[210] Only about 10% of the drug administered into the lungs by nebulization is retained — the degree of bronchodilation is dependent upon the systemic blood levels obtained.[207]

Isoproterenol is a powerful beta stimulator, without an alpha effect. Thus, it will cause vasodilation of the pulmonary mucosal vessels. This not only increases airway resistance, but results in an increased mucosal blood flow with consequent rapid absorption of the drug. The resultant effect is a relatively short persistence of the bronchodilating action with a marked tendency for cardiac beta-1 side-effects. Tachycardia, palpitation, and flushing of the skin are common side-effects of aerosolized isoproterenol and are often given as reasons for patients not tolerating IPPB therapy.

Our guideline for the IPPB maximum safe adult dose of isoproterenol that may be administered via an aerosol is 5 mg administered over a 10-minute period, repeated no more than each hour. The preparation comes in either a 1:100 or 1:200 solution. Since 1 ml of a 1:200 solution would contain 5 mg of isoproterenol, ½ ml of 1:200 isoproterenol would contain 2.5 mg — this is the routine recommended dosage diluted at least 3 times in the nebulizer. This is 50% of the IPPB maximum safe adult dosage and is extremely effective in most patients.

Isoproterenol is a potent and reliable bronchodilator, but demonstrates the pharmacologic principle of *tachyphylaxis*. This is the phenomenon of less and less response to increasing doses of a drug over a period of time. In addition, its action is far less effective when acidemia is present.[207]

ISOETHARINE (BRONKOSOL).—The recently introduced catecholamine isoetharine has become very popular because it has little beta-1 effect *in relation to isoproterenol*. However, it does have beta-1 effect and should not be considered a pure beta-2 stimulator since large doses result in tachycardia. It is a less powerful bronchodilator than isoproterenol but, nonetheless, is clinically effective.

Isoetharine is available in the United States under the trade name of Bronkosol, which contains 1% isoetharine. Our IPPB maximum safe adult dose of isoetharine is 5 mg given over a 10-minute period, repeated no more than each hour. It is recommended that ½ ml of Bronkosol be diluted 3–5 times in the nebulizer and administered every 2 to 4 hours.

METAPROTERENOL (ALUPENT, METAPREL).—Metaproterenol is the most recent aerosol bronchodilator to be introduced into the United States market. The drug has been used in Europe for many years and has proved itself a useful agent. Although a much less powerful bronchodilator than isoproterenol, it has a more prolonged effect. At the present time, metaproterenol is available in the freon cartridge and orally, but is not available in the liquid form for inclusion in IPPB therapy. Although metaproterenol has less beta-1 effect than isoproterenol, it is *not* a pure beta-2 drug.[210]

SALBUTAMOL AND TERBUTALINE. — Both salbutamol and terbutaline are drugs that have been used in Europe for several years and have proved to be superior bronchodilators. They are pure beta-2 stimulators and are effective by mouth as well as aerosol. Metabolism is much slower than with isoproterenol and, therefore, the effects are significantly prolonged. These are not presently available in the United States for aerosol administration.

Decongestants

RACEMIC EPINEPHRINE (MICRONEFRIN, VAPONEFRIN). — Racemic epinephrine is a mixture of the levo- and dextro-isomers of epinephrine in a 50:50 proportion. Compared with epinephrine, this agent has little beta or alpha effect. However, in aerosol it is a good mucosal decongestant. The beta-2 effect of the drug is mild — significantly less than isoproterenol — but the effect is prolonged because of the mucosal alpha effects.

Topical alpha stimulation causes mucosal vasoconstriction, and this is the prime value of the agent. It is an effective aerosol decongestant. Clinically, racemic epinephrine provides a near perfect routine additive to IPPB nebulization in the presence of tracheobronchial inflammation. The drug is an effective topical vasoconstrictor, a mild systemic bronchodilator, and a drug which has an extremely low incidence of cardiovascular side-effects. It must be emphasized that this agent is a *mild* bronchodilator and is not the agent of choice when severe bronchospasm is present.

Racemic epinephrine is commercially available in a 2.25% solution. It is administered as ½ ml of the drug in 3–5 ml of diluent. It may be repeated as often as every hour in the adult. The occurrence of cardiovascular side-effects is rare, but when they occur, they are the same as those for epinephrine.

PHENYLEPHRINE (NEO-SYNEPHRINE). — Phenylephrine is an alpha drug often used in conjunction with beta stimulators. Solutions of 0.25 to 1.0% may be administered in IPPB nebulizers, ½ ml diluted 3–5 times no more than each hour.

Mucokinetic Aerosol Agents

Mucus is composed of protein and sugar molecules bound together in extremely long chains. These "mucopolysaccharide chains" are bound by amino acid and sulfur bonds. The sulfur bonds are known as "sulfhydryl" bonds. When mucus is extremely thick and viscous, breaking the mucopolysaccharide chains creates smaller molecules that are less viscous.

HYPOVISCOSITY AGENTS. —*Water and weak electrolyte solutions* reduce the viscosity of sputum by diluting the mucopolysaccharide strands. The appropriate aerosol delivery of weak electrolyte solutions is by far the most effective of all the mucokinetic agents available.

Sodium bicarbonate makes the mucus alkaline. This tends to decrease its viscosity by making the amino acid bonds less stable.

Detergent agents have been used in the past for IPPB therapy. They have proved to be no more effective than water or sodium bicarbonate.

Glycerol and propylene glycol are sometimes used to stabilize aerosol particles. Ultrasonic nebulizers have erased the need for the addition of hydroscopic agents such as propylene glycol.

Alcohol is an agent that decreases surface tension and will theoretically decrease viscosity. Its use in respiratory care is best limited to pulmonary edema as a "defoaming agent."

MUCOLYTIC AGENTS. —*Pancreatic dornase* (Dornavac) is the most popular enzymatic mucokinetic. It is a particularly effective proteolytic enzyme, digesting the deoxyribonucleic acid (DNA) present in purulent sputum. It has little effect in nonpurulent sputum.

N-acetylcysteine (Mucomyst) is a chemical substance that destroys sulfhydryl bonds of mucopolysaccharide chains; it is an extremely effective mucolytic agent.[215] It will act on nonpurulent as well as purulent secretions. Acetylcysteine is administered in a 10% solution and has a very low incidence of bronchospasm; however, we still recommend that it be given with racemic epinephrine.

Steroids

Steroids are known to be potent, topical anti-inflammatory agents and it is only logical that they be tried in aerosol therapy to decrease tracheobronchial inflammation. Evidence indicates that there is little steroid absorbed systemically with properly administered aerosol. The prime systemic absorption of aerosolized steroids comes from swallowing the medication.[216]

Aerosolized steroids should never be a replacement for adequate systemic steroids. We believe that the primary use of aerosolized steroids is as an adjunct to systemic steroid therapy (aspiration pneumonia, glottic edema). In circumstances where chronic lung disease patients are steroid-dependent, adjunctive aerosolized steroids may decrease the need for systemic steroids.

Dexamethasone (Decadron) is the most widely used steroid compound for inhalation. Usually doses are ½ to 1 mg in 3 cc of diluent per IPPB treatment.

Antibiotics

Antibiotics have been widely used in aerosol form for the treatment of pulmonary infection.[217] It is doubtful that there is an advantage to this route over systemic injection and its use has precipitously diminished. Antibiotics work best by systemic absorption and there is no evidence of a decreased toxic effect when administered by the aerosol route. In addition, there is evidence that certain antibiotics topically administered may increase the incidence of sensitivity reaction to that drug. There is little rationale for the use of antibiotics in aerosol therapy.

14 • CLINICAL APPLICATION OF BRONCHIAL HYGIENE THERAPY

RETENTION OF secretions in the tracheobronchial tree is the forerunner of atelectasis, pneumonia, and lung abscess. This retention is frequently preventable and always treatable by bronchial hygiene regimen. The effectiveness of *individual* respiratory therapy modalities is poorly documented, but the intelligent and appropriate application of *combinations* of techniques appears to provide an effective means of reducing the symptom complex that results from retained secretions. In the previous chapters we have emphasized that the critical factor in bronchial hygiene is *how well the therapy is applied!* Bronchial hygiene is clinically effective when the patient's needs are carefully evaluated and the proper combination of respiratory therapy modalities applied.

In order to accomplish a rational bronchial hygiene program it is necessary to consider both the *formulation* and the *evaluation* of such a program. Intelligent formulation of a bronchial hygiene program necessitates (1) defining the clinical problem, (2) defining the therapeutic goals, and (3) selecting the techniques to accomplish the goals.

Defining the Clinical Problem

The respiratory care practitioner seldom comes in contact with a patient unless a physician has made the decision that respiratory care may be indicated. Thus, the initial approach becomes one of defining the clinical problem *in terms of respiratory care* so that a rational and intelligent consultation may be provided. This requires two essentials: (1) the obtaining of sufficient background information, and (2) the classification of a working diagnosis to establish the need for respiratory therapy.

Obtaining Background Information

To assure that all appropriate information is obtained, six steps should be followed. The steps need not be carried out in exact order, but are listed here as a means of helping the respiratory care practitioner organize his approach.

1. Read the medical history and review the medical chart. It is essential to have an appreciation of the length of the problem and its severity. A review of the physician's workup can provide essential background information and provide a reasonable estimation of the patient's physical status.

2. Obtain the results of the laboratory studies appropriate to respiratory care. These studies include, but are not limited to (1) screening *pulmonary function* measurements or complete pulmonary function studies — these document the existence of obstructive and restrictive components and quantify the general mechanical status of the pulmonary system; (2) *chest x-ray,* which may document the existence and general location of acute and chronic pulmonary disease; and (3) *arterial blood gas studies* which reflect the cardiopulmonary status in general and specifically help evaluate ventilatory, acid-base, and oxygenation status.

3. Interview and directly observe the patient to evaluate his ability and willingness to communicate and cooperate. This is an excellent opportunity to find out whether the patient produces sputum, coughs, has difficulty breathing, or is afraid of therapy. A history should be obtained concerning the amount, color, and consistency of sputum.

4. Observe the patient's mechanical ventilatory state. This should involve (1) observation of the ventilatory pattern; (2) observation of the time sequences of inspiration to expiration; and (3) use of accessory muscles of ventilation.

Mechanical parameters of breathing, such as tidal volume, frequency, and vital capacity, should be measured with a portable spirometer to quantitate the observations.

5. Examine the patient's chest, including auscultation, noting the presence and location of decreased breath sounds, rhonchi, rales, etc. Physical examination of the chest not only provides the respiratory care practitioner with excellent information, but also establishes a "laying on of hands" rapport between the therapist and the patient.

6. Evaluate personally the patient's mechanical ability to cough and breathe deeply. This usually entails the straightforward approach of asking the patient to take a maximum breath and do his best to cough. This is an invaluable observation and gives tremendous information

concerning the patient's ability or inability to maintain bronchial hygiene. The subjective evaluation of cough effectiveness may be substantiated by the measurement of vital capacity and inspiratory capacity (see Chapter 3), which are the most valuable bedside measurements to reflect the patient's ability to breathe deeply and cough.

Establish Need for Bronchial Hygiene Therapy

It is incumbent upon the respiratory care practitioner to decide what disease processes are creating a need for bronchial hygiene therapy support. The essential question is: Does the need for the bronchial hygiene therapy stem from pulmonary or nonpulmonary disease? This differentiation is essential because it determines whether the bronchial hygiene is for prophylaxis or therapeutics.

Prophylactic Bronchial Hygiene

Prophylactic therapy is the application of techniques for the *prevention* of inadequate bronchial hygiene. This assumes that the patient's pulmonary system is relatively free of *acute* disease. Some examples are neurologically diseased patients with weakened neuromuscular ability; comatose or semicomatose patients with central nervous system disease; postoperative patients with hypoventilation, splinting, and/or decreased vital capacity; and patients with trauma to the head, chest, or abdomen.

Therapeutic Bronchial Hygiene

Therapeutic bronchial hygiene therapy is the application of techniques for the *reversal* of inadequate bronchial hygiene: specifically, to mobilize secretions that are tending to be retained and thereby reinflate areas of absorption atelectasis and decrease the extent and longevity of infection. Since all pulmonary pathology is *not* accompanied by failure to adequately mobilize secretions,[218] the therapeutic indications for bronchial hygiene therapy must be based on the patient's ability to mobilize secretions—not on the severity of the pulmonary disease.

It is incumbent upon the respiratory care practitioner to consult with the physician after arriving at a working diagnosis to make sure that it is in keeping with the physician's concept of the patient's need for therapy.

Defining Therapeutic Goals

Defining bronchial hygiene goals involves evaluation of the two primary bronchial hygiene mechanisms: the mucociliary complex and the cough.

Mucociliary malfunction usually involves the mucous blanket becoming dried or abnormally tenacious. Of course, the ciliary function may be abnormal. These circumstances will result in an abnormally discontinuous mucous blanket and/or in ciliary action being ineffective in mobilizing the mucus. In either case, a mucociliary complex *mal*function should be improved by hydrating the mucus.

Disruption of the cough mechanism involves (1) the inability to breathe deeply, (2) the glottis, or (3) the abdominal muscles. The exact component causing malfunction must be evaluated and supported. The cough mechanism may also be disrupted by airway disease — such as bronchospasm, hyperemia (mucosal congestion) — or by retained secretions.

The therapeutic goals are to bolster or restore functions that are believed to be inadequate! The goals of aerosol, IPPB, chest physical therapy (CPT), and SMI therapy have been discussed previously. Table 14 – 1 outlines these goals. Note that SMI therapy is primarily a prophylactic technique.

Selection of Therapeutic Bronchial Hygiene Techniques

After the clinical abnormality and the goals of bronchial hygiene therapy are delineated, the next step in establishing a bronchial hy-

TABLE 14-1.—GOALS OF BRONCHIAL
HYGIENE THERAPY

I. Goals of Aerosol Therapy
  A. Aid bronchial hygiene
    1. Restore and maintain mucous blanket continuity
    2. Hydrate dried, retained secretions
    3. Promote expectoration
  B. Humidify inspired gases
  C. Deliver medication
II. Goals of IPPB Therapy
  A. Improve and promote cough mechanism
  B. Improve distribution of ventilation
  C. Deliver medication
III. Goals of Chest Physical Therapy (CPT)
  A. Aid bronchial hygiene
    1. Prevent accumulation of bronchial secretions
    2. Promote mobilization of bronchial secretions
    3. Improve the cough mechanism
  B. Improve efficiency and distribution of ventilation
IV. Goals of SMI Therapy
  A. Optimize lung inflation
    1. Prevent atelectasis
    2. Prevent accumulation of bronchial secretions
  B. Optimize cough mechanism
  C. Early detection of acute pulmonary disease

---

giene program is to choose the techniques that will best accomplish the goals. In essence, this means the application of aerosol, IPPB, and chest physical therapy either alone or in appropriate combinations for therapeutic purposes, and SMI therapy and CPT either alone or in appropriate combination for prophylactic therapy.

Aerosol Therapy

When there is disruption of the mucous blanket, the addition of water directly on retained mucus results in a thinning of the secretions. Thus, by appropriately applying aerosol therapy we hope to (1) restore and maintain mucous blanket continuity; (2) hydrate dried, retained secretions; and (3) promote expectoration. Systemic hydration (intravenous or gastrointestinal route) can prevent further dried and tenacious secretions from being produced, but will do little to hydrate the retained secretions already present in the airway.

Coarse rhonchi and expiratory wheezes throughout the chest usually mean that secretions are present in the larger airways and are located in areas where there is a good chance of depositing the aerosol. Another reliable sign of dried, retained secretions is the presence of a dry and unproductive cough. The cough reflex is active because there is irritation of the respiratory mucosa; however, the cough is unproductive because the mucus is not fluid. This is most commonly caused by inflamed pulmonary mucosa (bronchitis) or dehydration. A history of unproductive coughing does not mean that secretions are not being produced. It is more likely an indication that secretions are being produced but not mobilized.

An abnormally discontinuous mucous blanket may result in gas flow directly irritating mucosal cells. Such failure to protect mucosal cells from gas movement may result in hyperemia, edema, and ciliary malfunction. This may explain why symptoms of acute bronchitis and croup can be so dramatically improved by the application of aerosol therapy. The delivery of vasoconstricting or bronchodilating drugs may play a significant role in decongesting the mucosa, relieving bronchospasm and mobilizing secretion.

IPPB Therapy

IPPB therapy has no rationale for the patient who is capable of taking an adequate deep breath spontaneously. A FVC greater than 15 ml/kg essentially rules out IPPB therapy. In addition, IPPB must deliver *at least* a tidal volume exceeding 75% of the patient's FVC to be effective.

We have previously stated that IPPB must be applied and evaluated on its mechanical effects, i.e., to provide a deep breath and good peripheral distribution of gas to assist the cough. IPPB is also useful in manipulating the ventilatory pattern to improve ventilation distribution, which in turn may result in re-expansion of atelectatic alveoli.

IPPB therapy must *not* be thought of solely as a means for delivering medications. In circumstances involving mucosal decongestion, relieving bronchospasm, and delivering mucolytic agents, IPPB therapy may be adjunctive and beneficial to an over-all medical program.

IPPB therapy is almost always used to improve the cough! An example is the patient who has an inadequate inspiratory capacity (less than 12 ml/kg) because of (1) pain and decreased vital capacity following abdominal or thoracic operation; (2) nervous system and neuromuscular disease; (3) restrictive and obstructive pulmonary disease; (4) abdominal distention and pain; and countless other conditions.

Chest Physical Therapy

Manipulating the chest wall and utilizing gravity as a means of mobilizing secretions are invaluable modalities in promoting bronchial hygiene. The basic techniques of chest physical therapy that aid in bronchial hygiene are postural drainage, chest percussion and vibration, and cough instruction.

Postural drainage is used to mobilize secretions that the cough mechanism is not adequately mobilizing. Gravity is used to aid the movement of secretions from small peripheral airways toward larger airways. The importance of postural drainage in prophylactic respiratory care is without equal.

In our experience, the greatest benefit of chest physical therapy techniques is in the augmentation of aerosol, SMI, and IPPB therapy. Proper aerosol therapy includes coughing instruction and postural drainage. Appropriate SMI and IPPB therapy must include breathing and cough instruction.

The application of chest physical therapy techniques without aerosol and IPPB is appropriate in certain disease entities and in chronic home care programs. Patients with copious fluid secretions can accomplish bronchial hygiene with chest physical therapy alone. An example is *bronchiectasis*, a disease of sacular deformities of bronchi and bronchioles with the accumulation of secretion within these outpouchings. Postural drainage with percussion and vibration accomplishes mobilization of these secretions into the bronchi where they can be coughed up. *Cystic fibrosis* is another disease where chronic, long-term bronchial hygiene is well accomplished by chest physical therapy modalities.[552, 553] However, aerosol therapy is most helpful in these patients — especially when they have acute disease superimposed on their chronic states.

Aerosol – IPPB Therapy

Modern respiratory care has shown that where individual modalities of bronchial hygiene may not be therapeutically effective, an appropriate combination of techniques may be extremely effective. Since a great number of patients receiving bronchial hygiene therapy have dried, retained secretions *and* mechanical difficulties in distributing ventilation, it is not unusual to find a high incidence of intensive care patients needing *both* aerosol and IPPB. There is great debate about whether the aerosol should precede or come after the IPPB, or whether the aerosol should be given simultaneously. The answer becomes obvious when care is taken to evaluate the patient and define the goals.

1. Aerosol therapy followed by IPPB therapy seems to be the most widely used combination. The objective is to first provide proper aerosol therapy to maximally hydrate secretions and then administer the IPPB for effective coughing and appropriate medication delivery. In our experience, this has proved to be the most effective method of giving the combined therapy.

2. Many respiratory specialists prefer to have the IPPB therapy given first, the object being to deliver a bronchodilator to make optimal the distribution of the following aerosol therapy. We feel that the administering of a bronchodilating drug should not be inexorably attached to the IPPB therapy. Inhalation of bronchodilating drugs can be given by cartridge spray, or the drug can be given systemically. Documentation concerning the effectiveness of these methods is not available. We can only emphasize that the order should be used that best fits the patient, therapist, and physician.

3. "In-line" ultrasonic with IPPB is a very popular mode of therapy. The rationale is to get better delivery of the aerosol particles by using positive pressure. This is popular among respiratory therapists since it is possible to deliver both treatments in a shorter period of time. It has been our experience that there is a higher incidence of increased airway resistance and paroxysms of coughing with in-line ultrasonic with IPPB.

This method is felt to be an extremely effective mode of therapy when aerosol therapy is indicated but the patient is unable to provide a reasonable ventilatory pattern for effective penetration and deposition. When delivering in-line aerosol therapy, it is incumbent upon the therapist to carefully monitor the patient and discontinue the treatment if there are any signs of respiratory distress or increased airway resistance.

Aerosol-Chest Physical Therapy

Aerosol therapy in combination with chest physical therapy is often used for patients with retained secretions who have good mechanical ability to cough. The combination of aerosol and chest physical therapy is often used when very aggressive bronchial hygiene therapy is indicated. The treatment is usually given with the patient first receiving the aerosol therapy and breathing instruction, followed by postural drainage and percussion and vibration.

Evaluation of the Effectiveness

The effectiveness of a therapeutic program is evaluated by the degree to which the goals of the program are accomplished. In other words, the effectiveness of bronchial hygiene therapy must be evaluated solely by whether or not the goals were accomplished. This means that the success of prophylactic bronchial hygiene therapy is based upon the prevention of pulmonary complication. With therapeutic programs such as the treatment of atelectasis, the effectiveness is judged on whether or not the atelectasis is resolved.

It is obvious why the effectiveness of bronchial hygiene therapy is difficult to evaluate. It can be postulated that only a portion of the patients receiving prophylactic respiratory care would develop pulmonary complications if no respiratory care were applied. Therefore, we are always dealing with an unknown factor that provides uncertainty for the believer and ammunition for the nonbeliever. There are some *objective* criteria that can be used for the evaluation of effectiveness of bronchial hygiene therapy and these are (1) sputum; (2) auscultation; (3) work of breathing; (4) blood gas measurement; and (5) pulmonary function studies.

Sputum

It is not unusual for sputum production to be delayed as much as 48 hours after the onset of bronchial hygiene therapy. The evaluation of sputum production must be on a 24-hour basis.

Careful examination of sputum will reveal significant information concerning the disease state present and will document changes in that disease state. Sputum must be examined both grossly and microscopically. The gross examination is primarily for consistency and color. The normal consistency of sputum is a "watery-like fluid" with little tendency to "stick to things." Very tenacious mucus usually represents dehydration. Retained secretions have small, solid green or yellow "flecks" which may represent casts of bronchioles.

Color is very important in studying sputum. Sputum is normally white and translucent (allows light to come through, but does not allow you to see through). *Yellow* denotes pus, since white blood cells have a yellow color. *Green* usually means old, retained secretions, since proteolysis of mucopolysaccharides results in a green color. When the sputum is green and has a foul odor, it usually means a Pseudomonas infection. A *brown* color usually denotes old blood. *Red* sputum denotes fresh blood (racemic epinephrine may turn sputum *pink*).

When sputum contains blood (hemoptysis), it is important to note whether blood is well mixed with the sputum or whether the sputum is "streaked" with blood. Blood-streaked sputum usually denotes tracheal or upper airway bleeding. Remember, *sputum contains pharyngeal and nasal discharge as well as lower airway mucus.*

Microscopic examination reveals the presence of white blood cells—these denote inflammation or infection. Bacteria are *always* seen on properly stained sputum smears. Only intracellular (within white blood cell) bacteria are significant, since they denote that infection is present; i.e., the bacteria have been ingested by the white blood cells.

Auscultation

Physical examination of the chest often reveals objective evidence of respiratory therapy effectiveness. The appearance of breath sounds, where there were none previously, means that previously collapsed lung is aerating. The absence or improvement in rhonchi and wheezes following therapy is a significant finding.

Work of Breathing

The work of breathing may be significantly decreased when retained secretions are mobilized. This may be clinically evident after several days by reevaluating the ventilatory pattern and the use of accessory ventilatory muscles. Of course, one must realize that many other things are being done to and for the patient during the same period and improvement may be due entirely or partly to these other regimens.

Blood Gas Measurement

Blood gas measurements may or may not be helpful in the evaluation of respiratory care modalities, since blood gas measurements reflect the total cardiopulmonary system rather than the pulmonary system in particular. Certainly, improvement in the blood gas state following therapy is reflective of effective therapy. But the lack of improvement in blood gases does not necessarily mean that the therapy was not useful or effective.

Pulmonary Function Studies

Pulmonary function studies have long been applied as *the* objective assessment of the effectiveness of respiratory therapy modalities. However, it is well documented that even significant mobilization of secretions and clinical improvement may not be accompanied by improvement in pulmonary function studies.

Summary

The formation and evaluation of a bronchial hygiene program is one of the prime areas of respiratory care that requires the therapist's knowledge and expertise. Nothing is quite as satisfying to the respiratory care practitioner as successfully contributing to the total scope of medical treatment.

SECTION IV
AIRWAY CARE

15 • THE ARTIFICIAL AIRWAY

THE FIRST PRINCIPLE of resuscitation and life support is assuring a patent airway. In the absence of an adequate airway, the pulmonary system is incapable of appropriate gas exchange. Nothing is more crucial in intensive respiratory care than the appropriate assessment and management of the airway. The medical specialty of anesthesiology has thoroughly studied and evaluated the techniques of airway establishment and maintenance. The respiratory therapist and respiratory nurse specialist are the nonphysician health care specialists responsible for airway care in the modern hospital. In the emergency room, recovery room, and intensive care unit, these respiratory care practitioners must be competent in all areas of airway care. The overwhelming importance of the airway in acute respiratory care and critical care medicine makes a thorough understanding of airway management essential.

Upper Airway Obstruction

Upper airway obstruction may occur from two sources: *soft tissue* obstruction and *laryngeal* obstruction.

The most common airway emergency is soft tissue upper airway obstruction. This phenomenon is caused by the soft tissues of the pharynx impinging on the patency of the upper airway secondary to (1) loss of muscle tone from C.N.S. abnormality, e.g., the unconscious patient; (2) space-occupying lesions, e.g., edema, bleeding, tumors; or (3) foreign substances, e.g., vomitus, false teeth, foreign bodies. The common factor in all soft tissue upper airway obstruction is the lack of patency between the base of the tongue and the posterior wall of the pharynx (Fig 15–1). The recognition of upper airway obstruction depends upon close observation and a high index of suspicion.

Partial upper airway obstruction is usually accompanied by noisy inspiration that sounds like snoring. The noise is usually limited to inspiration and is of a low tonal quality. The greater the obstruction, the louder the noise.

Complete upper airway obstruction is accompanied by marked inspiratory efforts without air movement. Marked sternal, intercostal,

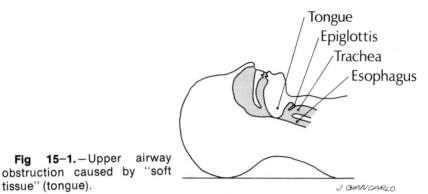

Tongue
Epiglottis
Trachea
Esophagus

Fig 15–1.—Upper airway obstruction caused by "soft tissue" (tongue).

and epigastric retraction is usually present along with strong contraction of accessory neck muscles of ventilation. If conscious, the patient will be obviously distressed and extremely anxious. If unconscious, the patient may appear "dusky," and the ventilatory attempts may become so violent that they appear to be "seizures."

The treatment of soft tissue airway obstruction is obvious. Relieve the obstruction! This should be accomplished with the simplest maneuvers possible.

Neck Extension and Chin Manipulation

The process of neck extension and elevating the chin (Fig 15–2) is effective in relieving soft tissue upper airway obstruction. This should be the first maneuver attempted. The unconscious patient can often be moved into a lateral position with neck extension so that gravity can clear the soft tissue obstruction. The lateral head position allows the tongue to move forward and open the airway. The mouth must always be inspected for foreign bodies, even after obstruction has been relieved.

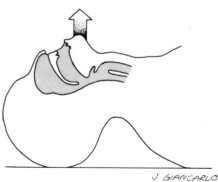

Fig 15–2.—Clearing of soft tissue upper airway obstruction by neck extension and chin elevation.

Oropharyngeal Airway

An oropharyngeal airway is a device designed for insertion along the tongue until the teeth and/or gingiva limit the insertion (Fig 15–3). The device lies between the posterior pharynx and the root of the tongue and thereby maintains a patent airway. It is designed so that a suction catheter can easily be passed to the laryngopharynx.

This type of airway frequently causes stimulation of the oropharynx and will activate the gag reflex if intact. Thus, an oropharyngeal airway is well tolerated by an unconscious patient, but as consciousness returns, the stimulation of this airway may produce gagging, vomiting, and even laryngospasm. In general terms, *the oropharyngeal airway is adequate for comatose patients only – and usually for limited periods of time.*

Nasopharyngeal Airway

The nasopharyngeal airway is a soft rubber tube constructed so it can be inserted through one of the nares and follow the posterior wall curvature of the naso- and oropharynx (Fig 15–4). Its terminal portion is positioned at the base of the tongue, separating it from the posterior

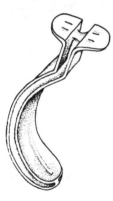

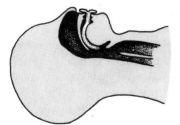

Fig 15–3.—The oropharyngeal airway (see test).

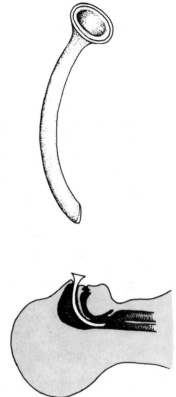

Fig 15–4. — The nasopharyngeal airway (see text).

J GIANCARLO

pharyngeal wall. Upon insertion, the nasopharyngeal airway may create bleeding which can be minimized if the tube is lubricated well.

The advantage of the nasopharyngeal airway over the oropharyngeal airway is that it is much better tolerated by the semicomatose and awake patient. In general, patients can better tolerate stabilized nasal airways that lie on the posterior pharyngeal wall than those inserted through the mouth. The nasopharyngeal airway provides an adequate means of preventing or relieving soft tissue upper airway obstruction in the semicomatose or alert patient for reasonable periods of time. Adequate suctioning of the pharynx is possible with an appropriately lubricated suction catheter passed through the airway. Even though the tube is flanged, a large safety pin placed at the outer tip or even taped to the side of the face will assure that the tube will not slip entirely into the nose and down into the larynx.

Artificial Airways

Definition

When the simple maneuvers just described are not adequate for relieving soft tissue upper airway obstruction, the establishment of an artificial airway must be contemplated. Although there are a variety of opinions about the exact definition of an artificial airway, we define it as *a tube inserted into the trachea that bypasses the upper airway and laryngeal structures as integral parts of the total airway.* In essence, we mean the establishment of an endotracheal tube or a tracheostomy tube. Accepting this definition, it is obvious that an artificial airway will relieve soft tissue and laryngeal obstruction, protect the lower airway from foreign body aspiration, and provide an easily accessible route for artificial ventilation and tracheal suction.

Indications

Since the establishment of an artificial airway is a serious step, the decision to do so cannot be made without rationale. It is essential to delineate definite criteria for establishing an artificial airway. Indications for establishing the airway may be divided into four categories: (1) the relief of airway *obstruction;* (2) the *protection* of the airway; (3) the facilitation of *tracheal suctioning;* and (4) the facilitation of prolonged *artificial ventilation.*

RELIEF OF AIRWAY OBSTRUCTION. — The establishment of an artificial airway guarantees the patency of the upper airway regardless of soft tissue or laryngeal abnormality.

PROTECTION OF THE AIRWAY. — The pharynx, vocal cords, and epiglottis play an important role in protecting the lower airway from aspiration of secretions and foreign bodies. These normal *airway protective mechanisms* are essential for the clinical evaluation of airway protection. There are four main airway protective reflexes. (1) *The pharyngeal reflex* has its afferent limb (sensory component) in the ninth cranial nerve and its efferent limb (motor component) in the tenth cranial nerve (vagus nerve). This reflex arc is responsible for both "gag and swallowing reflex." (2) *The laryngeal reflex,* neurologically described as a vagovagal reflex (afferent and efferent components are vagus nerves), will cause apposition of the vocal cords (laryngospasm) and an associated closing of the epiglottis. (3) *The tracheal reflex,* a vagovagal reflex, causes a cough when foreign body or irritation occurs in the trachea. (4) *The carinal reflex,* a vagovagal reflex, causes a cough with irritation of the carina.[97]

The protective airway reflexes are obtunded from the top down, i.e., first the pharyngeal reflex, then the laryngeal reflex, and then the tracheal reflex. This is true in all circumstances affecting depression of the C.N.S., whether by anesthesia, drugs, disease, or general "loss of consciousness." It is extremely unusual for the carinal reflex to be totally ablated, since this reflex persists to the deepest level of C.N.S. depression. Thus, one would expect to obtain some type of rudimentary cough reflex from stimulation of the carina even in deeply comatose patients.

When an individual awakens from general anesthesia or recovers from a state of unconsciousness, the airway protective reflexes will resume appropriate functioning from "the bottom up"; i.e., first the tracheal reflex will return, then the laryngeal reflex, and finally the pharyngeal reflex.

The establishment of an artificial airway is indicated whenever an individual cannot protect the lower airway due to alteration of the airway protective reflexes. This is an important indication for establishing an airway, since the most important element of supportive care in many disease states is to establish an airway to protect the lungs from aspiration (see Chapter 33).

FACILITATION OF SUCTIONING. — There are numerous disease states in which the patient's bronchial hygiene mechanism is inadequate. There are numerous methods for mobilizing secretions to the trachea, but mobilization from the trachea to the pharynx requires either an adequate cough or direct suctioning of the trachea. Although it is possible to insert suction catheters via the nose or mouth into the trachea, this is not always effective and can become an extremely traumatic and time-consuming process. In many circumstances, it is essential to establish an artificial airway for the purpose of facilitating removal of tracheal secretions by direct suctioning.

SUPPORT OF VENTILATION. — It is unfortunate that many physicians and respiratory care practitioners equate the need for establishing an artificial airway directly and exclusively with the need for support of ventilation. This is certainly an essential indication, but only one of four.

It is universally agreed that an artificial airway should be established in order to adequately support ventilation for any extended period of time. Ventilation by positive pressure can be adequately performed with a mask over the nose and mouth for short periods of time, but should *not* be attempted over long periods of time because (1) a tight mask fitted over the nose and mouth for long periods of time can become extremely uncomfortable and, in fact, cause skin inflammation and possibly necrosis; and (2) the opening pressure of the esophageal-cardiac sphincter may be exceeded, resulting in air filling the stomach. This may cause gastric distention which leads to nausea, vomiting, and ileus. We believe it is a fair statement that any patient requiring support of ventilation for other than extremely short-term periods requires and deserves the establishment of an artificial airway.

To summarize, there are four separate indications for establishing an artificial airway: (1) relief of upper airway obstruction; (2) protection of the airway; (3) suctioning of the airway; and (4) support of ventilation. Any single one or combination of factors is an adequate indication for establishing an artificial airway. It is incumbent upon the respiratory care practitioner to have clearly in mind his reasons and rationale for establishing and maintaining an artificial airway.

Hazards of Artificial Airways

There are significant hazards involved with the establishment and maintenance of artificial airways. Although many of the complications and hazards are dependent upon the type of airway and the appropriateness of care during maintenance, there are several *universal* problems that must always be considered by the respiratory care practitioner.

1. The establishment of an artificial airway bypasses the normal defense mechanisms that prevent bacterial contamination of the lower airway. The establishment of an artificial airway assures bacterial contamination of the tracheobronchial tree.

2. An artificial airway removes the effectiveness of the cough maneuver because the vocal cords are rendered nonfunctional. An endotracheal tube prevents the vocal cords from approximating; a tracheostomy bypasses the vocal cords.

3. The establishment of an artificial airway removes the patient's ability to vocally communicate. Not being able to communicate with those around you can be an extremely frustrating and frightening experience. Ill patients are understandably afraid of their environment, especially in the overwhelming atmosphere of the critical care unit. The respiratory care practitioner must always remember that the patient must be dealt with in an understanding and communicative manner when artificial airways are in place. A "magic slate" or writing pad should be provided for the patient to write messages to the staff and family, and appropriate answers should always be provided.

4. A fourth universal problem with the establishment of artificial

airways in the conscious patient is the loss of personal dignity. It is understandable and predictable that most patients will be extremely embarrassed and concerned about the fact that there are "tubes" keeping him from talking and allowing him to breathe normally. This feeling of loss of body and environmental control may be minimized if those individuals involved with the care of the patient are informative, understanding, patient, and, above all, humane.

The maintenance of airway patency, the protection of the lower airway from foreign body, the accomplishment of adequate bronchial hygiene, and the support of ventilation are overwhelming reasons for establishing airways when indicated. The support and maintenance of the life process must overshadow the potential complications. It is essential to remember that with proper care of the airway, the complications are seldom clinically significant.[219]

Establishing the Emergency Airway

An emergency airway is defined as one which *must* be established immediately; i.e., it is a matter of life or death. The emergency airway of choice is an oral endotracheal tube placed under direct vision. When presented with an unfamiliar patient under emergency conditions, direct vision for placement of an oral endotracheal tube is almost always the surest and safest way of establishing an emergency airway, even in the hands of someone relatively untrained and inexperienced in intubation.

Technique of Intubation

The *laryngoscope* is an instrument made specifically for intubation of the trachea. The anesthetist's laryngoscope differs from that of the otolaryngologist; the purposes are different. The otolaryngologist is primarily concerned with visualization of the glottis for obtaining appropriate biopsy samples and accomplishing other surgical procedures. He is far more concerned with adequate exposure than with the insertion of an endotracheal tube through the glottis. On the other hand, the anesthetist is far less concerned with total exposure of the glottis, since the primary purpose is the insertion of an endotracheal tube. In respiratory care, the laryngoscope that is used for establishment of airways is the anesthetist's laryngoscope.

Figure 15–5 illustrates the two basic types of laryngoscope blades used for orotracheal intubation: the straight blade and the curved blade. The straight blade is placed under the epiglottis and with an upward motion the glottis is exposed. The curved blade is inserted

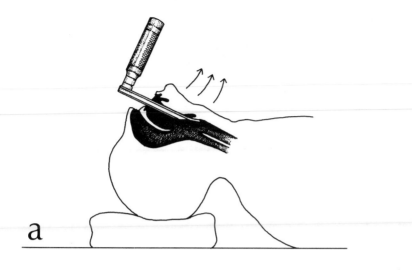

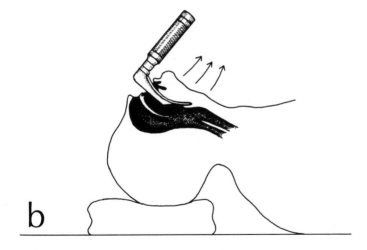

J. GIANCARLO

Fig 15–5.—The laryngoscope in orotracheal intubation. **A** depicts the *straight* laryngoscope blade—this blade is placed under the epiglottis to expose the glottis. **B** depicts the *curved* laryngoscope blade—this blade is placed between the base of the tongue and the epiglottis.

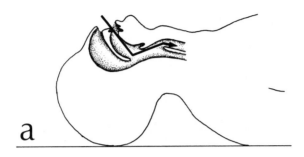

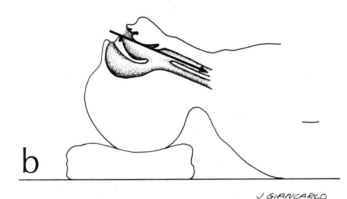

J GIANCARLO

Fig 15–6.—Head and neck positioning for orotracheal intubation. Neck extension alone is seldom adequate to provide good glottic exposure **(A).** Placing the head at a level above the shoulders allows better exposure **(B)** – called the "sniffing" position (see text).

between the epiglottis and the base of the tongue, and with a forward and upward motion, the epiglottis is raised and the glottis exposed.[220] The various nuances, sophistications, and modifications of these basic blades are primarily to meet special needs and desires of anesthesiologists. For the respiratory care practitioner who has only sporadic experience with intubation, it is best to simply categorize all blades as either straight or curved. The respiratory care practitioner should familiarize himself with both types of blades so that either can be used in an emergency circumstance. The technique of inserting the laryngoscope is extremely important since exposure of the glottis is rather simple if a few principles are followed.

Appropriate positioning of the head, neck, and shoulders must be assured. It is essential to have as straight a line as possible between the open mouth and the glottis to facilitate intubation of the larynx. As illustrated in Figure 15–6, exposure of the glottis will not be a straight line if the base of the skull is on the same plane as the shoulders after extension of the head and neck. On the other hand, if the extended head and neck are elevated to a plane above the shoulders, a reasonably straight line results from the mouth to the glottis. This position is known as the *sniffing position*. Even in the most emergent of circumstances, it is well worth the few seconds necessary to assure appropriate head, neck, and shoulder positioning.

Laryngoscopes are made for the right-handed person and, therefore, must be held in the left hand. This is an important factor, since the right-handed individual can best manipulate the insertion of the endotracheal tube with the right hand. If you are left-handed, you must learn to intubate the same as a right-handed individual.

Initial insertion of the laryngoscope blade on the right-hand side of the mouth allows the tongue to be moved to the left as the blade is brought to the midline (Fig 15–7). This will allow the mouth area on the right side of the blade to be free of soft tissue structures such as the tongue. This facilitates visualization of the appropriate structures and

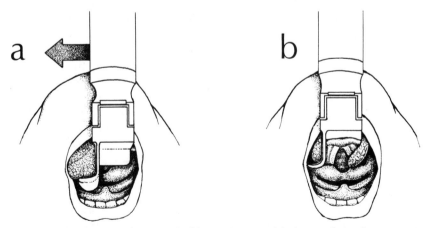

Fig 15–7. – Proper placement of laryngoscope blade requires placement to the right initially **(A)** and then movement to the midline. This maneuver moves the tongue out of the way.

B depicts what happens if tongue is not moved to the left. It will hang over and hinder the passage of an endotracheal tube (see text).

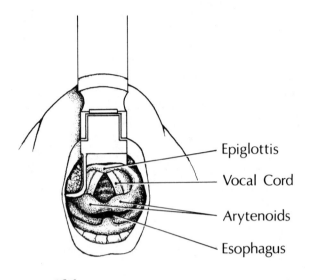

Epiglottis

Vocal Cord

Arytenoids

Esophagus

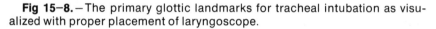

J GIANCARLO

Fig 15−8.−The primary glottic landmarks for tracheal intubation as visualized with proper placement of laryngoscope.

the placement of the endotracheal tube. The blade is advanced forward along the surface of the tongue with a slight "lifting" pressure until the tip of the epiglottis is visualized. Upon exposure of the epiglottis, the blade must be brought to the midline; this pushes the tongue to the left-hand side of the mouth and allows maximum exposure of the glottis when the laryngoscope is lifted upward.[220]

The primary glottic landmarks are the epiglottis and the arytenoid cartilages (Fig 15−8). Upon recognition of the arytenoid cartilages, the position of the vocal cords and, thereby, the opening of the glottis are known. It is not necessary to visualize *all* of the vocal cords. If the epiglottis and arytenoid cartilages can be seen, the only possible opening between these structures is the glottis. In addition, the esophageal opening can be seen below the arytenoid cartilage so that placement of the tube in the esophagus will not go unrecognized.

Insertion of the endotracheal tube can then be made. With the tongue on the left side of the mouth and the essential glottic landmarks exposed, the endotracheal tube is then manipulated through the right side of the mouth toward the glottis. By directing the endotracheal tube either in an upward or a downward direction, the tip of the tube can be manipulated to enter the glottis.

When the endotracheal tube enters the glottis, it should be advanced approximately two inches under direct vision. One should *visualize* the tube being inserted to assure that the tube is in fact entering the larynx and not the esophagus. Care must be taken *not* to insert the endotracheal tube as far as it will go. This will result in an *endobronchial* intubation – usually into the right main stem bronchus. The average adult trachea is 11–13 cm in length and can be easily traversed by an endotracheal tube. The tube must be inserted far enough to assure that the cuff is below the cords (to assure protection and sealing of the airway) without intubation of the bronchus.

The most important factor to remember while attempting intubation is *not to get excited!* If the first attempt at intubation is not successful, it should be momentarily discontinued, the airway cleared, and the patient ventilated and oxygenated with mask and bag. Try to evaluate why the intubation was not successful. Recheck the steps just outlined and make corrections. Then, with the patient appropriately ventilated and the airway cleared, a second attempt should be made to intubate.

Post-intubation Essentials

The immediate concern following the placement of the endotracheal tube is the assurance that the tube is within the trachea. The respiratory care practitioner must immediately inflate the cuff and listen to the chest with a stethoscope to make sure that the lungs are being ventilated *equally* and *bilaterally*. Even if the patient is breathing spontaneously, give a few deep breaths with a positive-pressure hand ventilator while listening to the chest. *YOU MUST BE POSITIVE THAT THE LUNGS ARE BEING EQUALLY VENTILATED!*

If the endotracheal tube is mistakenly placed in the esophagus and positive-pressure ventilation initiated, the air movement in and out of the stomach may easily be misinterpreted as lung ventilation. The stethoscope should be placed over the stomach to detect air movement in and out. If there is any question at all, the glottis must be re-exposed and assurances made that the tube is not in the esophagus. If there is any doubt about the location of the tube, the patient must be *extubated, ventilated,* and then re-intubated. *An inappropriately placed or nonfunctioning endotracheal tube is even more lethal than the patient's own poorly functioning airway!*

Once the airway is assured, the next concern must be the securing of the tube so that inadvertent extubation will not take place. Use of tincture of benzoin on the face where the tape will be placed aids in assuring that perspiration, secretions, or the movement of facial structures will be less likely to loosen the adhesive. We have found taping endotracheal tubes with a "head halter" technique extremely dependable.

There must be constant reevaluation of the placement of the emergency airway and constant reassurance that there is ventilation of the lungs. This is especially important during the rigors of cardiopulmonary resuscitation and in the early support of critically ill patients. There are usually many people gathered around the patient carrying out various functions. It is the prime concern of the respiratory care practitioner to assure appropriate establishment *and maintenance* of the airway.

Cricothyroidotomy

When emergency *surgical* entrance into the trachea is demanded, only the most skilled and experienced of surgeons should attempt an actual tracheostomy. The operative procedure of tracheostomy is difficult and dangerous even under optimal conditions. The *emergency* surgical entrance into the trachea is called the cricothyroidotomy. The *cricothyroid membrane* (see Chapter 1) is an easy landmark to find since it lies directly below the "Adam's apple." The membrane usually lies well above the large thyroid vessels and below the vocal cords. A midline incision through the cricothyroid membrane will allow entrance into the larynx below the vocal cords without interrupting major blood vessels.[221] Any type of tube may be inserted to maintain patency.

The advantages of this emergency surgical approach is that the landmarks are easily found under emergency circumstances. In addition, the incision site is well above the area where a definitive tracheostomy would be performed, allowing the definitive tracheostomy to be done electively without contamination.[222]

The cricothyroidotomy is a procedure that should not be performed without great concern by respiratory care practitioners. However, the technique must be understood so that if it is ever necessary to save a life, it can be appropriately and satisfactorily accomplished.

Emergency Airways in Cardiopulmonary Resuscitation

An essential responsibility of the respiratory care practitioner is to be involved in cardiopulmonary resuscitation. *The first priority is to ventilate.* The initial attempts should be made with bag and mask or mouth-to-mouth resuscitation. However, with prolonged closed chest massage or other resuscitative efforts, it becomes essential to establish and maintain an artificial airway. *The oral endotracheal tube is the emergency airway of choice!*

There have been many attempts to develop techniques that avoid the necessity for emergency endotracheal intubation by inexperi-

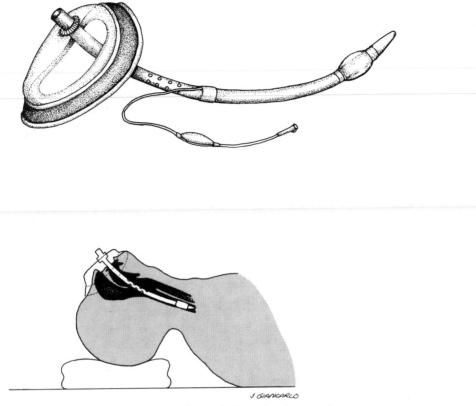

Fig 15–9.—The esophageal obturator (see text).

enced individuals. There is a new method—the esophageal obturator—which must be given due consideration. The authors wish to
emphasize that at the present time there has been only limited experience with this device; no absolute statement can yet be made as to its
effectiveness.

The esophageal obturator is schematically represented in Figure
15–9. It is composed of a mask that can be placed tightly around the
nose and mouth to provide an adequate seal. The tube itself has a
blind end and is meant to be inserted into the esophagus. With the cuff
inflated, regurgitation is theoretically prevented and the possibility of
forcing air through the esophagus into the stomach is theoretically
avoided. Holes in the tube are present at the level where it lies in the
oropharynx and, therefore, positive pressure placed on the tube will
cause positive pressure in the mouth. With all other outlets for the

escape of air occluded (nose, mouth, and esophagus), the air will be forced into the airway and the lungs.[223]

The use of the esophageal obturator is entirely dependent upon the assumptions that (1) the esophagus is easier to intubate than the trachea; (2) the inflated balloon will seal off the lower esophagus and stomach, avoid regurgitation, and prevent inflation of the stomach; and (3) an adequate mask seal can be maintained.

The greatest potential for using the esophageal obturator undoubtedly lies with paramedical individuals outside of the hospital or resuscitation teams not trained in endotracheal intubation.[224] It may prove a reasonable alternative to endotracheal intubation in those circumstances, but at the present time has not had widespread clinical trials. Animal studies indicate that the esophageal obturator does *not* provide as good ventilation as the endotracheal tube, but does a slightly better job than bag and mask, with the potential advantage of preventing regurgitation, which the bag and mask does not.[223] On the other hand, there may be regurgitation following the removal of the esophageal obturator and one must be ready to suction, turn the patient on his side, and intubate the trachea if necessary. *All attempts must be made to prevent aspiration.*

In summary, endotracheal intubation is the route of choice for ventilation during cardiopulmonary resuscitation.[225] Every effort should be made to train respiratory care personnel in this technique. However, in circumstances where there are personnel with limited training and in mobile coronary care and rescue units where endotracheal intubation may not be feasible, the esophageal obturator may be a desirable alternative to simple face mask ventilation.

Limitations of Emergency Airways

The oral endotracheal tube and cricothyroidotomy have been discussed as the choices for establishing emergency airways. The oral endotracheal tube is not ideal for *prolonged* (greater than 24 hours) periods because (1) it is usually poorly tolerated in the semiconscious or conscious patient; (2) it is extremely difficult to stabilize since the cheeks and tongue are freely movable; (3) inadvertent extubation is common; (4) to keep the patient from biting on the oral tube an oropharyngeal airway or some type of bite-block is usually inserted, which causes further discomfort to the conscious patient; (5) vagal stimulation may result from excessive movement of the tube within the pharynx and the trachea;[219] (6) it may be extremely difficult to suction because of its curvature and poor stabilization; (7) it is almost impossible to feed the patient orally; and (8) it is often difficult to attach respiratory therapy equipment to this poorly stabilized airway.

The limitations of a cricothyroidotomy are intuitive: (1) the incision is so close to the vocal cords that it is undesirable to keep the stoma cannulated for any length of time; and (2) the incision is usually made under less than sterile conditions and the chances of wound infection are high. *A cricothyroidotomy should be replaced with an appropriate airway as soon as possible!*

Non-emergency Airways

In respiratory care, non-emergency airways are defined as those that are essential for placement but are not an *immediate* life-and-death concern. This situation occurs under one of two conditions: (1) there is already an emergency airway in place which makes the placement of a more permanent airway less acute; or (2) the placement of the initial airway is elective since the problem is not one of immediate urgency of life and death.

Non-emergency airways in respiratory care are either nasotracheal tubes or tracheostomies and are *always* accomplished by fully trained and qualified personnel.

The Nasotracheal Tube

The placement of an endotracheal tube through the nose is termed nasotracheal intubation. This is accomplished "blindly" or under direct laryngoscopic vision. In either case, it should be placed *only* by skilled individuals. *Blind nasotracheal intubation* is indicated in alert patients who are capable of spontaneous ventilation for at least short periods.[97] The nose and pharynx can be adequately anesthetized so that the placement of a nasotracheal tube by a skilled individual is a reasonably atraumatic experience.

In respiratory care, the nasotracheal tube is most commonly accomplished after an emergency oral endotracheal tube has been placed. The anesthetist now has an unhurried opportunity to choose the largest tube that will comfortably go through the nose. After appropriate anesthesia and vasoconstriction (1% lidocaine spray and 1/4% Neo-Synephrine drops), the tube is placed through the nose and into the pharynx. Under direct vision, both the oral endotracheal tube entering the glottis and the tip of the nasal tube are visualized. With appropriate forceps, the tip of the nasotracheal tube is grasped and "steered" into the glottis after an aide has removed the oral tube (Fig 15–10). In skilled hands, this procedure is accomplished without the patient missing a single breath.[220]

The nasotracheal tube is better suited for long-term intubation than

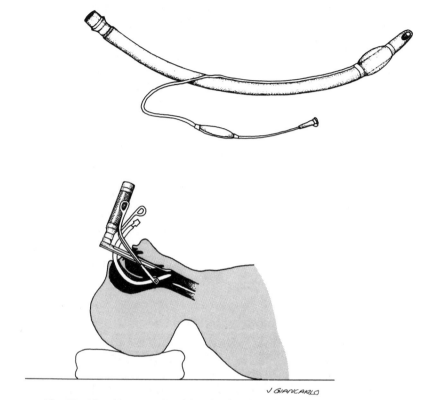

Fig 15–10. — Nasotracheal intubation by direct vision (see text).

the oral tube because (1) it is easier to stabilize, (2) it is easier to suction, and (3) it is safer for equipment attachment.

The nasotracheal tube is well lodged within the canal of the nose and can be firmly taped to the nose and face. These factors add great stability and diminish the chances of accidental extubation. The stability also results in less movement of the endotracheal tube with suctioning and ventilation, and therefore, less vagal stimulation and better patient comfort. The tube lies firmly along the curvature of the posterior pharyngeal wall and rapidly becomes well tolerated by most patients. Many patients will relate that an appropriately stabilized nasotracheal tube is no more irritating than a nasogastric tube.

The distal end of the nasotracheal tube will move with changes in head and neck position regardless of nose stabilization. Since the patient is constantly being moved and manipulated, one must be aware that there can be significant changes in position of the tip of the tube

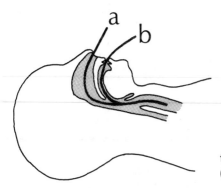

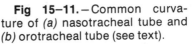

Fig 15–11.—Common curvature of *(a)* nasotracheal tube and *(b)* orotracheal tube (see text).

within the trachea. Appropriate placement is for the tip of the tube to lie in the middle third of the trachea when the head is in a neutral position. This should be documented by listening for bilateral breath sounds with the patient's head both flexed and hyperextended and by chest x-ray. With appropriate placement there is little chance that a main stem bronchus intubation or tracheal extubation will occur from changing the patient's position.

Figure 15–11 demonstrates that the curvature of the endotracheal tube is usually less severe in the nasotracheal tube than in the orotracheal tube. This lesser degree of curvature usually makes for easier insertion and removal of a suction catheter. The chances of the catheter getting "stuck" in the tube or requiring a great deal of "pushing" to pass down the tube are greatly diminished. Facilitation of suctioning means less chance of hypoxemia and other complications.

The nasotracheal tube presents certain limitations because of *pressure*. It is not uncommon for significant pressure necrosis to occur in the area of the ala nasi from pressure of the tube on the skin.[226] Great care must be taken to prevent the tube from exerting undue pressure against the tissue. This is best accomplished by appropriately supporting the attached equipment and tubing.

The nasotracheal tube within the nose can totally *obstruct the sinus drainage* and lead to acute sinusitis.[227] Often the patient is comatose or otherwise unable to complain of headache or pain in the sinus area. The only manifestation of acute sinusitis may be a very high fever. The treatment includes removal of the tube from that side of the nose.

The nasotracheal tube may block the opening of the *eustachian tube* in the nasopharynx. This obstruction may result in a middle ear infection (otitis media), and may lead to painful earache, fever, and mastoiditis.[228]

The external diameter of the nasotracheal tube plays a great role in the potential pressure in the nose. In respiratory care we advocate using large internal diameter endotracheal tubes to reduce airway resistance during mechanical and spontaneous ventilation. This should be weighed against the possible trauma that too large a tube will cause in the nose. The thinner the endotracheal tube wall, the more desirable the tube.

Other limitations of nasotracheal tubes: (1) The cuff may rupture during insertion of the tube through the nose, necessitating reintubation. (2) Significant septal deviation is common in adults and can cause an encroachment upon the lumen of the tube, which may not affect ventilation but may well affect the ability to pass a suction catheter. Occasionally a nasotracheal tube will have to be replaced with an orotracheal tube so that suctioning can be facilitated because of a deviated septum. (3) Feeding by the oral route is difficult while a nasotracheal tube is in place, but not impossible. Swallowing water can be a great morale booster to a critically ill patient and can be accomplished reasonably well with an indwelling nasotracheal tube. Maintenance feeding, however, is poorly tolerated with a nasotracheal tube.

Bleeding is seldom a problem during insertion or maintenance, but is often a problem following extubation. Occasionally, a posterior pack may be needed to control bleeding.

Tracheostomy (Fig 15–12)

There is little question that the tracheostomy tube is by far the most satisfactory artificial airway. It totally bypasses the upper airway and the glottis and, therefore, avoids any potential complication in those areas. It is far easier to stabilize, far easier to suction, and makes it far easier to properly attach respiratory therapy equipment. The patient can eat freely and there is rarely a problem of tolerating the airway. The tracheostomy is the most permanent and desirable of all airways, and when done by a skilled surgeon under ideal conditions carries minimal hazards.[229]

When the decision is made to perform a tracheostomy, it must be made with the knowledge that there are specific complications caused by the surgical procedure. Over-all mortality figures associated with tracheostomy have been reported anywhere from 0.9 to 5.1%.[230-232] It is understandable that there would be a high mortality rate associated with tracheostomies since most patients are critically ill when in need of the procedure. The complications of the procedure can be separated into three phases: immediate, late, and post-extubation. The post-extubation complications of tracheostomy will be considered later. We shall now discuss the immediate and late complications of tracheostomy.

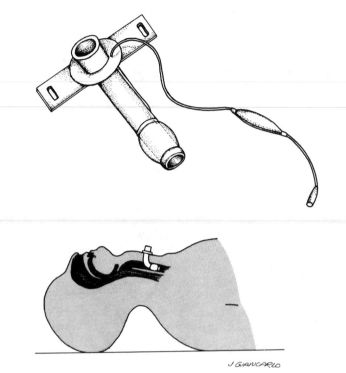

J. GIANCARLO

Fig 15–12. — A model tracheostomy tube (shown in detail) and its placement within tracheostomy stoma (see text).

Immediate complications are those occurring within the first 24 hours and are those associated with the surgical procedure. The major concern is *bleeding.* Most often the bleeding is due to inadequate hemostasis by the surgeon. Most non-arterial bleeding can be stopped by the application of adequate pressure for 24 hours. Arterial bleeding from the tracheal stoma must be evaluated by the operating surgeon. *Pneumothorax* may occur from lacerating the pleural apices which are close to the fascial planes of the neck. This occurs very often in children[233] and patients with chronic obstructive pulmonary disease. The incidence is much higher in patients who have unrelieved upper airway obstruction during the operative procedure. In such cases, an endotracheal tube should be placed prior to the surgical procedure. *Air embolism* may occur from the tearing of pleural veins. The subatmospheric pressure within the pleural veins can result in "sucking" of air through the wound into the veins and result in air embolism to the right ventricle.[234] *Subcutaneous and mediastinal emphysema* is of significance following tracheostomy.[233] Air under pressure must seek release of that pressure and will follow the path of least resistance. The fascial planes of the neck are contiguous with the mediastinum and offer little resistance to airflow. The subcutaneous tissues may offer an alternative route for air escaping the pleural space under pressure. Subcutaneous and mediastinal emphysema are not dangerous in and of themselves — the air will resorb. However, their presence must suggest the possibility of the potential hazard of tension pneumothorax and must be carefully investigated.

It is our experience that as long as tracheostomies are performed by experienced surgeons in unhurried and optimal conditions, the immediate complications associated with tracheostomy are less than 2%.

Late complications are those occurring after 24 to 48 hours. The over-all morbidity associated with tracheostomy may be as high as 40% in some series.[229-231] *Infection* is always a problem in surgical wounds. *Hemorrhage* is an ever-present problem following surgical procedures and has been reported to be as high as 4% following tracheostomy. Bleeding may be from the wound, the tracheal wall, secondary to tracheitis, or rarely from massive hemorrhage of erosion into the innominate artery.[235] *Airway obstruction* is a potential danger that exists constantly in every patient with a tracheostomy. Kinking of a softened tube, the cuff slipping down over the cannula opening,[236] and occlusion of a softened tube by pressure of an overdistended cuff[237] are all real possibilities.

Dysfunction of the swallowing process is not an uncommon complication of tracheostomy. The secondary and involuntary phase of the normal swallowing mechanism may be disrupted by the trachea being anchored to the skin by the tracheostomy tube.[238] This problem usually goes away when the tube is removed.

Tracheoesophageal fistula has been reported following tracheostomy and is primarily due to tracheal ischemia secondary to pressure of the tube and the cuff. Incidence of this complication has been reported as high as 0.5%.[239]

An extremely controversial practice is the routine changing of tracheostomy tubes. Many physicians state that tracheostomy tubes should be routinely changed as often as every 3 days to as infrequently as once a week. It should be remembered that these "routines" were established prior to the thorough understanding of the importance of appropriate humidification of the airway. There seems to be no evidence in the medical literature which would tend to support the routine changing of tracheostomy tubes in the presence of appropriate humidification. *Tracheostomy tubes need not be changed as long as they are functioning appropriately, the airway is being humidified appropriately, and there is no infectious process present in the airway or the tracheostomy wound.* If these conditions are not met, routine changing of the tracheostomy tube is advised at least once a week.[232]

Changing a tracheostomy tube within the first 48 hours after the operative procedure carries a high incidence of complication since the surgical canal is not well established and bleeding can be induced. When the tube is removed, the tissue layers may begin to approximate immediately along with the tracheal rings receding. This makes it difficult to recannulate the trachea. Changing a tracheostomy tube in the first 2 days should be done *only* as a last resort and only by the surgeon. Such procedures as checking the cuff well before inserting the tube and carefully avoiding tearing the cuff on insertion will help to avoid this significant airway emergency.

Modern Tube Materials

There must be appropriate concern for the various substances that are used to make endotracheal and tracheostomy devices. For many years, tracheostomy tubes were exclusively silver—a completely nonreactive substance when in contact with living tissue. These tubes were expensive and not very durable. The early endotracheal tubes were manufactured from naturally occurring rubber (elastomers) and were found to be rigid, nondurable, and difficult to clean. Also, these rubber substances were found to be far more irritating to tissue than plastic (polymeric) substances made available for medical use. In the last 10 to 15 years a variety of plastics have been used for the manufacture of artificial airways.

Endotracheal and tracheal tubes are in direct contact with body tissue, and, therefore, the ideal material for artificial airways would be one with no physical or chemical reactivity (no tissue toxicity, no allergic manifestation, and no carcinogenic potential). An ideal material would be soft and flexible, molding easily to the contours of the airway. If disposable, it would be inexpensive; if nondisposable, economical and safe to resterilize.

Federal standards have been set for testing tracheal devices. The symbols I.T. on a plastic tube stand for *implantation tested* which means the material is nontoxic and free from tissue reaction when implanted in rabbit muscle. The Z–79 present on artificial airways stands for *Z–79 Committee for Anesthesia Equipment for the American National Standards Institute,* which indicates the manufacturer has used a cell culture technique specified by the organization to establish that the device is nontoxic.[240]

The word *plastic* defines a property, not the content, of the material. Within each type of "plastic," there are wide varieties in physical properties as well as composition.

Synthetic materials commonly found in endotracheal and tracheal devices are teflon, nylon, polyethylene, polyvinylchloride, and silicone.

Teflon causes little body tissue reaction and is easily sterilized without physical damage by autoclaving. Its primary disadvantage is its rigidity and expense.

Nylon is degraded by moist heat and may become tissue toxic. Nylon tracheal tubes are rigid and can be physically irritating because of a comparatively rough surface. Impurities in nylon products can cause tissue toxicity. Nylon is seldom used for artificial airways.

Polyethylene is resistant to chemicals and moisture. The low density type of polyethylene is generally thought to be compatible with tissue as well as nontoxic. Volatile materials, such as anesthetics, penetrate polyethylene rapidly. Gas sterilization requires thorough aeration.[241, 245] Autoclaving might distort the material.

Polyvinylchloride (PVC) is the most widely used plastic for artificial airways. The PVC resin in its pure state may be formed into a rigid device, but various degrees of flexibility can be obtained through use of additives. PVC used in medical application should be a pure grade resin and not a commercial variety, since stabilizers have been a source of toxicity. In general, PVC endotracheal or tracheostomy tubes are composed of a PVC resin, a plasticizer, and a stabilizer. If all of the ingredients are properly prepared and evaluated, no tissue reaction as a result of chemical irritation should occur.[242] Flexibility to mold at body temperature to the curves of the airway, and tissue compatibility, are two advantages of PVC tubes. In addition, its low friction resistance makes passage of a plastic suction catheter easy.

The respiratory care practitioner must exercise caution in the re-use and sterilization of PVC tubes. Compounds are added to PVC to make the plastic more flexible and durable. These additives have been shown to react with ethylene oxide (ETO) gas to form toxic compounds.[242, 244] PVC products must be dried before processing with ETO to prevent the formation of tissue-toxic ethylene glycol. They must be *completely aerated* according to the manufacturer's specifications after sterilization. Autoclaving will deform PVC.

Advantages of *silicone* are that (1) it may be autoclaved; (2) it will not deteriorate with time; (3) body tissue does not adhere to it; (4) body fluids will not wet the silicone substance; and (5) it is nontraumatic to tissues. Its only real disadvantage is cost.[246]

Autoclaving is not applicable to most plastic airways because heat causes physical deformation and a decrease of longevity.

Gas sterilizing with ETO (ethylene oxide) has become extremely popular in respiratory care. Units are available with both hot and cold cycles, and aeration chambers are available to speed the aeration process. The length of time of aeration depends on the wrapping material used, the temperature, and the type of material being sterilized. Gas sterilization of some plastic artificial airways has been more limited by cuff structure than by the toxic potential of the plastic itself. The essential thing is that proper aeration time must be provided.

Chemical sterilization is effective as long as the chemical is not contaminated and the material is *thoroughly* rinsed with sterile water and packaged without contamination.

Gamma radiation by manufacturers to sterilize disposable products has aroused controversy because of studies reporting toxic levels of ethylene chlorohydrin following resterilization by ETO.[241] Some manufacturers of plastic airways have indicated there is little danger in using gas to sterilize plastics which have been gamma radiation sterilized, as long as the aeration time is sufficient. Until more research has been done, endotracheal and tracheostomy tubes labeled *gamma radiation sterilized* should not be resterilized.

The softness and flexibility of the plastic used in endotracheal tubes is an important consideration for the respiratory care practitioner. The ability of an endotracheal tube to mold to the contours of the pharynx and glottis plays a large role in glottic trauma. It has been shown that many stiff plastic and rubber tubes exert pressure on the arytenoids and the posterior half of the vocal cords as well as the dorsal wall of the trachea. Other materials, such as the new plastics and silicone materials, mold with body heat to the tissue contours and cause less trauma.

In summary, the various forms of plastics that are available today for endotracheal and tracheostomy tubes are safe and nontoxic to tissue when handled properly. As long as the respiratory care practitioner is aware of the appropriate steps that must be taken to assure proper sterilization and aeration, there will be few complications from the substances. The much publicized and studied circumstance of polyvinylchloride and ethylene oxide is of academic interest today since the precautions that must be taken are well known.

Such factors as the diameter of the tube, ability of the tube to mold appropriately to airway contours, and the movement of the tube against glottic and tracheal tissues seem to play a much greater role in pressure necrosis and post-intubation complications than does the material itself. Since the respiratory care practitioner has the primary responsibility for setting up and carrying out sterilization procedures, he must be aware of all the ramifications of this very important area.

16 • MAINTENANCE OF ARTIFICIAL AIRWAYS AND EXTUBATION

A MOST CONTROVERSIAL subject in the maintenance of airways is the question of endotracheal tube versus tracheostomy. There must be several general statements made prior to a discussion of this question. First, it has been thoroughly documented that patients can be maintained with endotracheal tubes for prolonged periods without serious complication.[246] The question is not whether prolonged endotracheal intubation is feasible, but whether it is *desirable* and of less hazard than tracheostomy. Secondly, a tracheostomy should be avoided when feasible. Even the most enthusiastic of tracheostomy supporters preface their remarks by stating that an unnecessary tracheostomy should never be performed. Thus, we can conclude that short-term airway management (up to 3 days) is best accomplished via nasotracheal (or orotracheal) intubation; long-term airway management (greater than 7 to 10 days) is best accomplished via tracheostomy.[247]

Endotracheal Tube versus Tracheostomy

The real debate centers around the "gray area" of from 3 to 10 days. What should the criteria be for making the judgment of whether or not a tracheostomy would be the most beneficial airway for the patient? This must be a physician's judgment made separately in each circumstance. A great deal of variation in judgment will take place from patient to patient, physician to physician, and institution to institution. There are no universally accepted criteria concerning the appropriateness of endotracheal versus tracheostomy airway management.

An important criterion for ending endotracheal intubation and performing a tracheostomy would be: How long can the larynx be intubated before there is a significant incidence of laryngeal trauma? Laryngeal granulomas have been found after 20 minutes of intubation. Countless patients have been intubated for as long as 6 weeks without occurrence of laryngeal granuloma. However, some investigators have shown a direct correlation between the severity of laryngeal and tra-

261

cheal lesions and the duration of intubation. They have suggested that maximal permissible times for safe laryngeal intubation in adults ranges anywhere from 8 hours to 1 week — in children anywhere from 2 days to 3 weeks.[248]

The authors believe that the maximum safe permissible time of endotracheal intubation should be that time at which the incidence of sequelae increases significantly in that institution. In our hands, most sequelae of glottic origin in adults occur after 3 days of endotracheal intubation. Tracheostomy is always performed by an experienced surgeon at an elective time. The patient always has an endotracheal tube in place. In our experience of over 700 tracheostomies done under these conditions, the complication rate is less than 2%, infection accounting for most of the complications. For any institution applying these modern respiratory care principles, the following *guideline* is safe and clinically applicable.

If there is a reasonable chance for the patient *not* to need an artificial airway in 72 hours or less, leave the endotracheal tube in place. This same evaluation is made every 24 hours. As long as it is our judgment that the patient may *not* need the airway in 72 hours, we will continue with the endotracheal tube. If it becomes our judgment that the patient will *definitely* need the airway for more than 72 hours, we will recommend a tracheostomy. We base this on our experience that when the judgment is made that the airway will be needed for more than 3 days, it usually is needed for significantly longer.

It should be emphasized that this guideline is in terms of adults only. The question of tracheostomy in small children and infants is a much more difficult problem. It is the authors' opinion that the decision for tracheostomy in infants and small children must be made almost entirely on the availability of pediatric surgeons with significant expertise. If such surgeons are not available, tracheostomy should be avoided if at all possible.

Contamination of the Airway

No bacteria exist below the level of the larynx in normal man. This is not true of the upper airway where there is "normal flora." The existence of bacteria in an area where they do not normally exist is known as *contamination*. Contamination does *not* necessarily mean there is infection in that tissue. *Infection* is defined as a tissue inflammation in response to an invasive organism. *Bacterial infection* is usually accompanied by numerous white blood cells that have come to the area to attempt to ingest (phagocytize) the bacteria. This accumulation of white blood cells is called *pus* and the process is termed *purulence*. Presence of bacterial contamination in the lower airway is *not* synonymous with the presence of clinical infection. A culture of bacterial organisms from the lower airway does *not* mean that a pulmonary infection is present.[250]

Diagnosis of Pulmonary Infection

How does one diagnose the presence of a pulmonary infection in the lower airway? Infection in the lower airway is diagnosed clinically by (1) the presence of white blood cells in the sputum and the presence of intracellular bacteria; (2) fever; (3) an increase in the white blood count (leukocytosis); and (4) x-ray and auscultatory evidence of new or progressive pulmonary infiltration. A combination of these factors must be present in order to make the clinical diagnosis of a pulmonary infection.

PURULENT TRACHEOBRONCHIAL SECRETIONS. — A sample of sputum must be obtained when pulmonary infection is suspected. Under the microscope, purulent secretions will be seen as numerous white blood cells. There may be numerous bacteria present in the sputum smear from the upper airway. This normal flora is *not inside* the white blood cells. The presence of *intracellular bacteria* denotes the fact that the white blood cells have been ingesting the bacteria in the airway. Sputum cultures will grow bacterial colonies after several days of incubation. This will allow for identification of organisms and their particular sensitivities to antibiotics.

Most sputum cultures will grow oral flora. Sometimes it is desirable to obtain a direct tracheal sample. This is accomplished by TLA (translaryngeal aspiration), which is done through the cricothyroid membrane. The respiratory care practitioner must be familiar with the examination of sputum smears under the microscope since these are immediately available, whereas cultures take several days to incubate.

FEVER. — Most pulmonary infections will be accompanied by increases in body temperature — a general body defense mechanism in response to infection. Pathogenic bacteria do not multiply well in temperatures above 37°C.; thus an increased body temperature is a helpful defense mechanism. Although pulmonary infection can be present without fever, this would be the exception rather than the rule.

INCREASED WHITE BLOOD CELL COUNT. — The usual response to an infection, and especially to a pulmonary infection, is to mobilize increased numbers of white blood cells from the bone marrow and other storage areas. These white blood cells are used to phagocytize the invading bacteria. An increase in the white cell count of blood is a helpful corollary to the diagnosis of pulmonary infection.

CLINICAL EXAMINATION OF THE CHEST. — Clinical examination of the chest will often reveal the presence of rales, rhonchi, or bronchial breath sounds when a pulmonary infection is present. Although these are helpful clinical findings, it must be emphasized that they may be absent when there is significant pulmonary infection.

CHEST X-RAY. — Chest x-ray may be extremely helpful in the diagnosis of pulmonary infection. The existence of new or progressive pulmonary infiltrates on the chest x-ray is excellent evidence of the existence of pulmonary infection.

It is essential to remember that the presence of bacteria within the lower airway does not mean there is infection present. Pulmonary infection is a *clinical diagnosis* and must be made on that basis. It is a serious error to confuse contamination of the airway with infection of the airway.

Incidence of Airway Contamination

Any interruption of the normal defense mechanisms of the lower airway for even a very short period of time will result in contamination of the lower airway. In spite of rigorous sterile techniques, endotracheal tubes inserted for periods as short as 30 minutes will result in a high incidence of contamination of the airway. *The placement of an artificial airway for more than 24 hours will result in contamination of the lower airway!* The respiratory care practitioner must understand that airway contamination is an *inevitable* result of artificial airway placement. This occurs regardless of how well the airway is maintained.

Common Airway Contaminants

The most common contaminants are *gram-positive organisms* — usually *Staphylococcus* or *Streptococcus*. These gram-positive bacteria are normal inhabitants of the upper airway. It is not surprising that they would contaminate the lower airway following the establishment of an artificial airway.

In debilitated patients, especially in intensive care areas, it is common to have *gram-negative organisms* contaminating the airway. In order of commonality they are: (1) *Klebsiella;* (2) *Pseudomonas;* (3) *Escherichia coli;* (4) *Enterobacter;* and (5) *Proteus.*[249] Gram-negative organisms are dangerous when they cause pulmonary infection because (1) they destroy lung tissue (necrotizing pneumonia); (2) they cause generalized sepsis (gram-negative shock); and (3) they require highly toxic antibiotics for eradication.

Prophylactic Antibiotics in Respiratory Care

Antibiotics have proved to be successful in treating pulmonary infection; however, their misuse can be as dangerous as their appropriate use is advantageous. There are numerous clinical circumstances in which the preventative or prophylactic use of antibiotics has proved to be of great benefit. In patients who have contaminated surgical wounds, the starting of antibiotic therapy prior to clinical infection plays a great role in decreasing morbidity and mortality. Although this principle has proved valid in many clinical circumstances, there is little evidence that prophylactic antibiotics are indicated in acute pulmonary disease.

The treatment of airway contamination with antibiotics results primarily in the suppression of the more common contaminating organisms, guaranteeing that if infection occurs it will be due to a potentially more dangerous gram-negative organism. The use of prophylactic antibiotics must always be a medical judgment based on each particular circumstance. We make the general statement that routine prophylactic antibiotic therapy for airway contamination is contraindicated because it may lead to dangerous and difficult to treat pulmonary infections. A clinical generality may be stated as follows: Pulmonary *infection* must be treated by appropriate antibiotic therapy, whereas airway *contamination* must be repeatedly evaluated, but not treated.

Nosocomial Infection in Respiratory Care

Nosocomial infection means infection that is transmitted to the patient by hospital equipment or personnel. This is a great danger in respiratory care, since we deal with equipment that is in direct communication with the airway. Aerosol therapy is a great source of nosocomial infection because bacteria are transported on water droplets. It is incumbent upon those in respiratory therapy to be sure that a patient's airway is not *cross-contaminated* by the respiratory therapy equipment. We cannot prevent the patient with an artificial airway from becoming contaminated, but we can protect him from becoming contaminated with other patient's bacteria via the respiratory therapy equipment. General equipment precautions must be followed, such as providing single patient units or circuits in aerosol and IPPB therapy, providing the appropriate filters on equipment, changing the parts of the equipment that come in contact with the patient at least every 24 hours, carefully draining condensate out of tubing so that the moisture is not stagnant, and carefully culturing the respiratory therapy equipment periodically to make sure that proper sterilization techniques are being carried out. Anyone caring for a patient with an artificial airway must maintain meticulous personal hygiene between patients. The simple technique of hand washing by those coming in contact with the airway will significantly reduce the possibility of cross-contaminants.[251]

Intensive Care and Airway Contamination

Positive sputum cultures may be due to one of three possibilities: (1) contamination of the specimen; (2) contaminating colonization of the tracheobronchial tree; or (3) clinical infection. In addition to the factor that an artificial airway practically guarantees contamination of the airway, there are numerous factors responsible for the high incidence of pulmonary infections in intensive care units: (1) extremely high patient density; (2) critically ill patients who have poor defense mechanisms to ward off infection; (3) contaminated respiratory therapy equipment; (4) injudicious use of antibiotics; and (5) improper technique by ICU personnel.

Summary

One must consider the insults to normal defense mechanisms produced by the placement of an artificial airway: (1) the inevitable contamination by bacteria of the lower airway; (2) the disruption of ciliary motion that occurs when a foreign body is placed within the trachea — this loss of normal ciliary motion greatly inhibits the functioning of the mucociliary escalator; and (3) placement of an artificial airway interferes with the most important protective mechanism in mobilizing retained secretions — the cough mechanism. Any patient with an artificial airway is greatly impeded in his ability to cough, and the chances of retaining secretions in the pulmonary tree are greatly increased. These overwhelming factors make the critically ill patient with an artificial airway vulnerable to pulmonary infection.

Colonization with pathogenic bacteria is universal in patients in whom endotracheal or tracheostomy tubes have been placed for longer than 24 to 48 hours. Bacterial cultures are difficult to interpret and must be considered intelligently. Inappropriate use of antibiotics can lead to more serious clinical infection. Although the prevention of bacterial colonization is a worthwhile area of investigation, it appears impossible to prevent.

The inevitability of contamination of the airway must not be interpreted as an excuse for poor technique in airway care. It is well known that poor technique leads to a much greater incidence of serious pulmonary *infection*. We must always strive for the best of sterile technique in both our equipment and airway care.

Suctioning the Airway

Since the patient with an artificial airway is not capable of effectively coughing, the mobilization of secretions from the trachea must be facilitated by aspiration (suctioning). Patients with copious secretions will require frequent suctioning. Serious complications, including cardiac arrest, may result from improper techniques of aspirating secretions from the trachea of critically ill patients.[252] Thus, it is essential for us to review the complications of suctioning and state the principles upon which proper techniques are based.

Complications of Airway Suctioning

The major complications of airway suctioning are (1) hypoxemia, (2) arrhythmia, (3) hypotension, and (4) lung collapse.

HYPOXEMIA. — Most patients with artificial airways are receiving some form of oxygen therapy; i.e., they are breathing enriched oxygen atmospheres that are essential for the maintenance of adequate arterial oxygenation. When a catheter is placed in the airway and a vacuum applied, oxygen-enriched gas is "sucked" out of the lungs and replaced by room air that enters around the catheter. Thus, we are replacing oxygen-enriched air with ambient air (21% oxygen), a circumstance that could result in severe hypoxemia.[253] One of the earliest discoveries in respiratory care units was that most of the cardiac arrests occurred either during or shortly following the suctioning process.[44]

Acute hypoxemia during the suctioning process will manifest heart-rate abnormalities in the critically ill patient. Most often there is an initial tachycardia without arrhythmia that reverts as soon as oxygenation is reestablished. Occasionally, the adult will manifest a bradycardia.

Any significant change in heart rate or rhythm during suctioning must be presumed to be due to hypoxemia. Ventilation and oxygenation must be immediately reestablished.

Pre-oxygenation is useful in avoiding hypoxemia during suctioning. Of greater importance is the technique of providing an oxygen-enriched atmosphere around the catheter so that room air does not enter the lung.[254]

ARRHYTHMIA. — Significant cardiac arrhythmias may occur during the suctioning process from two sources: (1) arterial hypoxemia leading to myocardial hypoxia[255] or (2) vagal stimulation secondary to tracheal irritation.[256] There still exists great debate about which of these two factors is most significant. They both play a potential role in the initiation of severe arrhythmia such as premature ventricular contractions during the suctioning process. True vagal stimulation may lead to profound bradycardias. These complications can best be avoided by appropriate technique.

HYPOTENSION. — Hypotension may occur from either of two circumstances: (1) profound bradycardia resulting from vagal stimulation; or (2) prolonged coughing maneuvers during the suctioning process. Tracheal irritation from the suction catheter may stimulate tracheal and carinal reflexes resulting in paroxysmal cough-like maneuvers which interrupt ventilation. These coughing maneuvers, along with bradycardia, can have a severe effect on both venous return and cardiac output.

Hypoxemia, arrhythmia, and hypotension are best avoided by suctioning techniques that (1) include pre- and intermittent oxygenation with high inspired oxygen concentrations;[255] (2) limit the suctioning process to 10 seconds or less;[257] and (3) include close cardiac monitoring.

LUNG COLLAPSE. — The insertion of a large suction catheter into a small diameter artificial airway results in inadequate space for air to readily "entrain" around the catheter.[258] Thus, when a vacuum is applied, the lung may collapse. This is avoided by using a catheter whose diameter is smaller than the radius of the artificial airway. A rule of thumb is that the suction catheter should not occupy more than one half the internal diameter of the tube being suctioned.

The Suction Catheter

The ideal suction catheter would (1) be made of a material causing as little trauma as possible to the tracheal mucosa; (2) have minimal frictional resistance passing through the artificial airway; (3) be long enough to easily pass the tip of the artificial airway (20–22 inches); (4) have smooth, molded ends to avoid mucosal trauma; and (5) have side holes to prevent mucosal trauma.[259]

The proximal end must have an opening that allows room air to enter and neutralize the vacuum in the catheter without turning off the suction apparatus. This allows the vacuum apparatus to remain on without subatmospheric pressure being transmitted to the catheter.

When suction is desired, the proximal hole is occluded with the thumb and the vacuum transmitted to the catheter. The proximal hole must be larger than the internal diameter of the catheter to prevent the Bernoulli principle from creating negative pressure when the hole is unoccluded.

Sterility of suction catheters is essential. We believe only disposable catheters should be used. The packaging should avoid "curling," so that removal from the package is easy and the suctioning process facilitated.

The adult left main stem bronchus originates from the trachea at a sharp angle. Straight catheters enter the left main stem bronchus less than 10% of the time regardless of head position. When left bronchus suctioning is required, coudé suction catheters may be used. These have a curved tip which facilitates easier passage into the left main stem bronchus.

Mucosal Damage from Suction Catheters

Autopsy findings in patients who received several days of tracheal suctioning reveal a high incidence of severe mucosal damage. Hemorrhagic and edematous mucosa is common. Sometimes the area is completely denuded.

Fiberoptic bronchoscopy has provided the means of observing the pathogenesis of these lesions. It appears that the mucosal hemorrhages and erosions are due to suction catheter trauma. Even with meticulous technique, this damage occurs consistently.[259]

Some suction catheters elevate the mucosa when vacuum is applied and invaginate the mucosa into the side or end holes of the catheter. These mucosal areas immediately become hemorrhagic and may erode. Vacuum in excess of -120 mm Hg facilitates this process, but even proper suctioning levels (-80 to -120 mm Hg) do not eliminate the process. Catheters made with "ring tips" or additional side holes seem to play a significant role in preventing such mucosal damage.[260]

The relationship between mucosal damage caused by suctioning and the incidence of tracheal infection is still in question. It would seem obvious, however, that the less damage one does to the tracheal mucosa during the suctioning process, the better it must be for the patient in relationship to comfort and possible infection control.

Suctioning Technique

Sterile technique must *always* be followed. This entails the use of a sterile glove for the hand that will handle the catheter, the use of a sterile suction catheter, and appropriate sterile rinsing solutions and container for clearing the catheter. The catheter must *never* be stored and re-used for suctioning an artificial airway.

Using the following procedure, the incidence of complications and mucosal damage will be minimized.

STEP 1. — Adequately pre-oxygenate the patient; this provides the greatest degree of oxygen reserve in the alveoli. Pre-oxygenation may be accomplished by hand ventilating with 100% oxygen or increasing the Fi_{O_2} to the spontaneously breathing patient (some ventilators have mechanisms for giving 100% oxygen prior to the suctioning process). The pre-oxygenation step will usually avoid arterial hypoxemia for appropriate suctioning periods.

STEP 2. — Insert the catheter *without vacuum* until it is obviously past the tip of the airway and approximately at the level of the carina. When a slight obstruction is felt, the catheter must be pulled back slightly and then intermittent suction applied while *rotating* the catheter between the thumb and forefinger during removal. This rotating movement and intermittent suctioning minimize mucosal damage and aspirate secretions more effectively.

STEP 3. — *DO NOT LEAVE THE SUCTION CATHETER IN THE AIRWAY FOR LONGER THAN 10 TO 15 SECONDS.* The total time from the beginning of the suctioning process to reestablishment of ventilation and oxygenation should never exceed 20 seconds. The electrocardiographic monitor must be watched during the suctioning procedure. With the onset of arrhythmias or other patient distress, the process must immediately be discontinued and the patient ventilated with 100% oxygen.

STEP 4. — Re-oxygenate and ventilate for at least 5 deep breaths and return to base-line vital signs before repeating the suctioning process.

The four steps should be repeated until all secretions have been aspirated and the airway appears clear. Following tracheal aspiration, the same catheter can be used to aspirate the oropharynx and the nose, but must never be re-used in the trachea.

Suctioning should never be done "routinely." Some evidence of tracheal secretions should be present, since unnecessary suctioning may irritate the mucosa[259] and stimulate secretion production.

Obtaining Culture Specimens

Routine artificial airway care includes the obtaining of tracheal secretion specimens for culture and sensitivity. The frequency of this routine varies from institution to institution. However, the respiratory care practitioner must be familiar with that institution's method of obtaining such a specimen. There are various sterile specimen containers that are easily attached to the line of a suction catheter. Following the normal sterile suctioning technique, without rinsing of the catheter, a specimen is obtained. We obtain our best specimens after ultrasonic treatments and postural drainage maneuvers.

It is our opinion that tracheal aspiration for culture should be obtained at least every 3 days for patients with artificial airways. In addition, cultures should also be obtained if the secretions change in color, consistency, or amount. Of course, one must change these guidelines for chronic or permanent artificial airways.

Humidification of the Airway

A patient with an artificial airway does not have the availability of the upper airway to heat and humidify the inspired air. This heat and humidity deficit must be provided by the tracheobronchial tree, unless otherwise provided. *It is essential that the gas delivered to an artificial airway be 100% humidified at body temperature.* Without appropriate humidification of the artificial airway, the incidence of obstruction caused by drying of secretions will be great. With appropriate heating and humidification of inspired gas, the incidence of crusting and obstructing of the airway by secretions is extremely rare.

For the spontaneously breathing patient with an artificial airway, an appropriate device to provide oxygen and humidification is a heated nebulizer and T-piece with a reservoir tubing on the exhalation limb. This provides a high-flow system which will allow complete control of humidity, temperature, and oxygen without adding resistance. In the longer-term patient or in circumstances where oxygen therapy is not critical, such devices as tracheostomy masks may be used.

Failure to properly humidify the inspired air will result in dried, retained secretions within the airway. The importance of humidification is dramatized by the following case history. A 27-year-old woman was admitted to a hospital with an original diagnosis of "stroke." An endotracheal tube was placed because of upper airway obstruction. Twenty-four hours after insertion of the endotracheal tube, the diagnosis of drug overdose was made, and the patient was transferred to our hospital for intensive respiratory care. She arrived in our emergency room 26 hours after intubation. For that entire period there had been no humidity added to the inspired air. She was noted to have signs of partial airway obstruction, and a suction catheter could not be passed through the tube. Upon removal of the endotracheal tube, there followed an almost perfect cast of the main stem and segmental bronchi (Fig 16–1). This was a thick, rubbery material, composed primarily of dried, re-

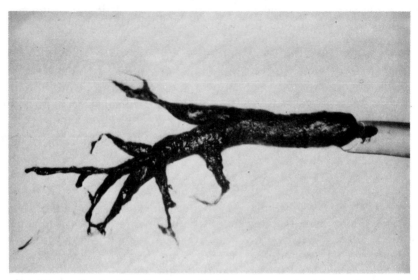

Fig 16–1.—Cast of tracheobronchial tree removed with extubation (see text).

tained secretions. Upon extubation, the patient's respiratory distress was dramatically cleared.

There used to be great concern for the frequent changing of artificial airways and the cleaning of inner cannulas every 3 or 4 hours to prevent crusting. Since the understanding of appropriate humidification and its role in maintaining airways, we seldom find problems with crusting or obstructing of the airways if humidification equipment is functioning properly. There should be no reason for routinely changing artificial airways. They should be changed only when there is an indication for such a change. The airway must be greatly respected — unnecessary extubation and intubation must be avoided.

Tracheostomy Wound Care

The respiratory care practitioner must be familiar with the basic principles of caring for a tracheostomy wound. After bleeding has been controlled, the major factor is to prevent the area from becoming grossly contaminated or traumatized. The wound should be cared for like any other surgical incision; i.e., it should be kept dry and as free from exudate and secretions as possible. The area should be cleaned routinely with 3% hydrogen peroxide, rinsed with sterile normal saline, and a sterile dressing applied. Cultures need only be taken if infection is suspected, since the area will most assuredly be contaminated with secretions. The tracheostomy "ties" should be securely fastened, using a knot to minimize the movement of the tracheostomy tube and prevent accidental decannulation. Care must be taken to prevent excessive pressure against the wound.

When reasonable attempts are made to keep the area clean and trauma to a minimum, there are seldom significant problems with tracheostomy wounds.

Cuff Care

The area of artificial airway care that has received great attention in the past decade has been that of positive-pressure cuffs. We shall discuss this question in great detail in Chapter 17. An essential part of the maintenance of airways is appropriate inflation and deflation techniques of these cuffs.

Inflation Technique

The object of proper inflation is to place the minimal volume of air in the cuff that will allow optimal sealing of the airway. This technique of inflation is called the "minimal leak technique" or "minimal occluding volume." This is based upon the assumption that during positive-pressure ventilation the tracheal diameter is maximal at the time of inspiration. Thus, if the cuff barely occludes during peak positive-pressure inspiration, there will be the least possible pressure on the tracheal mucosa during the expiratory phase where the diameter is the least. In other words, *a minimal leak should be present at the moment in the ventilatory cycle when the tracheal diameter is maximal.* Use of the minimal occluding volume (MOV) necessary to create an airtight seal will act to avoid undue pressure on the tracheal mucosa and, thus, keep ischemia at a minimum.[247] Recently, there has been interest in actually measuring the intracuff pressure and keeping it below 20 mm Hg.

Periodic Deflation

Periodic deflation of the cuff at various intervals is less beneficial than generally believed. In fact, this periodic deflation-and-inflation routine may cause the therapist and nurse to be less careful in properly reinflating the cuff. The original purpose of periodic deflation was to restore the blood flow to the tracheal mucosa. There has been no evidence to show that capillary blood flow is restored to the area in less than an hour, and certainly not in 5 minutes or less.[261] Another objection to periodic deflation is that many patients on controlled ventilation do not tolerate the deflation, PEEP cannot be maintained, and cardiopulmonary instability often results.

It is our procedure that once the inflation is made with a minimal leak technique and the patient is placed on airway pressure therapy, the cuff is *not* deflated routinely. A significant change in airway pressures would mean a significant change in the maximal tracheal diameter; under these circumstances the cuff should be deflated and reinflated. Many patients have high-peak airway pressures when first placed on ventilators, and then as they adjust to this procedure, or their disease process improves and the compliance and resistance of the lung and airway change, the peak pressures may diminish. Thus, a cuff volume that was producing a minimal leak when the airway pressures were high would be excessive after the airway pressures diminished — this calls for readjustment of the cuff volume.

There are some who advocate periodic deflating of the cuff in order to prevent secretions from pooling above the cuff site. We have found that this can be adequately prevented by appropriate postural drainage and pharyngeal suctioning.

If it is necessary to deflate the cuff, certain safeguards must be taken: (1) the trachea must be suctioned; (2) the area above the cuff should be suctioned as well as possible through the pharynx; and (3) the cuff must then be deflated, followed by immediate tracheal suctioning to assure that any secretions lodged above the cuff do not go down into the airways. Applying positive pressure with the cuff down helps "blow" secretions into the pharynx for easier suctioning and prevents a feeling of shortness of breath on the part of the patient.

Some years ago there were those who advocated using a tube with two cuffs to alternate the areas of cuff pressure. This results in a larger area of tracheal mucosal damage and appears to have no advantage over a single cuff.[278]

Artificial Airway Emergencies

An artificial airway must never be taken lightly. This is best illustrated by a discussion of the *immediate* artificial airway emergencies: (1) cuff leaks, (2) inadvertent extubation, and (3) obstruction.

Cuff Leaks

Ventilation must be maintained while preparation is being made for replacement of a tube with a faulty cuff. Often, no more is needed than increased tidal volumes to compensate for the gas escaping. In the case of a tracheostomy tube, it may be possible to support ventilation by bag and mask from above.

A leaky cuff should not prove a disastrous occurrence since the respiratory care practitioner should be capable of maintaining reasonable ventilation until a new tube can be placed. It is essential that a spare airway of the same size, appropriate intubation equipment, and a hand ventilator with mask be at the bedside of all acutely ill patients with artificial airways.

Inadvertent Extubation

Replacement of the endotracheal tube or tracheostomy tube should be attempted, but if it cannot be immediately accomplished, the tube should be completely removed. Ventilation must then be established by any means available. This may mean simple mouth-to-mouth (or mask and bag) ventilation with occlusion of the tracheostomy stoma. It is unusual when reasonable ventilation cannot be accomplished for short periods of time. The respiratory care practitioner is obliged to assure reasonable ventilation until preparation and personnel can be gathered for replacement of the artificial airway.

Obstruction

There is no greater emergency than being confronted with an artificial airway that is obstructed and prevents ventilation. When presented with this circumstance, there are five common etiologies that must be immediately thought of: (1) the tube may kink—slight manipulation of the head, neck, and tube will often correct the circumstance; (2) the cuff can slip or herniate over the end of the tube and cause complete occlusion—this most commonly occurs following positional changes of the head and neck and positional changes of the tube (Fig 16–2), and can be immediately relieved by deflation of the cuff; (3) plugs within the lumen of the artificial airway may cause partial or complete obstruction; (4) the tube may collapse—this is most common with nasotracheal tubes that are impinged on by a deviated septum; and (5) the bevel of the tube may impinge upon the carina, the wall of the trachea, or bronchus—this is often relieved by simple manipulation of the tube.

Obvious steps when confronted with airway obstruction are to (1) manipulate the tube, (2) deflate the cuff, and (3) attempt to pass a suction catheter. If none of these maneuvers are successful, the tube must be *removed!* Ventilation must then be established and a new tube placed.

When all of these maneuvers have been attempted and ventilation

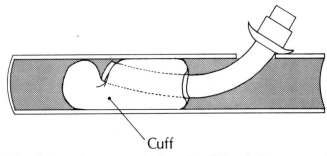

Fig 16–2.—Schematic representation of cuff herniating over end of tube and causing obstruction (see text).

is still not possible, one must think of the existence of a *tension pneumothorax.* This is a circumstance where there is air in the thoracic cavity under pressure and the lung parenchyma and great vessels are being compressed. A tension pneumothorax must be immediately relieved by opening the chest to the ambient pressure.

A rule that must never be broken in intensive care areas is that duplicate airways and appropriate intubation and ventilation equipment must be at the bedside at all times. *The best treatment for airway emergencies is prevention.* Have adequate and well-functioning equipment at the bedside, check all tubes and cuffs before placing them in the patient, and constantly reevaluate the function of the airway. When faced with a true airway emergency *ventilate any way you can, but ventilate!*

Discontinuing the Artificial Airway (Extubation)

The decision to extubate must rise from the general principle *that any airway is no longer needed when the indications for its placement are no longer present.* Therefore, evaluation for extubation must be made by judging whether or not there is still a need for the artificial airway.

OBSTRUCTION.—If the airway was placed for reasons of upper airway obstruction, the only sure way of testing whether or not the airway is needed is to extubate and watch for recurring signs of upper airway obstruction. Upper airway obstruction is most often due to C.N.S. obtundation—improvement in sensorium would be an indication for extubation.

PROTECTION OF THE AIRWAY.—Protection of the airway must involve the evaluation of the airway reflexes. The airway reflexes are obtunded from the top down, i.e., first the pharyngeal, then the laryngeal, then the tracheal, and finally the carinal. It is reasonable to assume that if a patient has a good swallowing mechanism (pharyngeal reflex) with the tube in place, the chances are that the laryngeal and tracheal reflexes are intact.

SUCTIONING. — The need for tracheal suctioning is greatly dependent upon the ability to cough adequately. This can be evaluated by measuring the vital capacity, the negative inspiratory force, and judging the level of consciousness. It is reasonable to assume that with an acceptable vital capacity and a cooperative patient, bronchial hygiene can be maintained without an artificial airway.

VENTILATION. — The patient must be free of the need for mechanical support of ventilation before the tube can be removed.

NO ONE SHOULD REMOVE AN ARTIFICIAL AIRWAY WHO DOES NOT POSSESS THE SKILL AND EQUIPMENT TO REPLACE THE AIRWAY! Whenever feasible, extubation should be accomplished during a period of the day when there is adequate personnel *both* to monitor and evaluate the patient as well as personnel who can replace the artificial airway.

Endotracheal Tube Extubation

When the decision has been made to extubate the patient with an indwelling endotracheal tube, there are some basic steps that should be followed:

STEP 1. — The procedure must be explained to the patient to the degree he is capable of comprehending. It is desirable to have the patient's cooperation during and after the extubation process.

STEP 2. — Secretions must be aspirated from the trachea and then from the oro- and nasopharynx.

STEP 3. — Increased inspired oxygen should be administered.

STEP 4. — The lungs should be completely inflated so that the patient will initially cough or exhale as the tube is taken from the larynx. This is accomplished in two ways: (1) the patient is asked to take the deepest breath he possibly can and at the very peak of the inspiratory effort the cuff is deflated and the tube is removed rapidly; or (2) positive pressure is administered with a hand ventilator and at the end of a deep inspiration the cuff is released and the tube removed.

STEP 5. — Appropriate oxygen is immediately administered.

STEP 6. — The patient's airway is immediately evaluated for signs of obstruction, stridor, or difficult breathing. The patient should be encouraged to take some deep breaths and to cough.

STEP 7. — The patient is not left unattended until there is no doubt of his ability to function without the artificial airway. Spare airway equipment must remain at the bedside for a reasonable period.

Laryngospasm

The most common significant problem confronted immediately after endotracheal extubation is spasm of the vocal cords causing obstruction of the airway. This *laryngospasm* is recognized by an inability of the patient to inspire or the inability to accomplish positive-pressure inspiration, in spite of adequate manipulations to clear the upper airway. Laryngospasm occurs far more commonly in infants and children than in adults.

Laryngospasm is usually of limited duration — some minor air exchange will usually ensue within 30 seconds. High oxygen concentrations with positive pressure may be adequate to maintain oxygenation during this period. If the laryngospasm persists it will be necessary to administer a muscle relaxant to paralyze the vocal cord musculature and allow the patient to be ventilated. Laryngospasm can be extremely hazardous in unskilled hands and its incidence must be kept in mind when contemplating extubation.

Tracheostomy Extubation

Since the tracheostomy is a far more permanent and better tolerated airway, the necessity for early extubation is not as pressing as with the endotracheal tube. However, the indications for removing a tracheostomy tube are precisely the same as for removing an endotracheal tube — when the indications and needs for the airway are no longer present. A greater degree of flexibility and variability in extubating techniques exists with tracheostomy than with the endotracheal tube.

One of the greatest advantages is that the patient can be given a trial at maintaining and using his own airway, without removing the tracheostomy tube, by using a "fenestrated" tracheostomy tube.

A *universal fenestrated tube* (Fig 16–3) is a tracheostomy tube in which a "window" or fenestration has been cut into the posterior wall of the outer cannula. It is possible to have the patient breathe around the tube and through the fenestration without actually removing the tube. This is accomplished by removing the solid inner cannula and placing a cork in the opening of the outer cannula.[262] Thus, one can evaluate the patient's ability to breathe without obstruction, handle

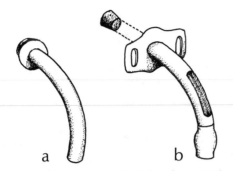

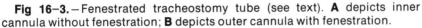

a   b

Fig 16-3. — Fenestrated tracheostomy tube (see text). **A** depicts inner cannula without fenestration; **B** depicts outer cannula with fenestration.

his own secretions, protect his own airway, and ventilate. A tremendous psychologic advantage is that the patient can talk with the fenestrated tube.

Numerous types of fenestrated tracheostomy tubes have been described. It is helpful to have a readily available "universal" fenestrated tube which can be placed immediately when it is felt the patient may be able to maintain himself without the tube. This allows a standard tracheostomy tube system to be reestablished simply by replacing the inner cannula (which is unfenestrated) and inflating the small emergency cuff. The inner cannula can also be replaced for suctioning, if necessary. This is not intended to be a long-term airway device, but rather a method for testing the ability of the patient to exist without the airway in a safe and reversible manner.

Commercially available fenestrated tubes have the disadvantage of small fenestrations. The manufacturers believe that larger fenestrations will threaten structural integrity when the plastic material warms; thus, it may be necessary to place a smaller size fenestrated tube in these circumstances. It is imperative to observe closely for signs of respiratory distress or airway obstruction for several hours after insertion of a fenestrated tube.

It may be desirable to keep patent the channel between the skin and the trachea, e.g., if replacement of the tracheostomy tube is contemplated at a later date. This would be beneficial if future surgery is contemplated or if the patient has a recurring disease that may necessitate the reestablishment of an airway. Various types of *tracheal buttons* have been designed with this in mind (Fig 16-4). They allow the stoma to be maintained open and allow suctioning through the button if necessary. These types of appliances are indicated in patients where it is felt the tracheostomy tube will be needed at some future

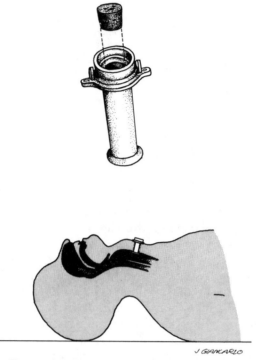

Fig 16–4. – The tracheal button (see text).

time or where suctioning may be required intermittently. Most "trach buttons" are temporary appliances. A teflon prosthesis is commercially available which consists of both an outer-hollow cannula and an inner-solid cannula. The proper-sized button is selected by placing a probe into the stoma and measuring the distance between the skin and the anterior wall of the trachea. The tracheal button is then fitted to the stoma, corked, and can remain for indefinite periods with routine skin care.[263]

It should be anticipated that the stoma will be completely sealed within 48 hours of extubation. Epithelialization of the canal is rare and occurs primarily when infection is present at the time of extubation. In general, the stoma heals quite well without any suturing. The patient may have to place pressure over the stoma area to have an effective cough while the stoma is closing. Reassurance should be given that the stoma will be closed in several days.

17 • LARYNGEAL AND TRACHEAL COMPLICATIONS OF ARTIFICIAL AIRWAYS

THE UPPER AIRWAY complications of endotracheal intubation have been discussed in the previous chapter. Here we shall consider the laryngeal complications of endotracheal intubation and the tracheal complications of tracheostomy and endotracheal tubes.

Laryngeal Complications of Endotracheal Intubation

The severity and incidence of complications from endotracheal intubation depend upon numerous circumstances. These can be discussed as three general factors: decisive, predisposing, and adjunctive.[219]

Decisive factors are those factors which by themselves can cause sequelae. We can primarily associate these with the trauma of intubation. Trauma to the pharynx and larynx during intubation and maintenance affects the complication rate — the greater the trauma, the greater the incidence of complications. Other factors such as duration of intubation, external diameter of the tube, shape of the tube, movement of vocal cords, cuff pressure, and construction material may all be considered decisive factors.

Proper airway care is very significant in decreasing complications. Variability in airway care undoubtedly accounts for much of the disparity in published complication rates.

Predisposing factors are those of the patient population. Age is an important predisposing factor; e.g., children appear to tolerate prolonged tracheal intubation better than adults. Post-intubation sore throat and granulomas are far more common in women than men. The unfortunate practice of using oversized tracheal tubes in females may be responsible.

Adjunctive factors refer to the individual patient's status. Chronic or debilitating states, such as anemia, hypovitaminosis, hypoproteinemia, prolonged steroid therapy, and alcoholism, affect the healing process and, therefore, increase the complication rate. Hyperhydration and allergies favor edema formation; dehydration diminishes mucous secretions and makes the laryngeal and tracheal mucosa more susceptible to trauma. The presence of upper respiratory tract infections increases the complication rate because of contaminated secretions that pool in the pharynx. Iatrogenic (physician-caused) adjunctive factors, such as nasogastric tubes, increase the incidences of complications. These tubes cause laryngeal edema by placing excessive pressure on the arytenoid area.

In summary, the incidence and severity of complications depend upon factors in the general population, in the particular status of the patient, and in the technical facility with which airways are placed and maintained. These factors must be kept in mind whenever the complication rate of endotracheal intubation is discussed.

Sore Throat and "Hoarse" Voice

Minimal damage to the pharyngeal and laryngeal epithelium occurs with even the most skillful intubations. This damage involves a disruption of the basement membrane from the submucosa and may lead to a "sloughing" of the epithelial lining. This denuding process is usually "spotty" and completely heals within 2 to 3 days; sequelae are extremely rare.

The patient experiences a sore throat and some "hoarseness" of voice. The treatment is reassurance and adequate humidity. The healing process will usually progress without incident if the traumatized mucosa does not become dry.[264]

Glottic Edema (Fig 17-1)

The glottis is defined as the superior opening of the larynx. Edema in this area is the most common complication of endotracheal intubation and is seldom severe. It is far more common in children than adults. The necessity for re-intubation is uncommon when edema is recognized early and appropriately treated.

Glottic edema is most commonly caused by (1) trauma during intubation and maintenance; (2) insertion of oversized endotracheal tubes; (3) poor technique of endotracheal tube care; (4) toxic material from improperly sterilized endotracheal tubes; and (5) allergic responses.

The cardinal clinical sign of glottic edema is *inspiratory stridor*—a high-pitched musical sound on inspiration caused by a narrowed glottic opening. The edema occurs in loose connective tissue located be-

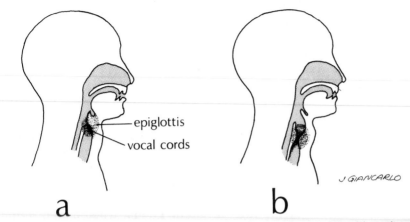

epiglottis

vocal cords

J GIANCARLO

a   b

Fig 17–1.—Glottic edema. In **A,** shaded area outlines general location of supraglottic and glottic edema; in **B,** shaded area outlines general location of subglottic edema (see text).

low the epithelium of the epiglottis, retroarytenoidal area, aryepiglottic folds, and vocal cords (see Fig 15–8). If this "submucosal space" edema occurs on the surface of the epiglottis and/or the aryepiglottic folds, the glottic opening will be impinged upon. If the edema occurs in the retroarytenoidal area, the abduction (spreading apart) of the vocal cords will be limited on inspiration. Either condition may cause marked ventilatory obstruction.[219]

The glottic area lies extrathoracic, so the glottic opening will be narrowest during spontaneous inspiration. When more than half of the normal glottic opening is restricted because of the edema, the symptomatology of inspiratory stridor and respiratory distress may develop. It should be obvious that edema in a small glottis will have significantly more obstructive effect than in a large glottis.

The clinical pathophysiology of glottic edema is important to understand. The submucosal swelling begins upon removal of the endotracheal tube and progresses gradually for as long as 24 hours. It must be realized that while the tube is in place, the pressure prevents the submucosal space from swelling significantly. Upon extubation the swelling may be rapid. It usually takes several hours for the edema to reach its maximum.

Inspiratory stridor present upon extubation must be considered serious, since the edema will progress over the next several hours. On the other hand, inspiratory stridor that becomes evident several hours after extubation is of less concern. In general, the absence of inspiratory stridor following extubation does not guarantee that glottic edema will not develop. The presence of inspiratory stridor following extubation is a warning that severe obstruction may develop.

Most post-extubation glottic edema is treated with reassurance, careful observation, and aerosol to prevent mucosal drying. Pharmacologic therapy for clinically significant edema that does not necessitate re-intubation falls into two categories: topical decongestion and steroid therapy.

The application of a vasoconstrictor directly to the edematous area has been recognized as the treatment of choice for glottic edema. The rationale is that a topical alpha-adrenergic drug will decrease the hyperemia and edema. The drug of choice is *racemic epinephrine* which may be administered by a simple hand atomizer or by IPPB machine using high-flow rates.[265] *Steroids* are potent anti-inflammatory agents and may decrease the severity of glottic edema when administered topically or by systemic route. Dramatic responses have been reported immediately following the I.V. injection of steroid compounds.[266]

In our institution, the treatment of post-extubation glottic edema is high-flow IPPB administration of a combination of racemic epinephrine and steroid: (1) ½ ml of 2.25% racemic epinephrine; (2) 1 mg of dexamethasone (Decadron); and (3) 3 ml of saline. A mouthpiece or mask is applied while a high-flow rate provides turbulent flow. This turbulence will "spray" the drugs on the glottic area. The duration of a treatment may be as little as 5–7 minutes, since the goal is the topical application of the drug on the glottis — not peripheral distribution.

The use of such techniques is believed to have reduced the incidence of re-intubation significantly. When the symptoms appear severe and re-intubation is contemplated, the administration of intravenous steroids seems justified.

Subglottic Edema (see Fig 17–1)

Subglottic edema is the most serious type of post-extubation edema; it is the one most commonly necessitating re-intubation or tracheostomy. Subglottic edema is more common in infants and children because of the small internal diameter of the larynx. In the newborn, a one millimeter edema in the subglottic area will reduce the cross-sectional area by 35%.[219]

The subglottic region is subject to trauma because of the fragile epithelium, loose submucosal connective tissue, and the complete cartilaginous cricoid ring which prevents any external expansion. In the small child and infant, the cricoid ring has the smallest diameter in the larynx and trachea and is subject to maximal trauma during intubation.

If a post-extubation edema does not respond to routine measures, subglottic edema must be assumed — this is a potentially life-threatening problem. The response of subglottic edema to intravenous steroid therapy is controversial. However, most would agree it should be administered. The definitive therapy is reestablishment of an artificial airway.

Ulceration of Tracheal Mucosa

Next to hoarseness, sore throat, and edema of the glottis, the most common complication following endotracheal extubation is ulceration of the tracheal mucosa. This usually occurs at the site of the cuff or on the anterior wall where the tip of the tube has abraded the epithelium. Pain with coughing is common; tracheitis is not uncommon; hemoptysis is rare. Conservative therapy consisting of aerosol and reassurance is adequate; sequelae are rare.

Vocal Cord Ulceration, Granuloma, and Polyp

Vocal cord ulceration, granuloma, or polyp is suspected when hoarseness persists for more than a week. The lesions are usually unilateral and are believed to be caused by (1) intubation trauma; (2) tubes that fit tight in the glottis; (3) protracted cough; (4) excessive movement of the tube, head, or neck during intubation; and (5) allergic reactions to the tube or lubricant. The diagnosis is readily made by indirect visualization of the glottis. The incidence is virtually unknown. The therapy is surgical excision.[268]

Vocal Cord Paralysis

Vocal cord paralysis is another lesion of unknown frequency. *Unilateral cord paralysis* occurs with surgical intervention in the neck and upper chest secondary to recurrent laryngeal nerve damage. *Bilateral cord paralysis* has been reported following endotracheal intubation and many causative factors have been suggested, including the possibility of ethylene oxide sterilization. At the present time the relationship between endotracheal intubation and vocal cord paralysis is unknown! Respiratory care practitioners must accept the fact that some relationship may exist; however, the incidence and causative factors are not clear.[220]

Laryngotracheal Web

Necrotic tissue at the glottic or subglottic level can lead to fibrin formation which combines with cellular debris and secretion to form a "membrane" or "web." These membranes may occupy as much as two thirds of the opening between the vocal cords or subglottic lumen before obstructive phenomena become clinically manifest. The onset of ventilatory difficulty is usually sudden because of a portion of the membrane freeing itself and *totally* obstructing the airway.[219]

The treatment is simple and successful when recognized early — aspirate the web with a suction catheter. There are some rare circumstances in which surgical removal may be necessary, but in almost all cases aspiration of the web will cure the condition.

Laryngeal webs are most often seen 4 to 5 days after tracheal extubation, but they have been reported to occur as late as 2 months to 2 years post-extubation. When *sudden* airway obstruction occurs several days following extubation, this phenomenon should be suspected. The membrane is often seen by direct visualization during the process of re-intubation. Aspiration is essential because the web may obstruct an endotracheal tube or be pushed into a main stem bronchus.

Post-extubation Tracheal Stenosis

Tracheal stenosis is a lesion that occurs from 1 week to 2 years following endotracheal intubation or tracheostomy. It is a "scarring" of the trachea caused by the healing process that results in stricture of the airway. A concomitant problem is *tracheal malacia*—the destruction of tracheal cartilage—resulting in collapsing of the trachea during inspiration. Malacia and stenosis often occur together. Stenosis often occurs alone; malacia seldom occurs alone except in infants.

Twenty years ago, post-extubation tracheal stenosis was rarely a problem since few patients survived ventilator care. This fact provides the proper perspective through which this problem must be viewed. Tracheal stenosis is a real and serious complication of tracheal intubation; everything possible must be done to decrease its incidence and severity. However, tracheal stenosis is *never* a contraindication for intubating or using cuffs on artificial airways when indicated for proper airway care!

Much of the literature concerning post-extubation tracheal stenosis is confusing, controversial, and misleading. Although the authors have attempted to present the most universally accepted viewpoints on this subject, the controversy is so vast, and the facts so scanty, that personal opinions based on clinical experience are difficult to avoid. We encourage the reader to make liberal use of the reference material. However, we feel confident that the following presentation is a clinically useful and dependable guideline for the respiratory care practitioner.

Incidence

The incidence of tracheal stenosis following tracheostomy with *uncuffed* tubes has been reported to be less than 2%;[230] with *cuffed* tubes the incidence has been reported in the range of 5%.[269-272] The real value of these statistics is to establish that tracheal stenosis is a significant complication of endotracheal or tracheostomy procedures with or without cuffs.

The significant lesions resulting from ventilator support through cuffed tubes are usually found a few centimeters below the stoma (at the cuff site). In patients receiving mechanical support of ventilation with cuffed tracheal tubes, studies report an incidence of tracheal stenosis in the range of 1–20%.[273] This variability is due to the different methods used to make the diagnosis. In studies where the criteria were the symptomatic presentation of dyspnea, loss of exercise tolerance, stridor, and recurrent pulmonary infection, the incidence was significantly lower than in prospective studies utilizing techniques such as laminagrams, bronchograms, and bronchoscopy.[274] A tracheal obstruction of less than 50% seldom results in clinical symptoms.[274] In our experience, the incidence of *symptomatic* tracheal stenosis requiring surgical repair is approximately 0.5% to 2% in patients receiving ventilator support with cuffed tubes.

Causal Factors

The incidence of significant tracheal stenosis at the site of the tracheostomy *stoma* seems to be less related to respiratory care factors than cuff site stenosis.[275] Although the authors do not wish to understate the importance of stenosis at the stomal site, it is recognized that a great responsibility for decreasing that incidence belongs to the surgeon.[276] Respiratory care factors which may contribute to stoma complications are too large a tube, excessive movement, and trauma from the tube. It has been shown that regardless of the type of incision made in the trachea, the ultimate loss of cartilage at the stoma is directly proportional to the diameter of the tracheostomy tube employed.[277]

The respiratory care practitioner must be primarily concerned with those factors involved in the prevention of tracheal stenosis at the site of the cuff. It appears there are six factors that play a significant role in the incidence of post-extubation tracheal stenosis at the site of the cuff: (1) cuff pressure; (2) time; (3) perfusion; (4) infection; (5) movement; and (6) toxicity.

1. *Cuff pressure* is the factor that has received the most attention in recent years.[278] The realization that cuff pressures are significant in tracheal stenosis has led to a variety of cuffs designed to decrease the pressure exerted on the tracheal mucosa.

2. *Time* has been *assumed* to be a factor. It seems intuitively correct that the longer a foreign body exists within the trachea, the higher would be the incidence of complications. There is evidence to support the assumption that the incidence of tracheal stenosis increases with time over the first several days;[279] however, in our opinion, there is a questionable relationship between the severity of tracheal damage and the duration of tracheal intubation.[275]

3. *Perfusion,* or circulatory instability, is common in critically ill patients needing mechanical support of ventilation. Up to 60% of patients receiving artificial airways and mechanical support of ventilation have significant episodes of hypoperfusion while cuffs are inflated. It is believed that hypoperfusion states are extremely significant in causing damage to the tracheal mucosa at the site of cuff inflation.[272, 273]

4. *Infection* has been postulated as a significant etiologic factor in tracheal stenosis.[277, 280] *Contamination* of the trachea by bacterial colonization is unavoidable; actual tracheal infection is uncommon with proper care. Tracheal contamination does *not* play a significant role in the etiology of tracheal stenosis, whereas infection is a well-documented contributor to the incidence of tracheal stenosis.[275]

5. *Movement,* weight, or tension on the tracheostomy or endotracheal tube may lead to higher incidences of stenosis. This is undoubtedly due to (1) increased tissue pressure on the stoma; (2) increased movement of the cuff; and (3) irritation to the tracheal mucosa. The role that movements of the vocal cords and trachea play in increasing post-extubation sequelae both in the spontaneously breathing and ventilator patient is not exactly known, but it has been documented that patients who are well sedated and do not resist the ventilator are less likely to suffer such damage.[281] The use of lightweight, swivel-type connectors and tubing for the respiratory care equipment is mandatory. Patient movement must be accomplished smoothly to avoid excessive tugging on the tracheostomy or endotracheal tube.

6. *Toxicity* from chemical irritation of tube material has been named as an aggravating factor, particularly following ethylene oxide sterilization. If this oxidizing agent is not completely aerated from polyvinyl plastics, tissue toxicity may result. Prospective studies using ethylene oxide sterilization techniques *with proper aeration* have revealed an absence of toxicity to tracheal tissue.[275] Allergic reactions are rare, but must be considered a type of toxic reaction.

Pathophysiology of Tracheal Wall Pressure

The intra-arterial pressure in blood vessels within the adult tracheal wall is approximately 30 mm Hg (42 cm of water).[267, 277] The venous end of the capillary bed has a perfusing pressure of approximately 18 mm Hg (24 cm of water).[282] These pressures are similar to airway pressures normally reached during positive-pressure ventilation. Thus, it is possible that during positive-pressure inspiration, the airway pressure may impede venous and/or arterial mucosal blood flow. Certainly, *any cuff pressures that exceed these tracheal mucosal circulating pressures will interrupt mucosal blood flow!*

In the normal adult it is reasonable to conclude that (1) pressures on the tracheal wall in excess of 30 mm Hg will completely stop arterial-capillary blood flow; (2) tracheal wall pressures in excess of 18 mm Hg will cause venous flow obstruction; and (3) tracheal wall pressures in excess of 5 mm Hg will cause lymphatic flow obstruction. Lymphatic flow obstruction will cause *edema;* venous flow obstruction will cause congestion; and arterial flow obstruction will cause ischemia.

The ideal cuff pressure would permit sealing of the airway during positive-pressure ventilation at the lowest possible tracheal wall pressure. It seems reasonable to assume that if cuff pressures do not exceed 15 mm Hg (21 cm of water), arterial and venous flow would be present throughout the ventilatory cycle. Pressures below 5 mm Hg (7 cm water) would allow even lymphatic flow and avoid edema, Obviously, any condition decreasing the perfusion state will potentially embarrass blood flow to the tracheal mucosa.

Numerous attempts have been made to document the day-to-day changes that occur in the tracheal mucosa when subjected to increased pressures.[271, 274, 277, 278, 283] These studies are primarily in dogs, and there is question as to how applicable the findings are to man. We believe that a reasonable correlation can be made by combining the dog study findings with those observed in man through the fiberoptic bronchoscope. With the subject on positive pressure, assuming a normal perfusion state, an uninfected trachea, and cuff pressures in excess of 50 mm Hg, the following events usually occur: (1) Within 24 hours, mucosal edema and erythema (redness) can be seen with varying degrees of interrupted capillary blood flow. This edema and congestion appear uniform throughout the mucosal area subjected to the cuff pressure. (2) Within 48 hours, there are areas of epithelial ischemia and necrosis. This necrosis is spotty and rarely causes circumferential lesions at this time. (3) Within 72 hours, there are spotty patches of sloughed mucosa resulting in denuded submucosa and/or cartilage. This sloughing is usually not circumferential. (4) Within 5 days, there is evidence of necrotic cartilage—again this is usually not circumferential.

This description is general and the authors have exercised significant "poetic license"; however, the description is useful as a clinical guideline and is in agreement with most of the literature. The essential fact to understand is *the entire process is completely reversible!* There seems to be no correlation between the extent of injury and repair without sequelae. The only consistent correlation is that when a circumferential sloughing of mucosa exists, the incidence of tracheal stenosis is nearly 100%.[274, 275, 277] Short of circumferential lesions, however, there is no apparent correlation between the degree of observed tracheal mucosal damage and tracheal stenosis. Again, we must emphasize that these generalities are true in the absence of perfusion problems and infection with tracheal wall pressures over 50 mm Hg.

The electron microscope has allowed studies of mucosal damage from cuffs and tubes. Regardless of minimal pressures, cilia are damaged within 2 hours and take up to 1 week to regenerate.[267] Therefore, we must not take false security in knowing cuff pressures are low—damage occurs as long as the foreign body is present.

Summary

The pathophysiology of tracheal wall changes from pressure are greatly dependent upon the cuff pressures, the perfusion state, the presence or absence of infection, among other predisposing factors. We have observed significant damage to tracheal epithelium within 3 days even with cuff pressures limited to 20 mm Hg. The degree of severity of observed damage seems to have no *direct* correlation with the incidence or severity of tracheal stenosis, except when circumferential necrosis is present. Incidence of permanent damage greatly increases with (1) suboptimal airway care; (2) cuff pressures above 20 mm Hg; (3) tracheal infection; and (4) hypotension.

Intermittent deflation of cuffs for 3–5 minutes has no proved advantage as far as mucosal damage is concerned. Routine deflation and inflation tend to lead to careless reinflation technique and possible higher cuff pressures.

Physics of Tracheal Cuffs

A positive-pressure tracheal cuff is the same as a balloon. As a volume of air is introduced into the cuff, the elastic forces of the balloon will be overcome and the cuff will expand. Intracuff pressures will

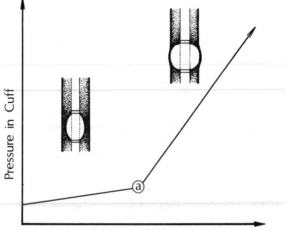

Fig 17–2. — Cuff pressures in relation to cuff volume. The drawings represent standard high-pressure cuffs. Point *a* represents (1) point where standard high-pressure cuffs make contact with the tracheal wall or (2) the point where high residual volume cuffs become fully distended and are in contact with tracheal wall.

increase slowly as the volume is increased, until the sides of the cuff touch the tracheal wall. At this point, an additional volume of air will cause a sharp rise in the cuff pressure. Thus, in standard high-pressure cuffs, as soon as the small portion of the cuff touches the sides of the tracheal wall, the pressure will increase sharply for even a small increase in volume (Fig 17–2).

In *high residual volume cuffs,* the effects of the elastic forces are extremely low because the material is essentially "stretched out." They are designed so that even when they are inflated and in contact with the tracheal wall, in most cases they will still be somewhat wrinkled and not fully distended. Under these circumstances, the intracuff pressure is equal to the cuff-to-tracheal wall pressure.[284] This means that for an increase in volume, there will be a small increase in pressure. However, it must be understood that if this cuff becomes completely distended, it may have the same exponential rise in cuff-to-tracheal wall pressure as the high-pressure balloons.[283, 285]

These physical facts dictate that it is far better to have a high residual volume cuff than a low residual volume cuff. It is generally agreed that it would be optimal to have a high residual volume cuff that could maintain an adequate seal at a resting tracheal mucosal pressure of 15 mm Hg.[286] In the authors' opinion, it would be ideal to maintain an adequate seal at less than 5 mm Hg cuff-to-tracheal wall pressure.

Low Residual Volume Cuff

The narrow, low residual volume cuff was standard in respiratory care until a few years ago. Made of latex or plastic, its characteristics are such that high intracuff pressures (at times exceeding 300 mm Hg) are the rule.[292] Cuff-to-tracheal wall pressures will exceed safe limits by virtue of the low residual volume. Tracheal wall contact is quite narrow, and small increments of air added after tracheal wall contact is made cause sharp increases in pressure at the tracheal contact area.

Although still commonly used in emergency rooms and operating rooms, the use of low residual volume cuffs is fading in respiratory care because they can be tolerated for only brief periods of time before causing significant tracheal damage.[287] These low residual volume cuffs are commonly referred to as *high-pressure cuffs. THEY HAVE NO PLACE IN MODERN RESPIRATORY CARE.*

High Residual Volume Cuffs

High residual volume cuffs are large cuffs made of pliable material which tends to inflate evenly and conform to the tracheal contour. Contact is made with a significantly large area of trachea. When properly used, these cuffs produce significantly less tracheal wall pressure than the low residual volume cuffs. They have become known as *low-pressure cuffs.*

"Floppy Cuff"

The *floppy cuff* is typical of a high residual volume cuff. It is cylindrical in shape and large in diameter. Made of latex, it has an unstretched (residual) volume of 12 ml to 15 ml. This type of cuff has been successfully modified to disposable tubes of excellent quality.

Cuff Size

A cuff diameter too small to drape freely on the tracheal wall will assume the characteristics of a high-pressure cuff. A useful rule of thumb is that if the intracuff pressure necessary for no-leak ventilation exceeds 20 mm Hg (measured during exhalation), the cuff is too small.[286]

Tracheal Dilatation

A common problem in *all* air blown cuffs is the phenomenon of "chasing the trachea" which is seen with *positive-pressure no-leak ventilation.* This occurs because a cuff inflated to seal during peak inspiratory airway pressure is overinflated during the exhalation phase. This "overinflation" results in tracheal dilatation. Maintenance of no-leak ventilation then requires the addition of another increment of air to the cuff. As the cycle repeats itself, tracheal dilatation progresses.[288] The problem of tracheal dilatation is not as significant in spontaneous breathing patients because intratracheal pressure changes are minor.

The clinical significance of tracheal dilatation with no-leak positive-pressure ventilation is not known. It has been suggested that if dilatation is sufficiently prolonged, the result will be lack of tracheal wall tone with loss of sealing effectiveness. This may help account for the phenomenon of aspiration in the presence of cuffed tracheostomy tubes. Tracheal dilatation may lead to esophageal compression, which may contribute to the incidence of aspiration, difficulty in swallowing, and ulcerations caused by nasogastric tubes.[289] It would seem reasonable that tracheal perforation at the cuff site would be preceded by dilatation or ballooning of the trachea.

Obstruction

Another danger peculiar to some high residual volume cuffs is total airway obstruction that occurs if the cuff "balloons" over the lumen (See Fig 16–2). A cough maneuver which partially ejects the tube while the cuff remains stationary may be sufficient to produce lumen occlusion. Overinflation may also result in a similar mishap.

Prestretched Cuffs

Prestretched cuffs are of historical interest only. Originally this was a method of converting a standard plastic high-pressure cuff to a high residual volume cuff.[290] There were numerous problems involved with the procedure.[291] It is no longer necessary to prestretch cuffs, since most plastic tubes are now commercially available with a high residual volume cuff.

The Shiley Tube

The Shiley tracheostomy tube became popular primarily because of features such as disposability, inner cannula, and swivel adapter. The new cuff is of thinner material and has a control pressure valve. This new cuff appears to be a high residual volume, low-pressure cuff.

The Kamen-Wilkinson Fome Cuff

The Kamen-Wilkinson Fome Cuff utilizes an entirely new concept. A large diameter, high residual volume cuff is composed of polyurethane foam covered by a silicone sheath. When suction is applied to the pilot port, the foam contracts. When the negative pressure is released, the cuff expands until stopped by the tracheal wall. The pilot port remains open to the atmosphere; therefore, the intracuff pressure is ambient.[292]

The degree of expansion of the foam determines the mean cuff-to-tracheal wall pressure. The more the foam is expanded, the lower will be the tracheal wall pressure; as the foam is compressed, the pressure increases. The foam must be markedly compressed to exert more than 25 mm Hg tracheal wall pressure.[293]

The open pilot port allows alternate compression and expansion of the foam during the ventilatory cycle. Therefore, when used properly, tracheal dilatation is negligible.[288] No-leak ventilation and aspiration protection can be accomplished with the proper size tube in the trachea. The advantages of the silicone material and the foam cuff make this an extremely promising concept, since the least damage to glottic and tracheal wall structures should result.

The Lanz Tube

The Lanz tube is also a recent innovation in artificial airways. It has a high residual volume, cylindrically shaped cuff with a "pressure regulating system" controlled by a specially designed external balloon reservoir and a pressure-regulating valve. After air is injected into the external pressure-regulating valve and balloon reservoir, the internal pressure of the reservoir and the cuff are theoretically equal. When used properly, the external reservoir is designed to achieve a pressure of 22 mm Hg.[294] It is claimed that large volumes of air may be injected into the reservoir without exceeding this pressure.[295] The valve system between the reservoir and cuff allows air to enter the cuff with ease, and if the syringe is left in the valve, air can go from the cuff to the reservoir freely. However, when the syringe is removed, it is more difficult for cuff air to re-enter the reservoir.

As the airway and cuff dilate during the inspiratory phase of IPPV, air tends to move from the reservoir to the dilated cuff. On expiration, the cuff may be unable to empty completely that increment which entered during inspiration. This repetitive process may eventually lead to tracheal dilatation.[288]

Other Disposable Tubes

In recent years a significant number of disposable endotracheal tubes have been developed with high residual volume, low-pressure cuffs. This means that the respiratory care practitioner now has the advantage of utilizing disposable artificial airways with the preferred type of cuff to prevent tracheal damage.

Summary

We have attempted to present an accurate review of the literature in conjunction with our own clinical observations. The authors recommend that respiratory care practitioners read the joint statement of investigators, inventors, and manufacturers on *Recommended Performance Specifications of Cuffed Endotracheal and Tracheostomy Tubes*. This paper is an outgrowth of a two-day symposium held for this purpose.[296]

SECTION V

CLINICAL ASSESSMENT OF ACUTE RESPIRATORY FAILURE

18 • DEFINING ACUTE RESPIRATORY FAILURE

Defining Respiratory Failure

RESPIRATION HAS BEEN DEFINED for almost one hundred years as the movement of gas molecules across permeable membranes.[297] The single cell animal very simply acquires oxygen from the environment and expels the carbon dioxide metabolite. In this organism the entire process of respiration requires nothing more than simple diffusion across the cell membrane. In man, respiration depends upon the *cardiopulmonary system* — two distinct capillary beds interfaced with the pulmonary and cardiovascular systems. This cardiopulmonary system is responsible not only for ensuring the prime requisite of cellular metabolism — oxygenation, but also for the moment-to-moment control of metabolite excretion (carbon dioxide) and, thereby, acid-base balance.

Homeostasis is the capability of physiologic systems to maintain internal stability by altering their responses to any situation or stimulus tending to disturb their normal condition or function. Thus, *cardiopulmonary homeostasis* would depend upon the ability of its components to alter their function when presented with disease processes tending to disturb normal functioning. *Adequate respiration in man depends upon the ability of the cardiopulmonary system to respond to stress by increasing its output and thus its work.*

An operational definition of organ failure is "the failure of an organ system to meet the metabolic demands placed upon it by the organism." In keeping with this definition, heart failure may be considered the failure of the heart to meet the metabolic demands of the body with respect to tissue perfusion. This concept makes no reference to the volume of cardiac output; that is, nothing is stated as to whether the heart is pumping more blood, less blood, or the normal amount of blood. In fact, high-output cardiac failure is not only possible, but quite common.

In terms of respiration, failure denotes the inability of the cardiopulmonary system to maintain adequate homeostasis. Although respiration may fail to meet metabolic demands at the tissue as well as the pulmonary level, tradition and practicality dictate that the term respiratory failure in clinical parlance refers to *failure of adequate gas exchange at the pulmonary level.* Failure of adequate gas exchange at the tissue level is commonly referred to as "hypoperfusion" or "shock." Thus, we shall limit the definition of respiratory failure to *the inability of the cardiopulmonary system to meet metabolic demands at the pulmonary level.*

Defining Acute Respiratory Failure

The cardiopulmonary system possesses a substantial ability to adjust to distinctly "abnormal" internal conditions if the change from normal is gradual. We refer to such "compensated" homeostatic states as *chronic.* Cardiopulmonary disease that is progressive and insidious will eventually result in "chronic respiratory failure." This means that although the system is unable to maintain "normal conditions," the "abnormal" state has been compensated and the result is an adequate milieu to sustain life.

Whenever a cardiopulmonary disease develops rapidly or whenever the cardiopulmonary system is incapable of compensating, the result is a life-threatening respiratory abnormality. *Acute respiratory failure denotes a direct life-threatening inability of the cardiopulmonary system to maintain adequate gas exchange at the pulmonary level.*[201]

Defining Acute Respiratory Care

The acutely decompensating cardiopulmonary system will ultimately result in the organism's death unless gas exchange is supported. The organism that is unable to maintain adequate vital organ function without supportive therapy is termed "critically ill."[56] *Acute respiratory care is the discipline devoted to the maintenance of adequate gas exchange through support of the cardiopulmonary system.*[67, 346] Thus, application of acute respiratory care depends upon a diagnosis of the existence of acute respiratory failure or the threat of impending acute respiratory failure (acute respiratory insufficiency).

Defining Acute Respiratory Insufficiency

When gas exchange is maintained at an adequate or minimally acceptable level at the expense of a significant increase in cardiopulmonary work, the increased work becomes obvious to the clinician even though acute respiratory failure is not present. The homeostatic balance is potentially threatened since the cardiopulmonary system cannot increase its work indefinitely. *Acute respiratory insufficiency* is the circumstance in which gas exchange is maintained at an acceptable level only at the expense of significantly increased work of the cardiopulmonary system.[298] The clinical significance of acute respiratory insufficiency is that acute respiratory *failure* will ensue when the cardiopulmonary system becomes incapable of maintaining the increased work.

Diagnosing Acute Respiratory Failure

Well-established acute respiratory failure is neither subtle nor difficult to diagnose. The patient can best be described as well into the process of dying! The therapy for such an extreme state of acute respiratory failure is *resuscitation*—the process of attempting to restore a decompensated cardiopulmonary system to an acceptable level of function. Resuscitation in well-established acute respiratory failure seldom leads to a successful outcome. Thus, intervention with supportive measures prior to the total collapse of cardiopulmonary homeostasis has become an important aspect of acute respiratory care.

When acute respiratory failure is developing, the diagnosis is best made by serial measurement of arterial blood gases. Severe oxygen deficit (hypoxemia), significant decreases in alveolar ventilation (increased arterial P_{CO_2}'s) in conjunction with decreased pH's, or a combination of both oxygen and carbon dioxide gas exchange abnormalities ultimately confirms the diagnosis of acute respiratory failure.[347] The need to differentiate the particular gas exchange problem so that the appropriate supportive measures may be instituted necessitates separating ventilatory, oxygenation, and acid-base imbalances.[35]

An even greater challenge to the clinician is to quantitate the degree of acute respiratory insufficiency. In physiologic terms, the challenge is assessment of the remaining cardiopulmonary reserves so that a judgment can be made as to when the stress may initiate cardiopulmonary decompensation. In other words, as important as the actual diagnosis of acute respiratory failure may be, the ability to properly assess *cardiopulmonary reserves* is of even greater importance. Indeed, the clinical diagnosis of acute respiratory failure or insufficiency depends upon appropriate assessment of cardiopulmonary reserves.

19 • ASSESSMENT OF CARDIOPULMONARY RESERVES

ACUTE RESPIRATORY FAILURE is related to the severity of disease *and* the inadequacy of cardiopulmonary reserves. Therefore, the decision to intervene with supportive care must be based on an evaluation of the disease process in relation to the *reserves* of the cardiopulmonary system. The clinician must answer the question: How capable is this patient's cardiopulmonary system of maintaining adequate function while challenged by the present or anticipated physiologic stress? The respiratory care practitioner may readily assist in the assessment of cardiopulmonary reserves by evaluating three entities at the bedside: (1) pulmonary reserve; (2) cardiovascular reserve; and (3) gas exchange capability. The entire scope of evaluation is listed in Table 19–1.

Pulmonary Reserve

Ventilation is defined as the movement of gases in and out of the pulmonary tree in a cyclic fashion.[41] The purpose is to present fresh gas to alveoli for molecular exchange with pulmonary blood followed by removal of that gas from the alveoli. This to-and-fro movement of gas within the pulmonary tree is reflected by spirometric pulmonary function testing. These measurements may be used to grossly estimate the *efficiency* of ventilation. The clinical challenge is not limited to assessment of ventilatory efficiency at the time of measurement, but also requires an assessment of the capability to maintain efficient ventilation in the presence of acute physiologic stress (disease).

Bedside evaluation of pulmonary reserve involves (1) clinical observation of the patient's spontaneous ventilatory pattern, plus (2) appropriate interpretation of two spirometric measurements—vital capacity and FEV_1.

The Ventilatory Pattern

The ventilatory pattern is composed of (1) a tidal volume; (2) a ventilatory rate; and (3) an inspiratory-to-expiratory (I : E) ratio.

302

TABLE 19-1.—ASSESSMENT OF CARDIOPULMONARY RESERVE

Pulmonary Reserve	Cardiovascular Reserve
I. Clinical observation	I. Non-invasive
II. Ventilatory pattern	A. ECG
A. Tidal volume	B. Blood pressure
B. Rate	C. Clinical observation
C. I:E ratio	D. Perfusion
III. Vital capacity	II. Invasive
IV. FEV$_1$	A. Cardiac output
V. Intrapulmonary shunt	B. A-V$_{O_2}$ difference
VI. Deadspace ventilation	C. Preload
	D. Afterload
	III. Contractility status

Respiration

I. Alveolar ventilation
II. Acid-base
III. Oxygenation
   A. Arterial P$_{O_2}$
   B. Mixed venous P$_{O_2}$

Tidal volume is defined as the air breathed in or out of the airway during the breathing process. Measurement of tidal volume is a simple procedure (described in Chapter 5); however, most clinicians fail to make the measurement because they falsely assume that they can accurately estimate air movement. It is mandatory that tidal volume *measurements* be carried out with critically ill patients. Although quantitative tidal volume measurement is important, *the simple observation of the ease with which the patient maintains that tidal volume* is equally essential; i.e., an estimation of the energy being expended to breathe is as important as the quantitative measurement itself.

A normal predicted tidal volume is 6–7 ml/kg (3–4 ml/lb) of ideal body weight. In the average adult, tidal volumes of less than 300 ml (*hypopnea*) or greater than 700 ml (*hyperpnea*) are abnormal and require further evaluation, especially when oxygen therapy is administered (see Chapter 7).

Ventilatory rate should be counted for 1 full minute. The normal adult ventilatory rate is 12–18 times per minute. Ventilatory rates above normal are termed *tachypnea;* rates below normal are termed *bradypnea.*

Minute volume (MV) is the product of exhaled tidal volumes multiplied by the ventilatory rate. This calculation is important in considering oxygen therapy and estimating work of breathing.

The *I:E ratio* refers to the time relationship between inhalation and exhalation. Normally the relationship is approximately 1:2; i.e., the time for exhalation is twice as long as that for inhalation. Inspiratory time may significantly affect the delivery of fresh gases to the alveoli. Expiratory time may significantly alter the degree to which the elastic lung and chest wall forces interact with airway dynamics to accomplish movement of gas out of the alveoli. *Tachypnea primarily encroaches upon expiratory time.* Since obstructive pulmonary disease requires longer expiratory times, tachypnea is extremely detrimental. *Irregular ventilatory patterns* are abnormal and usually reflect C.N.S. or myocardial malfunction. These may be considered "forerunners" of worse things to come.

Vital Capacity

The interrelationships of vital capacity, ventilatory pattern, and the work of breathing were discussed in Chapters 3 and 5. These principles can be summarized as follows: (1) The work of breathing is increased as the portion of the vital capacity utilized for tidal volume increases. Thus, *an acutely decreased vital capacity reflects a decreased ventilatory reserve.* (2) Under these conditions, the energy expended in increasing ventilatory rate is less than the energy required to increase tidal volume. (3) The organism will choose the ventilatory pattern that produces the necessary minute ventilation at the *least* expenditure of energy. Thus, when faced with decreased ventilatory reserve, the organism generally chooses to increase the ventilatory rate and decrease the tidal volume. This provides the needed minute volume for the least expenditure of energy.

Bedside assessment of ventilatory reserve is most reliably reflected in the *forced* vital capacity measurement. For over twenty years forced vital capacity has been measured in critically ill patients, and the "test of time" has produced the following reliable guideline: *A previously healthy adult requires a minimal vital capacity of 15 ml/kg to assure an effective cough and to adequately deep breathe.* When an acutely ill patient is unable to meet this minimal vital capacity requirement, he must be considered *limited* in his capability to maintain an undiseased pulmonary system; i.e., there exists a great likelihood for retained secretions, atelectasis, and pneumonia.[44] Of course, a vital capacity above 15 ml/kg does *not* unequivocally guarantee the maintenance of clear lungs. Another useful guideline is that a previously healthy adult with a vital capacity acutely less than 10 ml/kg *may not* be able to spontaneously maintain adequate ventilation for a prolonged period.

Remember that a bedside vital capacity measurement is prone to error because both a tight airway seal and the patient's cooperation are required. Even with cooperative patients, the measurements may vary according to the "forcefulness" with which the procedure is imposed. However, all errors will give values *less* than the actual, since patients can never provide a vital capacity greater than their true vital capacity.

Negative Inspiratory Force (NIF)

In patients who are unresponsive, comatose, or obtunded, the concept of *negative inspiratory force* was devised to estimate ventilatory reserve.[76] The NIF maneuver has been described in Chapter 5. In normal, healthy individuals, the NIF is well in excess of negative 80 cm of water within 10 seconds.

The NIF measurement can be clinically useful as long as its limitations are recognized and the results are not misinterpreted. Clinical experience has demonstrated that an individual who can generate an NIF of *negative 20 cm H_2O within 20 seconds* can be assumed to have a vital capacity of 15 ml/kg or greater. In other words, a negative inspiratory force of better than negative 20 cm H_2O within 20 seconds means that the *minimum* vital capacity requirements for maintaining adequate ventilation over a prolonged period of time are most likely present. The measurement may be used for no more than this! Since this is a static measurement, any element of preexisting lung disease such as increased resistance, decreased compliance, or actual loss of lung volume makes the measurement even more unreliable.

FEV₁

The measurement of forced expiratory volumes has been discussed in Chapter 3. A decrease in the FEV_1 generally reflects a significant increase in airway resistance. This is not an appropriate test for detection of *early* or subtle small airway disease.[4] The very fact that this measurement reveals only significant clinical disease is its greatest asset in respiratory care. A patient with an abnormal FEV_1 will require significant energy expenditure to increase ventilation in response to stress. The pulmonary physiologist prefers to consider FEV_1 in terms of the patient's *predicted* ability to expire gas in the first second. In respiratory care, the FEV_1 is expressed as a percentage of the patient's *actual* forced vital capacity; this is believed to be more reflective of the patient's reserves that are available to meet stress. A %FEV_1/FVC of less than 50% is generally interpreted to reflect airway resistance of sufficient magnitude to significantly diminish ventilatory reserve (see Chapter 31).

Cardiovascular Reserve

Traditionally, the cardiovascular system has been primarily supported by pharmacologic means. In spite of the technical advances of cardiac assist devices and membrane oxygenators, the application of these devices in most patients has not provided improved survival or decreased morbidity. Therefore, *primary* cardiovascular support in critical care still rests on pharmacology, fluid therapy, and proper acid-base balance. In many circumstances, significant stabilization of cardiovascular function is accomplished by relieving the patient of the work of breathing and by augmenting his pulmonary gas exchange. Oxygenation techniques and mechanical support of ventilation may often be applied primarily to aid and maintain cardiovascular function.

The respiratory care practitioner must be able to evaluate the cardiovascular system, since it is impossible to support the pulmonary system appropriately without an appreciation of cardiovascular function and reserve.[56] Often, the primary limitation to mechanical support of the pulmonary system is embarrassment of the cardiovascular system.

Minimal bedside evaluation of cardiovascular reserve depends upon a clinical assessment of (1) heart rate; (2) blood pressure; (3) the heart as a pump; and (4) perfusion.

Heart Rate and Rhythm

An acceptable heart rate and rhythm are essential for proper cardiovascular functioning (see Chapter 2). A rate that is too rapid will not allow adequate filling of the ventricles and, therefore, the cardiac output will diminish. In addition, rapid heart rates (shorter diastolic time periods) mean less time for effective coronary blood flow and increased myocardial oxygen consumption. It is generally agreed that adult heart rates above 140 per minute (160–180 in young, healthy persons) embarrass adequate mechanical function. Heart rates below 50 per minute are also generally detrimental. An adult heart rate above 100 is termed *tachycardia;* a rate below 50 is termed *bradycardia.* Rhythm irregularities represent potential interference with mechanical function and inadequate cardiac output. Therefore, constant evaluation of the ECG monitor is essential to assure that there are an acceptable heart rate and rhythm.

Blood Pressure

Blood pressure has been discussed in Chapter 2. The basic relationship of pressure being equal to flow times resistance ($P = F \times R$) must be kept in mind since an increase in blood pressure can be the result of increased peripheral vascular resistance as well as an increased cardiac output. It must be realized that *blood flow and tissue perfusion maintain life;* a blood pressure measurement does not always reflect flow and tissue perfusion in the critically ill.

The Heart as a Pump

This function of the heart must be evaluated in the critically ill. Such evaluation depends on an assessment of (1) myocardial contractility; (2) ventricular preload; and (3) ventricular afterload. These factors are discussed in detail in Section VII.

Perfusion

Perfusion is primarily assessed by clinical observation: (1) *Urine output* is a guide to the adequacy of renal perfusion. The kidney cannot produce urine if there is inadequate perfusion; however, the lack of urine output may reflect primary kidney malfunction and not perfusion deficit. (2) *Skin* that is warm and dry in the extremities is indicative of sufficient total body perfusion. Cold and clammy extremities are early general indicators of a precarious and perhaps insufficient general perfusion status. (3) *Capillary fill* (a gross approximation of tissue perfusion) is evaluated by pressing down on the nail bed and making it blanch. Upon release there should be immediate "filling," with a reddish pink appearance. (4) *Sensorium* may be a reflector of perfusion. The cerebral brain function (consciousness) is extremely sensitive to a decrease in perfusion (oxygenation). A change in the state of consciousness (obtundation, confusion, agitation) occurs with a decrease in cerebral perfusion. (5) Characterization of *peripheral pulses* may be helpful. In times of extreme physiologic stress, muscle and skin are less well perfused than vital tissues. Therefore, arteries such as radials, dorsalis pedis, and posterior tibials are often weak and thready, and the tissues normally perfused by these vessels are cold, blanched, and often clammy.

Poor peripheral perfusion is a clinical sign that should suggest the probability of poor total body perfusion; however, one must not be misled by assuming that because the skin is well perfused, vital organs are being adequately perfused.

The essentials of adequate tissue perfusion are related not only to blood volume but to adequate red cells (hemoglobin) and oxygen content. An appropriate amount of protein is necessary to assure an adequate colloid osmotic pressure (COP) (see Chapter 29). Serum electrolytes must be maintained within reasonable balance for adequate cellular functioning. Acid-base balance is important in vascular function since acidemia causes profound changes in the vascular system secondary to both central and peripheral effects. These changes affect arteriolar distribution of blood as well as the microcirculation itself.

Gas Exchange – Respiration

The final step in the clinical evaluation of cardiopulmonary reserves is to assess the status of gas exchange, both at the systemic and pulmonary levels.

Alveolar Ventilation

Alveolar ventilation is defined as that portion of the minute ventilation that undergoes blood-gas exchange, i.e., that portion of ventilation that respires.[35] Assuming a constant metabolic rate (and therefore a constant carbon dioxide addition to the venous blood), the arterial carbon dioxide tension ($PaCO_2$) is a direct reflection of the adequacy of pulmonary gas exchange in relation to blood flow. Based on this logic, the arterial PCO_2 may be considered a reflection of the adequacy of alveolar (physiologic) ventilation. (1) An arterial PCO_2 below 30 mm Hg is considered clinically significant alveolar hyperventilation in the critically ill. Alveolar hyperventilation is secondary to either a need for better oxygenation, a response to metabolic acidosis, or a malfunction of the C.N.S.[35] (2) An arterial PCO_2 above 50 mm Hg is considered a significant alveolar hypoventilation reflecting inadequate alveolar ventilation. This is defined as ventilatory failure (respiratory acidosis).[35] (3) An arterial PCO_2 within the 30–50 mm Hg range is considered an *adequate* clinical ventilatory state in the critically ill patient.[35]

Deadspace Ventilation

Deadspace ventilation is that portion of total ventilation that does not undergo molecular gas exchange with blood, i.e., the portion of ventilation that does *not* respire. Increased deadspace ventilation represents the need for increased work of breathing if adequate alveolar ventilation is to be maintained. At a basal metabolic rate, a normal cardiopulmonary system with a normal minute ventilation results in an arterial PCO_2 of 40 mm Hg. In the absence of abnormal deadspace, doubling the minute volume without increasing metabolic rate produces an arterial PCO_2 of approximately 30 mm Hg; a minute volume of 4 times normal produces an arterial PCO_2 of about 20 mm Hg (Table 19–2). Thus, a significant *minute ventilation-to-PCO_2 disparity* must reflect deadspace disease when metabolic function is normal.[35] Since total ventilation is composed of two parts: gas that exchanges with

TABLE 19-2.—EXPECTED MINUTE VOLUME-
TO-ARTERIAL CARBON DIOXIDE TENSION
RELATIONSHIPS IN THE NORMAL
NONEXERCISING MAN

MV	Pa_{CO_2} (mm Hg)	RANGE (mm Hg)
Normal	40	35–45
Twice normal	30	25–35
Quadruple normal	20	15–25

pulmonary blood (alveolar ventilation) and gas that does not exchange with pulmonary blood (deadspace ventilation), the clinical significance of deadspace ventilation is that the organism has to expend energy to move air that has no physiologic advantage. If the deadspace ventilation is significant, the organism will have to expend a tremendous amount of energy to move additional air so that a normal alveolar ventilation can be maintained. This is obviously an inefficient situation and is not well tolerated for long periods of time.

A co-equal factor in the efficiency of pulmonary gas exchange is pulmonary blood flow. Inadequate pulmonary blood flow will result in increased deadspace ventilation because there is inadequate blood flow through the lung to exchange with air (ventilation in excess of perfusion).

Arterial pH

Arterial pH is a measurement of the acid-base status of the blood. This must be taken into consideration when evaluating physiologic ventilation, since an acute (sudden or recent) change in the ventilatory state will be accompanied by a corresponding change in the acid-base state (respiratory acidosis and alkalosis). The arterial measurement of acid*emia* or alkal*emia* must not be confused with the pathophysiologic conditions of metabolic acid*osis* and alkal*osis,* which reflect the overall imbalance of acids and bases in the body tissues.

Acidemia and alkalemia lead to changes in the vascular system and cell membranes that may result in precarious oxygenation of myocardium, brain, and other vital organs. In addition, acidemia may decrease the effectiveness of various pharmacologic agents, as well as decrease the predicability with which these drugs affect target organs.

Oxygenation

The oxygenation status of tissue is not clinically measurable (see Chapter 6). The measurement of arterial oxygen tension levels is valuable in determining the arterial blood's *potential* for delivering oxygen to tissue.[35] Arterial oxygen tension does *not* guarantee adequate tissue oxygenation because it is only one factor in oxygen transport. The assumption that an adequate arterial oxygen tension means that there is adequate tissue oxygenation is erroneous and dangerous. Nevertheless, inadequate arterial oxygen tension (hypoxemia) is certainly a distressing factor and one that should be supported in the critically ill patient. However, *hypoxemia* is not synonymous with inadequate tissue oxygenation. If the cardiovascular system is capable of making up for the hypoxemia, or if oxygen-carrying capacity is increased (increased hemoglobin), adequate tissue oxygenation can still be maintained.

With the availability of *pulmonary* artery blood gas measurement, further evaluation of tissue oxygenation is possible through appropriate interpretation of mixed venous oxygen tensions, arterial-venous oxygen content differences, and intrapulmonary shunt measurements (see Chapter 28).

20 • PULMONARY PATHOPHYSIOLOGY LEADING TO ACUTE RESPIRATORY FAILURE

RATIONALE FOR SUPPORTING inadequate gas exchange at the pulmonary level must be based on some schema that allows multiple factors to be evaluated and treatment modalities to be monitored in an organized fashion. Pulmonary function criteria provide a convenient and well-established base upon which to build a rational, logical, and practical schema for approaching the common pulmonary pathophysiologic pathways of acute respiratory failure.[304] Following is a brief review of the basic pulmonary physiology and pulmonary function factors essential to our schema. These factors have been discussed in detail in Chapters 3 and 4.

Airway resistance accounts for a major portion of the normal work of breathing. Gross changes in airway resistance may be reflected in expiratory flow spirometry, e.g., FEV_1, MMEFR. In addition, regional differences in airway resistance may dramatically alter the distribution of ventilation. *Lung and chest wall compliance* are major factors in determining (1) the transpulmonary pressures required to inspire a given tidal volume; (2) the work of breathing; and (3) the FRC. *Vital capacity* is a gross reflection of ventilatory reserve. *Total lung capacity* is comprised of four lung volumes and is measurable in the pulmonary laboratory in a cooperative patient.

Functional Residual Capacity

FRC is the combination of residual volume (RV) and expiratory reserve volume (ERV). It represents the end-expiratory lung volume and, thereby, the lung volume at which inspiration must begin. FRC is measurable without requiring the patient's active cooperation since it is non-effort dependent. This factor makes the measurement reasonably reliable in acutely ill patients.[359] Presently the bedside measurement of FRC is a research tool; however, new technology and methodology may well provide for routine bedside measurement in the future.[299, 300]

FRC may reliably be used as a direct reflection of total lung capacity since (1) *a decreased FRC almost inevitably reflects a decreased TLC;* and (2) an increased FRC most probably reflects an unchanged or increased TLC. Thus, acute obstructive or restrictive pulmonary pathology may be grossly diagnosed and evaluated via FRC measurement. Acute decreases in FRC have predictable affects on compliance and V/Q relationships (see Chapter 4). *As FRC acutely decreases* (1) *lung compliance decreases,* and (2) *V/Q imbalance occurs (increased deadspace and shunt effect).*

Obstructive Lung Disease

Increased total lung capacity and decreased expiratory flow rates are the hallmarks of obstructive pathology.[41] The common denominator is *increased airway resistance* from which exhaled gas flow is impeded to a greater degree than inhaled gas flow. The resultant increase in FRC ("air trapping") leads to an increased lung compliance.

Acute obstructive pathology (asthma, bronchitis, bronchiolitis) is believed to be the most common acute pathologic pulmonary process encountered in the United States other than pneumonia.[298] These diseases are usually self-limiting and seldom life threatening. Treatment is primarily pharmacologic, i.e., bronchodilators, antibiotics, vasoconstrictors, and anti-inflammatory agents. Acute obstructive pathology is an *un*common cause of acute respiratory failure!

Chronic obstructive pathology is usually a combination of emphysema (loss of lung elastic tissue and interalveolar septae) and chronic bronchitis. Most common in elderly patients, chronic obstructive pulmonary disease (COPD) represents a significant diminishment in pulmonary reserves and may result in chronic respiratory failure (see Chapter 32). In terms of repiratory care, these patients must be viewed as having a tenuous base-line function and may not be able to maintain homeostasis when confronted with acute pathology. They require careful monitoring and early therapy. With COPD, acute respiratory failure may result from any physiologic stress and commonly does.

Restrictive Lung Disease

Decreased total lung capacity and decreased vital capacity are the hallmarks of restrictive pathology.[41] *Chronic* restrictive abnormality is usually the result of some form of pulmonary fibrosis or chest wall abnormality.[4] These patients must be considered at high risk for acute respiratory failure when confronted with an acute pathologic stress.

Acute Restrictive Lung Disease

Acute restrictive pathology is by far the most common pulmonary cause of acute respiratory failure in the United States! It has been our experience that more than 80% of potentially salvageable patients requiring acute respiratory intensive care have an acute restrictive pathologic process. *The common denominator of acute restrictive pulmonary pathology is an acutely decreased functional residual capacity!*[303]

Certain generalizations pertaining to acute restrictive pathology may be stated as follows: 1. Decreased compliance of the lung-thorax complex must be present and, therefore, the patient's cardiopulmonary system must provide for an increased work of breathing. 2. The vital capacity is acutely diminished; however, the degree to which the vital capacity is affected is highly variable. Therefore, varying degrees of ventilatory reserve exist in patients with acute restrictive pathology. 3. Ventilation-perfusion relationships are always abnormal, but the composition of these imbalances (i.e., deadspace and shunting) is highly variable.

In summary, any acute restrictive pulmonary pathology will lead to some increased work of breathing, some diminishment of ventilatory reserve, and some inefficiency of pulmonary gas exchange (V/Q imbalance). It is the combination of these adverse factors that so often leads to acute respiratory failure.

Three Variations of Acute Restrictive Pathology

There appear to be three separable types of acute restrictive pathology commonly confronted in critical care medicine (Fig 20–1). All three have decreased total lung capacities, vital capacities, and functional residual capacities. However, they differ in the degrees to which various lung volumes are affected and, thereby, manifest very different therapeutic requirements.

Equal Diminishment of All Lung Volumes
(see Fig 20–1, Type A)

This may occur in the presence of a normal lung or be due to primary lung pathology. In either case both vital capacity and FRC are diminished significantly. When primary lung pathology is the cause, there is usually a significant "true shunt" (refractory hypoxemia) that compounds the stress. The most common pulmonary pathology causing this type of problem is atelectasis; the most common *non-*

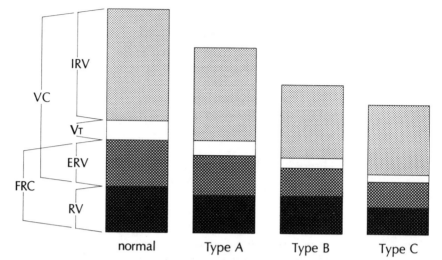

Fig 20–1.—Bar graphs of the three types of acute restrictive pathology commonly confronted in critical care medicine. RV = residual volume; ERV = expiratory reserve volume; V_T = tidal volume; IRV = inspiratory reserve volume; FRC = functional residual capacity; VC = vital capacity. *Type A* = equal diminishment of all lung volumes commonly seen with acute atelectasis, CNS depression, and neuromuscular disease (see text); *Type B* = major diminishment in vital capacity commonly seen in the postoperative patient (see text); *Type C* = major diminishment in FRC commonly referred to as the adult respiratory distress syndrome *(ARDS)* (see text).

pulmonary pathologies are (1) C.N.S. depression and (2) neuromuscular disease.

Atelectasis

The collapsing of lung tissue is defined as atelectasis. When this occurs in a random pattern ("patchy or miliary" atelectasis), it is not discernible on chest x-ray. However, most atelectasis of clinical concern involves contiguous areas of lung (usually segments or lobes) and is readily discernible on chest x-ray.

When lung is externally collapsed, it is termed *compression* atelectasis and is usually secondary to pleural fluid, pneumothorax, or space-occupying lesions of the thorax. Primary therapy of compression atelectasis is usually of a surgical nature and does not directly involve respiratory therapy techniques.

Absorption atelectasis is the most common type of acute lung collapse and is usually due to retained secretions (see Chapter 8). Pooling of secretions exists not only in major airways but also in the bronchioles and small bronchi. The latter are poorly mobilized with bronchoscopy or segmental suctioning; therefore, bronchial hygiene techniques of respiratory therapy are the first line of defense in the prevention and treatment of absorption atelectasis secondary to retained secretions (refer to Section III).

Segmental or lobar collapse results in an *acute* decrease in TLC even though eventual hyperinflation of adjacent lung is common. In the majority of cases there is reasonably uniform infringement on the various lung volumes. Although there is decreased pulmonary blood flow to an acutely collapsed area of lung, there is by no means a total absence of blood flow.[301] This results in a "true physiologic shunt" (unventilated, perfused lung). The arterial hypoxemic affect of such a shunt will depend on the amount of blood traversing the shunt units and on the oxygen content of the pulmonary artery blood.[35] The hypoxemia of true shunting is poorly responsive to oxygen therapy (see Chapters 6 and 7) and requires significant compensatory work from the cardiovascular system. This partially explains why acute atelectasis is usually accompanied by tachycardia, mild hypertension, and tachypnea.

Acute atelectasis secondary to retained secretions is a common problem in critically ill patients. The atelectasis decreases both blood and lymph flow in the area, thereby hindering two major defense mechanisms for preventing infection. In addition, pooled secretions are rich in nutrients (sugars and proteins) essential for bacterial growth. The inevitable result is *stasis pneumonia*—a serious and common complication of critically ill patients.

C.N.S. Depression

Obtundation of the C.N.S. is commonly due to (1) primary C.N.S. disease, (2) drugs, (3) hypoxemia, and (4) diminished cerebral perfusion. The obtundation generally results in (1) diminished C.N.S. response to ventilatory stimuli; (2) ablation of the periodic variation (sighs) of normal breathing pattern; and (3) diminished stimulation to the diaphragm and intercostal muscles. These factors are believed to lead to hypoventilation and decreased chest wall and diaphragm muscle tone, which results in acute restrictive pathology with all lung volumes fairly equally diminished.[41] Since few alveoli actually collapse and lung is not primarily diseased, arterial oxygenation is readily maintained with minimal supplemental inspired oxygen.

In addition to the restrictive pulmonary pathology, a potential threat to all obtunded or unconscious patients is aspiration and upper airway obstruction secondary to interference with the airway protective reflexes (see Chapters 33 and 34). An inescapable conclusion is that basic principles of acute respiratory care are applicable to all unconscious and obtunded patients. The expertise with which these techniques are applied may well be the most important aspect in supportive care of the unconscious patient.[302] Airway evaluation, adequate oxygenation, and ventilation must be assured! Steps to prevent atelectasis and early treatment of lung collapse are essential!

Neuromuscular Disease

Disease processes that temporarily or permanently weaken the ventilatory apparatus will initially result in a diminished total lung capacity that uniformly affects all lung volumes. Table 20–1 outlines the most common neuromuscular disease entities encountered in the United States. Such patients often have potentially reversible disease. They present a great challenge in respiratory supportive care—especially ventilator care![305] The goal is to maintain clear lungs throughout the disease course. Close monitoring of ventilatory reserve and airway competence allows appropriate and timely intervention. Aggressive prophylactic pulmonary care may often prevent the need for ventilator support.

Major Diminishment of Vital Capacity
(see Fig 20–1, Type B)

When lung remains free of pathology while an injury or insult is sustained that limits movement of the diaphragm and/or chest wall, an

TABLE 20–1.—NEUROMUSCULAR
DISEASES COMMONLY REQUIRING
RESPIRATORY INTENSIVE CARE

I. Spinal cord disease
   A. Trauma
      1. Quadriplegia
      2. Paraplegia
   B. Poliomyelitis
II. Motor nerve disease
   A. Acute idiopathic polyneuritis
      1. Guillain-Barré syndrome
      2. Landry's ascending paralysis
   B. Tick bite paralysis
   C. Porphyria
III. Myoneural junction disease
   A. Myasthenia gravis
   B. Myasthenic syndrome
IV. Muscle-wasting disease
   A. Muscular dystrophy
   B. Congenital myotonia
V. Tetanus

acute restrictive pathology results in which the vital capacity is dramatically diminished while the residual volume is minimally affected. This would lead to an increased work of breathing (attributable to the decreased ventilatory reserve) and to some degree of V/Q imbalance (due to the decreased FRC). A mild hypoxemia (shunt effect) is present and responsive to moderate increases in inspired oxygen. This pathophysiology is most commonly encountered in patients following abdominal and thoracic surgical procedures. This is discussed in detail in Chapter 31.

Major Diminishment of FRC (see Fig 20-1, Type C)

Significant decreases in lung compliance result in a severe restrictive pathology. Total lung capacity and vital capacity are significantly diminished; however, the greatest insult is the diminishment in functional residual capacity. This type of primary decrease in lung compliance results in profound increases in the work of breathing and profound V/Q imbalance (true shunting, shunt effect, and deadspace ventilation). Since RV and ERV are so greatly affected, there exists a far better IRV (and therefore vital capacity) than would be anticipated for that degree of restrictive pathology. Thus, the ventilatory reserve is better than expected for the degree of restrictive pathology present.

The clinical manifestations are (1) refractory hypoxemia, (2) increased work of breathing, and (3) an excellent ability to achieve the increased work necessary to maintain adequate or low $PaCO_2$. This type of acute restrictive pathology is commonly encountered as the adult respiratory distress syndrome (ARDS) and is discussed in detail in Chapter 30.

SECTION VI
AIRWAY PRESSURE THERAPY

21 • DEFINING AIRWAY PRESSURE THERAPY

NORMAL GAS MOVEMENT in and out of the pulmonary system occurs in response to pressure gradients that exist between the alveoli and the upper airway. Thus, it is reasonable, convenient, and traditional to use *airway pressures* as a reference point when discussing support of the pulmonary system. Whenever airway pressures are discussed, the reference or base-line pressure is always *atmospheric or ambient pressure,* since it is this pressure to which the upper airway is normally exposed. For ease of reference, it is traditional to refer to the atmospheric pressure as zero (0). It should be realized that this does *not* imply an absence of pressure (as exists in a vacuum) but, rather, refers to atmospheric pressure as a "base line." References to *negative pressures* are always in relation to this defined base line; thus, a negative pressure of 10 is in reality a pressure 10 units below atmospheric. It is traditional to refer to airway pressures in centimeters of water (cm H_2O) rather than millimeters of mercury (mm Hg). Thus, throughout our discussion it is assumed that we are referring to airway pressures in terms of centimeters of water and cardiovascular pressures in terms of millimeters of mercury. Airway pressures are assumed to be measured at the level of the trachea unless otherwise specified.

Pulmonary Pressure Gradients

Since normal mechanisms of breathing are dependent upon pressure gradients, it is imperative to understand the nomenclature applied to pressure gradients within the pulmonary system (Fig 21–1). The pressure difference between the airway opening (mouth, endotracheal tube, or tracheostomy tube) and the alveolus is referred to as *transairway pressure* or *"driving pressure."* This is the pressure gradient that will directly result in movement of gas molecules into or out of the pulmonary system. *Transpulmonary pressure* refers to the pressure difference between the airway opening and intrathoracic (intrapleural) pressure.

Alveolar Distending Pressure

Alveolar distending pressure refers to the pressure difference between the alveolus and the pleural space. At FRC (end-expiratory

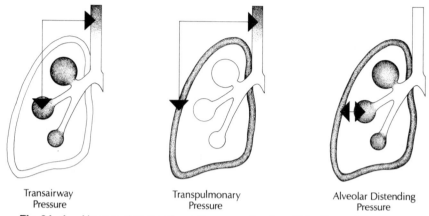

| Transairway Pressure | Transpulmonary Pressure | Alveolar Distending Pressure |

Fig 21–1.—Nomenclature of pressure gradients within the pulmonary system. *Left, transairway pressure*—pressure gradient between airway opening and alveolus; *center, transpulmonary pressure*—pressure gradient between airway opening and pleural space; *right, alveolar distending pressure*—pressure gradient between alveolus and adjacent pleural space.

lung volume), the alveolar volume is maintained because the alveolar elastic recoil forces are opposed by an equal "alveolar distending force." Since alveolar and ambient pressures are equal at FRC, the alveolar to intrapleural pressure gradient (alveolar distending pressure) is equal to the airway to intrapleural pressure gradient (transpulmonary pressure). Therefore, *at FRC the alveolar distending pressure and transpulmonary pressure are equal.*

Airway Pressure Cycle (Fig 21–2)

Inspiratory driving pressure is generated by the muscles of ventilation (primarily the diaphragm) rapidly increasing the chest volume, thereby creating a decrease in intrapleural and alveolar pressures (Boyle's law). This drop in alveolar pressure creates a *transairway pressure gradient,* which results in gas flow from airway opening to alveolus. For any given transairway pressure gradient, the primary factor determining the flow of gas to the alveolus is the airway resistance.

Inspiration ends when flow ceases. Thus, at the end of inspiration the ambient, airway, and alveolar pressures are equal and, therefore, transairway pressure equals zero.

The expiratory driving pressure is primarily the result of the elastic recoil of the lung tending to return the lung volume to its resting state (FRC). These elastic forces create an increased pressure within the

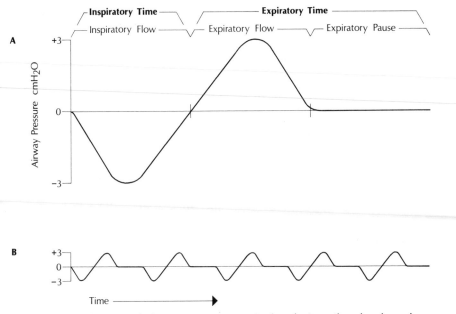

Fig 21–2.— A, normal airway pressure cycle. Inspiratory time begins when airway pressures fall below ambient (see text). Flow into lungs results and continues until airway pressure returns to ambient. Expiratory time begins when airway pressures rise above ambient (see text). Flow out of lungs ceases prior to next inspiration, providing an expiratory pause; i.e., the latter portion of the expiratory time in which airway pressure is ambient and, therefore, no flow is occurring. **B,** five consecutive breathing cycles. Note consistency of expiratory pause.

alveoli, producing a transairway pressure in the reverse direction. This results in flow out of the lung. The rate of expiratory flow will be primarily affected by airway resistance factors, although lung compliance and chest wall compliance also play a role.

Expiration ends when the next inspiration begins. Note that the airway pressure normally returns to ambient (atmospheric) prior to the end of expiration. That portion of time at end expiration when airway pressures are ambient reflects a period of absent or near absent flow. This is often referred to as the "expiratory pause."

Defining Airway Pressure Therapy

Acute respiratory intensive care is concerned with manipulation of airway pressures to provide improved ventilatory mechanics and physiologic gas exchange.[57] Such airway pressure therapy includes inspiratory maneuvers (primarily ventilator care) and expiratory maneuvers (primarily PEEP therapy). The discipline of applying airway pressure therapy to the critically ill patient is confusing and frustrating to most clinicians. A great deal of this confusion is attributable to the complex physiology, physics, and technology that must be understood. However, much confusion exists because of the "alphabet soup" that has developed pertaining to airway pressure therapy nomenclature.

Terminology in respiratory care is so confusing and contradictory that it is often impossible to separate differing ideas from differing nomenclature. It would be naïve and presumptuous for us to purport that our particular preferences in terminology should or would be accepted by everyone. However, to teach clinical application of airway pressure therapy we must "arbitrate" terminology. The following is presented solely for the purpose of clarifying how *we* define various terms, and how these terms are consistently used throughout this text. We believe our terminology is consistent with the present mainstream of respiratory care and find no *major* differences between our terminology and that adopted by such organizations as the American Thoracic Society and the American Association for Respiratory Therapy.

IPPB (intermittent positive-pressure breathing) – inspiration by positive airway pressure; expiration is passive; airway pressure returns to ambient prior to next inspiration.

IPPV (intermittent positive-pressure ventilation) – IPPB applied in a repetitive manner for the purpose of mechanically supporting ventilation.

IMV (intermittent mandatory ventilation) – spontaneous ventilation intermittently augmented by positive-pressure ventilation at *mandatory* intervals.

IDV (intermittent demand ventilation) – spontaneous ventilation intermittently augmented by positive-pressure ventilation on patient demand, i.e., in synchrony with the spontaneous pattern; also referred to as SIMV (synchronized IMV) and IAV (intermittent assisted ventilation).

PEEP (positive end-expiratory pressure) – an expiratory airway pressure maneuver in which the airway pressure is maintained above atmospheric at the end of expiration.

CPPV—IPPV and **PEEP;** the combination of mechanical support of ventilation and PEEP; may also be referred to as "the ventilator with PEEP" or "IMV with PEEP."

CPAP (continuous positive airway pressure)—spontaneous ventilation and PEEP; the most widely used technique for applying PEEP to the *spontaneously* breathing patient. The apparatus must allow for inspiratory airway pressures to be maintained above atmospheric; i.e., the entire breathing cycle must have positive airway pressures.

EPAP (expiratory positive airway pressure)—a *technique* for applying PEEP to the spontaneously breathing patient in which inspiratory airway pressures are *required* to fall below atmospheric in order for inspiratory gas flow to occur.

The following four chapters discuss the physiologic and clinical principles of airway pressure support and their complications. For ease of reference and discussion, three broad interrelated areas are discussed separately: (1) inspiratory airway pressure support to augment ventilation (ventilator care); (2) positive end-expiratory pressure (PEEP); and (3) combinations and complications of these airway pressure maneuvers.

22 • PRINCIPLES OF VENTILATOR CARE

History

CONSISTENTLY SUCCESSFUL TECHNIQUES for artificial ventilation were first developed in the 1920s in conjunction with anesthetic administration.[306] These were positive-pressure techniques that developed parallel with capabilities for endotracheal intubation. The development of ventilatory support outside the operating room simultaneously developed in a different direction primarily because of the unavailability of endotracheal intubation, the desire to avoid tracheostomy,[307] and the fact that the necessity for ready access to the patient's body was far less necessary than in the operating room. Therefore, the negative-pressure ventilator (iron lung) gained enormous popularity.[308] Applied almost exclusively to the polio victim, the iron lung provided reasonable support of ventilation without the necessity for tracheostomy or endotracheal intubation.

The effectiveness of negative-pressure ventilators came into serious question during and following World War II. The Scandinavian polio epidemics of the early 1950s clearly demonstrated that survival was better with positive-pressure techniques;[309, 310] the superiority of positive-pressure ventilatory support was generally accepted and the modern era of respiratory care begun. Over the past thirty years it has remained true that the power and capabilities of positive-pressure machines far exceed those of negative-pressure machines. And it has remained true that following the establishment of a secure airway, the positive-pressure machinery can be placed a distance from the patient, allowing appropriate monitoring, therapy, and nursing care. However, it has *never* been true that the positive-pressure ventilator is *physiologically* advantageous—to the contrary, the physiologic *dis*advantages are numerous.

Disadvantages of Positive-Pressure Ventilation (PPV)

The disadvantages of positive-pressure ventilation may be divided into two broad categories: (1) problems related directly to increased airway pressures; and (2) variance in the distribution of ventilation in relation to pulmonary perfusion.

326

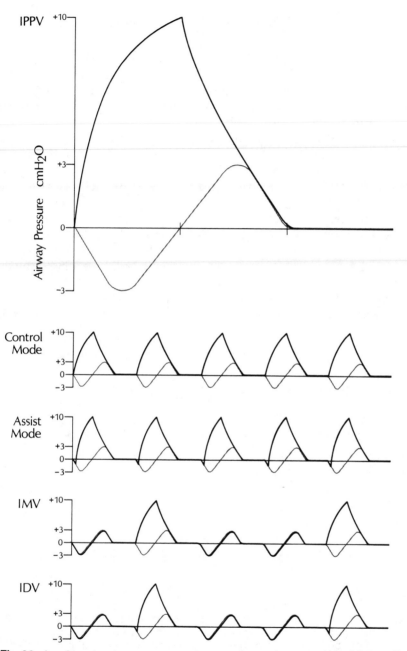

Fig 22–1.—Classic airway pressure curves for various modes of intermittent positive-pressure ventilation *(IPPV)* superimposed on the normal spontaneous airway pressure curves. *IMV* = intermittent mandatory ventilation; *IDV* = intermittent demand ventilation.

Increased Airway Pressures

When compared to the spontaneously breathing individual, PPV *must* result in increased mean airway pressures (Fig 22–1). These increased airway pressures *must* result in increased intrapleural (intrathoracic) pressures. Although these relationships are not always linearly related and may vary quantitatively with pulmonary disease, the effect of positive-pressure ventilation can be generalized as follows: *the increased airway pressures result in increased intrathoracic pressures.*[155] This increase in intrathoracic pressure is potentially harmful to cardiovascular function, since the return of venous blood to the right heart is dependent on the pressure gradient from the peripheral veins to the right atrium.[153] Since increased intrathoracic pressure leads to increased intra-atrial pressure, the "driving pressure" from the extrathoracic veins to the atrium of the right heart is diminished (Fig 22–2). This phenomenon is known as a *reduction in venous return* and will be discussed in detail in Chapters 26 and 27.

Thus, increased airway pressures have a potential to cause a de-

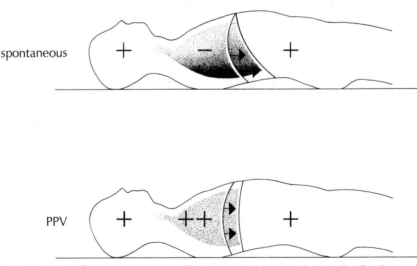

Fig 22–2. — Spontaneous ventilation provides optimal distribution of ventilation in relation to perfusion due to mechanics of the spontaneously contracting diaphragm. In addition, venous return is optimized because intra-abdominal and intracranial pressures are more positive than intrathoracic pressures. Positive-pressure ventilation *(PPV)* results in greater air distribution to the non-gravity-dependent portions of lung and potentially hinders venous return because intrathoracic pressure is more positive than intra-abdominal or intracranial pressure.

crease in venous return; which may lead to a decrease in cardiac output. This is perhaps the greatest single detriment to placing patients on positive-pressure ventilation! Venous return embarrassment is a physiologic phenomenon that the respiratory care practitioner must thoroughly understand, monitor, and react to appropriately. It is of no benefit to the patient to have the process of improving ventilation result in decreased circulation of blood to the lung and body.

Distribution of Pulmonary Perfusion

The increased alveolar pressures resulting from positive-pressure ventilation tend to favor pulmonary blood flow even more toward gravity-dependent portions of lung than with normal alveolar pressures. This process potentially results in greater areas of lung being well ventilated but poorly perfused. Thus, *positive-pressure ventilation usually results in increased deadspace ventilation,* even when adequate cardiac output is maintained.[312, 319]

Distribution of Ventilation

The spontaneously breathing supine individual (see Fig 22–2) demonstrates a relatively greater diaphragm excursion posteriorly than anteriorly.[329] This is advantageous since posterior lung is better perfused than anterior lung in this position. With positive-pressure inspiration, the diaphragm is essentially passive, and the tidal volume tends to distribute to areas of better compliance, i.e., distribution of ventilation is favored to the non-gravity areas.[313, 320, 321] This tendency for positive-pressure inspiration in the supine position to result in increased aeration of anterior portions of lung makes deadspace ventilation and physiologic shunting more prevalent than with spontaneous ventilation. These relationships are believed to be present in all positions; i.e., positive-pressure ventilation tends to favor distribution of ventilation to non-gravity-dependent areas of lung.

The above factors lead to a general clinical statement: *it is physiologically advantageous to breathe spontaneously to whatever extent is consistent with maintenance of cardiopulmonary homeostasis.* This physiologic and clinical truism, along with the technical capability for providing augmented means of ventilation, has recently provided a significant improvement in ventilator care.

Ventilators Are Not Respirators

The general classification of positive-pressure ventilators has been presented in Chapter 3. It must be stressed that *these machines are ventilators and not respirators!* The machines do *not* ensure molecular gas exchange at the pulmonary level (respiration); rather, they provide movement of gases into and out of the pulmonary system (ventilation). Since true respirators are presently available (e.g., extracorporeal membrane oxygenators and heart-lung bypass machines), it becomes essential to realize that although it is traditionally acceptable to refer to ventilators as "respirators," they are *not* truly respirators and *provide only ventilatory support.*

Physiologic Capabilities of PPV

It cannot be assumed that all patients in acute respiratory failure or acute respiratory insufficiency will benefit from mechanical support of ventilation. Only when physiologic *respiration* can be improved or maintained is it logical to consider application of positive-pressure ventilation. Since the ventilator is a machine that only alters inspiratory airway pressures, a rationale for its application must be based upon delineating the conditions in which such airway pressure alteration may be physiologically advantageous.

It may be generalized that a positive-pressure ventilator may beneficially alter physiologic gas exchange by performing three tasks: (1) to provide the *power* to maintain physiologic ventilation; (2) to manipulate inspiratory airway pressures and flow patterns to improve distribution of ventilation; and (3) to manipulate the ventilatory pattern to improve gas exchange.

Power

Inspiration is a process requiring muscular energy (oxygen consumption). When the ventilatory muscles are incapable of providing the needed power, or doing so is detrimental to the organism, a ventilator can provide all or part of the required energy.[314]

Inspiratory Flow Pattern

Inspiratory flow patterns may have significant affect on the manner in which inspired gases distribute, especially in the presence of pulmonary disease.[315, 317] Modern ventilators have significant flexibility in altering inspiratory pressures and flow patterns. The most significant of these maneuvers appears to be the end-inspiratory pause (see Chapter 23).

Ventilatory Pattern

Inspiratory-to-expiratory ratios, ventilatory rate, and tidal volumes greatly affect respiration.[312, 318] Ventilators can partially or completely control (or modify) these factors.

Ventilator Commitment

Based on acceptance of the generalizations stated to this point, it is reasonable to discuss the clinical rationale for placing a patient on a ventilator. As medicine and surgery increase their ability to cure and palliate disease, an increasing number of patients are becoming candidates for mechanical support of ventilation. Mortality and morbidity are believed to be significantly decreased when *early* commitment to ventilatory support is initiated. Ventilator commitment is best avoided when unnecessary; however, if commitment is indicated, it is best instituted prior to cardiopulmonary collapse and resuscitation. Such "early" or semi-elective commitment to ventilator support makes it incumbent upon the respiratory care practitioner to insure that the procedure is performed in the safest possible manner.

Ventilator care places a great responsibility on the physician and the respiratory care practitioner. The physician must accept the procedure as a complex and demanding commitment and create the milieu in which all health care personnel can provide the highest quality of care. The physician must be prepared to make whatever commitments are necessary and indicated; "halfway" ventilator care is worse than none.

Ventilator care is never curative! It is a supportive technique that demands the presence of potentially reversible pathophysiology. The ventilator can accomplish no more than maintain cardiopulmonary homeostasis within acceptable physiologic limits for a period of time. It is a disservice to the patient, his family, and society to commit or continue the use of mechanical support of ventilation when disease reversibility is not possible.

The recent sophistication and general acceptance of ventilator care have led to moral, religious, legal, and philosophic problems that must be dealt with by the entire health care delivery system and society. It is neither the intent nor the scope of this text to discuss these aspects of the subject. The authors simply wish to emphasize that all criteria and rationale for the institution and maintenance of ventilator care must be based on the clinical assertion that a potentially reversible disease process exists!

Indications for Mechanical Support of Ventilation

It would be futile to categorize indications for mechanical support of ventilation by disease entity. Not only would this result in endless lists, but with each disease, it would have to be stated that it is not the disease itself that necessitates the ventilator but rather the degree to which the disease's physiologic stress impinges upon cardiopulmonary reserves. The clinical indications for commitment to a ventilator are best stated in terms of cardiopulmonary pathophysiology. There are four such categories that have universal application in the clinical setting: (1) apnea; (2) acute ventilatory failure (acute respiratory acidosis); (3) impending acute ventilatory failure; and (4) oxygenation.

Apnea

Absence of spontaneous ventilation necessitates mechanical support of ventilation.

Acute Ventilatory Failure (Acute Respiratory Acidosis)

The patient's minute ventilation may have little correlation with his effective (physiologic) ventilation. Inadequate alveolar ventilation may be due to an increased physiologic deadspace in which case the patient usually has an increased minute ventilation. Therefore, simple clinical observation or measurement of minute ventilation does not necessarily reflect the adequacy of physiologic ventilation. Assessment of the adequacy of physiologic ventilation can be accomplished only by blood gas analysis![35] Inadequate alveolar ventilation (arterial carbon dioxide above an acceptable limit) reflects a failure to adequately remove carbon dioxide via the lungs. When such a "ventilatory failure" is accompanied by acidemia (arterial pH below an acceptable limit), the failure must be of recent origin (acute) and, therefore, a direct threat to cardiopulmonary homeostasis. Thus, an increased arterial P_{CO_2} with a decreased pH is acute ventilatory failure (acute respiratory acidosis).[35] In such a circumstance, mechanical support of ventilation is indicated unless some other effective treatment is immediately available.

Impending Acute Ventilatory Failure

Clinical assessment of the work of breathing, the pathogenesis of the disease process, and the patient's cardiopulmonary reserves may result in the clinical judgment that acute ventilatory failure is inevitable or extremely probable. This is sometimes referred to as the patient "tiring" or "fatiguing." This is often a debatable and unclear clinical problem necessitating careful monitoring and sound clinical judgment. It can be most classically documented when sequential blood gas analysis reveals consistently increasing P_{CO_2} and decreasing pH values.

Oxygenation

When the patient is breathing room air, hypoxemia will be present with apnea, acute ventilatory failure, and usually impending acute ventilatory failure. In fact, most ventilatory problems are accompanied by poor arterial oxygenation. However, restoration of adequate physiologic ventilation usually improves the hypoxemia and thereby enhances tissue oxygenation.

With modern capabilities of airway pressure support, oxygen therapy, and intravenous fluid therapy, it is no longer reasonable to consider most primary oxygenation deficits as indications for ventilators. Most primary oxygenation deficits are best supported by oxygen therapy, cardiovascular support, PEEP therapy, bronchial hygiene therapy, or combinations of these techniques. Although any of these may be administered in conjunction with the ventilator, none of them *requires* the use of a ventilator. Thus, modern indications for ventilatory support do *not* include most primary oxygenation deficits unless they are directly attributable to a deleterious work of breathing or ventilatory pattern. If oxygenation may be improved by decreasing the work of breathing,[314] or if cardiac function may be improved by decreasing the work of breathing,[316] a ventilator may directly improve the oxygenation status.

Summary

It is essential for the physician and the respiratory care practitioner to have a clear understanding of both the indication for commitment to mechanical ventilation and the "working diagnosis" of the potentially reversible process. Appropriate maintenance and discontinuance of ventilator care may be accomplished only in the context of clear-cut criteria for commitment. For example, if a patient has been placed on a ventilator for apnea, it is obvious that when the patient begins to make ventilatory efforts, the need for the ventilator must be reevaluated. On the other hand, if a patient is placed on a ventilator for acute or impending acute ventilatory failure, he is usually breathing quite actively at the time of commitment. In such circumstance, efforts to breathe while on the ventilator should not be necessarily interpreted as signs for reevaluation of the need for ventilator support. Modern ventilator care demands clear-cut clinical goals, clear-cut indications, and a thorough knowledge of the cardiopulmonary pathophysiologic process. Under these circumstances, safe and intelligent commitment may be undertaken.

The Five Steps of Ventilator Commitment

Presentation of the following material is meant as a *guideline* for the respiratory care practitioner in the process of ventilator commitment. It is meant to be neither an exclusive, dogmatic statement nor a complete list of all possibilities. The authors believe that if the following steps are used as a general guideline, they will serve well in the safe and orderly conduct of ventilator commitment.

Step #1.—Establish the airway and manually support ventilation

The safe establishment of an artificial airway to facilitate the support of ventilation and protect the lungs from aspiration of foreign substance is the first and most important factor in ventilator commitment. The respiratory care practitioner must be capable of assisting the physician in appropriate airway establishment and able to assume responsibility for ventilation once the airway is established.

Initial support of ventilation should be accomplished by "manual ventilation." A self-inflating bag with a one-way valve system is appropriate. Most commercially available manual ventilators have capacities of approximately 1.5–2 liters and will deliver approximately 40–80% oxygen concentrations when connected to oxygen sources. Manual ventilation offers the advantages that (1) it is immediately available; (2) it can be easily varied from moment to moment to meet the patient's demands; (3) it is reasonably free of technical and mechanical complexities; and (4) it offers the clinician direct moment-to-moment contact with airway patency, system compliance, and patient effort.

Step #2.—Cardiovascular stabilization

Establishment of the airway and institution of positive-pressure ventilation in a critically ill patient may initially add to cardiovascular instability (hypotension and arrhythmia). Too often, hypotension following the establishment of an airway and positive-pressure ventilation is assumed to be due to such factors as (1) stress of intubation; (2) delay in accomplishing successful intubation; (3) pharmacologic agents used to facilitate intubation (e.g., muscle paralyzants, narcotics); and (4) inappropriate support of ventilation. Although any of these factors are possible (especially when improperly applied), hypotension often occurs when none of these factors is present and in spite of the highest degree of skill. Most often hypotension and arrhythmia are secondary to either (1) decreased sympathetic tone; (2) decreased venous return; or (3) a combination of these factors.

Decreased sympathetic tone. —The autonomic nervous system in a patient requiring ventilator commitment is usually experiencing significant stimulation (e.g., hypoxemia, hypercarbia, acidemia) while attempting to maintain cardiopulmonary homeostasis. In conscious patients the physiologic stress is usually compounded by a state of anxiety and fear. These factors result in a significant degree of arterial and venous constriction as well as myocardial stimulation. Since support of ventilation usually relieves the work of breathing and significantly reverses hypercarbia, acidemia, and hypoxemia, the patient "relaxes" and may enter a state of "sleep" for several hours. Also, it is not uncommon for a state of unconsciousness to be induced pharmacologically.

The combination of loss of consciousness, relief of work of breathing, and improved ventilation and oxygenation often leads to a *profound and sudden decrease* in sympathetic stimulation to the cardiovascular system. This decrease in sympathetic tone often results in arteriolar and venous relaxation, leading to a rapid and significant increase in the vascular space. The sudden "relative hypovolemia" may not be immediately compensated because the patient is unable to mobilize extravascular fluid rapidly. In addition, the relative hypovolemia is significant because the intrathoracic positive pressure created by the ventilator accentuates interference with venous return.

Decreased venous return. — Most patients committed to ventilator care have limited cardiopulmonary reserves. The combination of relative hypovolemia and positive-pressure ventilation often results in hypotension. This should be anticipated and dealt with rapidly and efficiently. It is imperative to be aware of the potential for hypotension following the establishment of positive-pressure ventilation.

The cardiovascular system is primarily stabilized by correcting the relative hypovolemia (see Chapter 27). When hypotension is severe, the patient should immediately have both lower extremities elevated 20–30° from the horizontal position. This is a form of "autotransfusion" in which lower extremity and pelvic blood drainage is facilitated by gravity. The transient increase in "core" blood volume should improve venous return to the heart.

The eventual correction of the relative hypovolemia is accomplished by appropriate intravenous fluid administration (see Chapter 27). During this period manual ventilation can be varied to be synchronous with the patient's efforts and allow long expiratory periods. The patient must not be allowed to "fight" the positive pressure and unduly increase intrathoracic pressure.

Step #3. — Establish appropriate monitors and base lines

Prior to commitment, or as soon as possible after airway establishment and positive-pressure ventilation, a cardiovascular base line (blood pressure and pulse) must be recorded and followed. An adequate intravenous line should already have been established. As soon as possible, an ECG monitor, arterial line, and other appropriate monitors should be evaluated.

Step #4. — Establish ventilatory pattern

The patient's spontaneous breathing should initially be augmented by manual ventilation. Usually patients will gradually relax and adopt the preferred slower and deeper positive-pressure ventilatory pattern. They can then be completely controlled or smoothly augmented. At this time the mode of ventilator support must be decided upon and the anticipated machine pattern mimicked by hand ventilation. If the patient will not tolerate the anticipated pattern by manual ventilation, he most likely will not tolerate being placed on the machine. The transfer from manual ventilation to machine should involve as little physiologic change as possible.

   Step #5. – Connection to the ventilator
   A ventilator is for maintenance! Emphasis must be placed on the fact that commitment to positive-pressure ventilation involves preparing the patient for the machine! Throughout all of ventilator care, the respiratory care practitioner must remember that whenever there is instability or mechanical problems, the patient should be manually ventilated. Thus, once the patient is connected to the mechanical ventilator, the process of ventilator maintenance has begun.

Ventilator Modes (Figure 22–1)

Definitions

   Spontaneous ventilation is defined as the patient's completely controlling ventilation and providing all the necessary power; i.e., the patient is initiating and providing the power for inspiration as well as such efforts as determining the frequency and depth of tidal volume. *Controlled ventilation* is defined as the patient taking *no* physiologically significant role in the ventilatory cycle; i.e., the machine initiates inspiration, provides the power for inspiration, and determines the rate of ventilation and depth of tidal volume. In essence, whatever ventilatory efforts the patient may be making, they are of no physiologic significance to cardiopulmonary homeostasis. *Augmented ventilation* is defined as both the patient and machine being actively involved in physiologically significant roles directed toward maintaining ventilatory homeostasis.

   It must be clearly understood that *the apparatus to which the patient is attached is not the sole determinant of the mode of ventilatory support*. In other words, because a machine is *capable* of augmenting ventilation does not mean that the patient is necessarily receiving augmented ventilation. In many patients it is difficult (and somewhat arbitrary) to distinguish control from augmented modes. The following clinical *guideline* is helpful: tidal volumes of 15 ml/kg or greater in conjunction with ventilator rates of 8 per minute or more are deemed control mode ventilation (CMV); rates of less than 8 per minute are deemed an augmented mode of ventilation *if* the patient is making significant efforts to breathe. If the patient is not making significant breathing efforts, even rates under 8 per minute are deemed control mode. Whatever the particular point of delineation in differentiating control from augmented modes of ventilation, *the determination must be based on the patient's physiology and not the equipment's capability.*

Control Mode

Since the advent of intermittent mandatory ventilation (IMV),[322] and thereby the technical capabilities of providing a physiologically sound method of augmenting ventilation, the use of control mode ventilation (CMV) has significantly decreased. However, it is our experience that the most unstable patients require at least an initial period of control ventilation, whereas those patients in whom the ventilatory support is required because of C.N.S. malfunction usually need prolonged control mode. Also, CMV provides the best *model* upon which clinical guidelines for all positive-pressure ventilation may be based.

Ventilatory Pattern

Inspiratory time and expiratory time may be manipulated to obtain desired physiologic effects. The relationship of inspiration to expiration (I:E ratio) and the frequency of the ventilatory cycle constitute the ventilatory pattern. The success and adequacy of control mode ventilation are more dependent on manipulation of the ventilatory pattern than on any other single factor.[307, 317, 318, 323]

With control mode IPPV, the airway pressure is lowest during expiration (see Fig 22–1). It may therefore be inferred that intrathoracic pressures are lowest during expiration. Inspiratory flow rates, volumes, and time play important roles in determining mean airway pressure;[324] however, keeping inspiratory dynamics constant, *the longer the expiratory time, the lower will be the mean airway pressure.* Since mean airway pressure will have a direct effect on the degree of embarrassment of venous return, relatively slow rates (less than 12 per minute) seem optimal for control mode ventilation. Large tidal volumes (above 10 ml/kg) minimize the effects of anatomic and physiologic deadspace while aiding the maintenance of adequate alveolar ventilation.[326] *Tidal volumes between 10 and 20 ml/kg delivered in a time span of 0.5–1.5 seconds show minimal variations in mean inspiratory airway pressures.*[325]

Incorporating large tidal volumes with slow ventilatory rates theoretically optimizes maintenance of adequate physiologic ventilation while minimizing the potential for compromising venous return. There are two additional advantages to such a ventilatory pattern: (1) the incidence of miliary atelectasis (and all atelectasis) appears to be decreased when large tidal volumes are utilized,[182, 187] and (2) large tidal volumes usually are better tolerated by the conscious patient on positive-pressure ventilation. There seems to be a need for the conscious patient to be aware of the ventilator's expanding the chest since, when this occurs, the patient is usually more comfortable.

In the absence of chronic restrictive pathology, *a reasonable initial ventilator tidal volume is 15 ml/kg at a rate between 8 and 12 per minute and flow rates that provide an inspiratory flow time of 0.5 – 1 second.* Final adjustments of the ventilatory pattern ultimately depend on blood gas analysis and other physiologic monitoring.

"Fighting" the Ventilator

A patient is "out of phase" with the ventilator when he is attempting to end the inspiratory cycle by exhaling while the machine is still in the inspiratory phase. When a patient is out of phase, he is said to be *fighting* the ventilator. This results in greatly increased intrathoracic pressure and decreased alveolar ventilation.[312, 324] Fighting the ventilator cannot be justified in any mode of ventilation!

A simple method to restore control of the ventilatory pattern is to use the technique of manual ventilation. The patient's ventilation is initially augmented and then tidal volumes are gradually increased while the rate is gradually decreased. Often the patient will relax and eventually allow the desired ventilatory pattern to be accomplished.

Faster rates and/or deeper breaths may be necessary to control ventilation. Assuming that venous return is not embarrassed significantly, deadspace tubing may be added to the ventilator circuit to assure eucapneic (normal PCO_2) ventilation. This technique will often facilitate control of the desired ventilatory pattern, but utilization of ventilatory circuit deadspace tubing must be used *only in control mode ventilation!*

Some patients will attempt to make ventilatory efforts during the expiratory phase of the ventilator. This is termed "breathing around or between" the ventilator and has little detrimental physiologic affect; in fact, it may be physiologically beneficial in many circumstances. It is important for the respiratory care practitioner to have clearly in mind the difference between the patient's being out of phase in distinction to simply breathing around the ventilator. In general, a patient who·is out of phase with the ventilator must be manipulated to come into phase; the patient breathing around the ventilator usually may be left alone if an IMV circuit is provided.

Augmented Modes

Between spontaneous and controlled ventilation exists the spectrum where both patient and machine play a physiologically significant role in the maintenance of cardiopulmonary homeostasis. The physiologic advantages of spontaneous over positive-pressure ventilation have already been discussed. Ever since positive-pressure ventilation was introduced, the clinician has been seeking an appropriate way of augmenting ventilation, i.e., allowing the patient to do whatever spontaneous breathing he is capable of (without detriment to homeostasis) and then having a machine augment the remainder of the ventilation. *The preferred mode of supporting ventilation is augmentation* — it is only when augmentation is neither possible nor desirable that control mode ventilation should be instituted.

Assist Mode

The assist mode (see Fig 22–1) has been available for over thirty years because its technology was developed early in the era of modern respiratory therapy. The mechanism allows the patient to control ventilator *rate,* since inspiration will begin when the patient creates a subatmospheric pressure in the circuitry. Initially developed for pressure-cycled ventilators, the patient had "some" control over tidal volumes and/or flow rates. However, with the advent of volume- and time-cycled machines, the assist mode controls only rate.

Over the past thirty years, use of assist mode has been far more attributable to its availability than to its desirability. The superficial concept that a patient is better off "triggering the machine" is one that holds little physiologic or clinical rationale.

In addition to the physiologic advantages of minimizing positive-pressure ventilation, true and effective augmented ventilation also should minimize the necessity for aggressive pharmacologic intervention such as the narcotization and paralysis so common with control mode. Thus, for the past thirty years there has been a constant search for a technically feasible and universally applicable method of truly augmenting ventilation.

Intermittent Mandatory Ventilation (IMV)

With IMV the patient is allowed to breathe spontaneously through the ventilator circuit, and at predetermined intervals a mandatory inspiration is provided by the ventilator. It is technically simple and

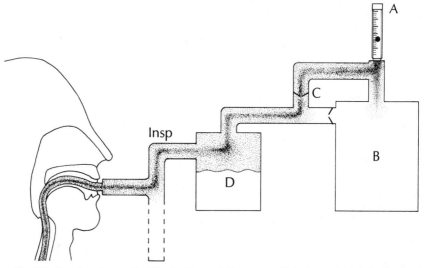

Fig 22–3.—A schematic illustration of the essentials for administration of IMV/IDV. Only the inspiratory limb is shown while spontaneous inspiration is taking place. *A* represents the common gas source so that all inspired gas has the same FI_{O_2}; *B* represents a volume- or time-cycled ventilator; *C* represents the spontaneous breathing circuit with appropriate one-way valve; *D* represents the humidifier through which all inspired gas must flow.

universally adaptable (Fig 22–3). All gas inspired, whether spontaneous or positive pressure, has the same temperature, humidity, and oxygen concentration. The mandatory positive-pressure breath takes place completely independently of the patient's own ventilatory pattern (see Fig 22–1). Since its reintroduction into clinical medicine in 1973,[322] it has proved to be a most significant improvement in airway pressure support. Although initially introduced as a weaning technique, it has been clearly established that the greatest use for IMV is as a maintenance mode.[330]

We consider our patients to be *receiving* IMV only when they are clinically accomplishing significant ventilation on their own. If they are receiving a ventilatory rate of 8 or more per minute with tidal volumes of 10 ml/kg or greater, we consider this to be control mode ventilation despite the patient's efforts. IMV is the basic methodology by which a physiologic *mode* of ventilation (augmented) is accomplished. As such, it should be clinically defined in terms of the patient's homeostasis rather than in terms of the mechanical apparatus attached to the patient.

Excellent as IMV has proved to be, it is *not* the answer for all patients. If our definition of CMV is applied, even those centers claiming no use of control mode ventilation are actually controlling at least 20% of their patients.[331] In our experience, 80–85% of patients requiring ventilatory support are maintained primarily on augmented ventilation (IMV, IDV). Thus, only 15–20% of patients require CMV for the major portion of their ventilator course. Although many patients are on CMV for the initial 3 to 12 hours of their course, they are rapidly changed to an augmented mode following cardiovascular stabilization.

Intermittent Demand Ventilation (IDV)

Intermittent demand ventilation is a mode of augmentation in which the patient is allowed to breathe on his own through the ventilator circuit, and at predetermined intervals the next spontaneous breath is "assisted" by the machine (see Fig 22–1).[332] Intermittent demand ventilation has been used for decades by the anesthetist who allows the patient to breathe on his own while "augmenting" every second, third, or fourth breath by compressing the anesthesia reservoir bag. Thus, an additional volume of gas is delivered *in phase* with the patient's efforts, i.e., on patient demand.

Various techniques have been developed to provide IDV, namely synchronized IMV (SIMV) and intermittent assisted ventilation (IAV). We prefer that the term IDV be used to distinguish the physiologic concept of augmenting on *demand* from augmentation at mandatory intervals (IMV). At present, IDV has not been documented to be of significant advantage over IMV. IDV may prove to have significant technical *dis*advantages, and at best should be considered a sophistication of IMV. The authors strongly urge the respiratory care practitioner *to consider the primary mode of augmented ventilation to be intermittent mandatory ventilation (IMV)* and to keep an open mind as to the future application of the IDV concept.

Control Versus Augmented Modes

There are essentially two modes of ventilator maintenance: control and augmented. Whenever clinically feasible, the augmented mode should be instituted since the patient should be allowed to do as much of his own work of breathing as is consistent with homeostasis. In general, the patient should be capable of assuming more spontaneous ventilation as the disease process improves. Decreasing the ventilator rate in an augmented mode is *not* a weaning process; rather, it should be considered an ability to maintain the patient at a lesser augmented rate due to an improvement in the underlying disease process.

In our experience, patients maintained on augmented mode have a better survival rate than those maintained on control mode. This must *not* be interpreted to mean that IMV must be used *at all costs!* Remember, most patients requiring CMV are severely C.N.S. diseased or are severely unstable cardiovascularly. Therefore, most patients who are capable of being appropriately maintained on augmented ventilation have an intact C.N.S. and reasonable cardiovascular reserves. Although augmented ventilation is desirable and is an encouraging prognostic sign, one should not withhold CMV when required.

Ventilator Discontinuance

Since all airway pressure support is theoretically instituted for the purpose of correcting a pathophysiologic process, adequate reversal of that underlying pathology would automatically dictate discontinuance of the therapy. With appropriate maintenance and medical care, *there is nothing magic about the way a ventilator can be manipulated to "tease" a patient away from the support before reversal of pathophysiology warrants.*[243] Although the dictionary defines the word *wean* as "to withdraw," the common connotation of the term is "to gradually tease away." This slow, gradual concept is unfortunate when applied to ventilator discontinuance. Therefore, the term "weaning from the ventilator" is purposely avoided in this text because, in the vast majority of patients appropriately committed and maintained on ventilators, the ventilator may be discontinued when the disease process has been adequately reversed.

In our experience over 80% of patients successfully discontinued from ventilators do not require a weaning process; rather, they are discontinued from the ventilator within several hours. We prefer to use the term "weaning" only in reference to those 20% of patients who cannot be discontinued from ventilatory support without *gradual* maneuvers for more than 12 hours.

Mechanical support of ventilation must be discontinued at the earliest possible time consistent with patient safety. This does not mean early weaning attempts without rationale, since this usually results in unnecessary cardiopulmonary stress without shortening the ventilator course. Everyone is anxious to "get the patient off the ventilator" as soon as possible. What must be realized is that the shortest ventilator course is accomplished by proper maintenance for the necessary period of time.

A major consideration for ventilator commitment—and a constant consideration during maintenance—is the establishment and evaluation of a working diagnosis, i.e., of the underlying disease process that necessitated the support of ventilation. *The cardinal guideline for discontinuance of ventilator care is evidence of significant improvement or reversal of the underlying disease process.* Numerous pulmonary and cardiovascular measurements supply objective criteria useful in making this clinical judgment; however, these measurements alone are not sufficient! An over-all clinical evaluation of the patient's condition is mandatory.

No dogmatic rule or guideline can be made regarding the timing or duration of a discontinuance process. The rapidity of the process will be determined by the patient. When a patient does *not* maintain an adequate cardiopulmonary status with spontaneous breathing, it is essential to distinguish physiologic from psychologic causes. Once it is reasonably established that the patient should be physiologically capable of independence from the ventilator, the patient's psyche becomes primary and the ensuing weaning process is aimed primarily at that factor.

Estimating Physiologic Capabilities

The procedure of ventilator discontinuance should begin once the following determinations have been appropriately assessed: (1) the underlying disease process is significantly reversed; (2) mechanical measurements of the cardiopulmonary reserves are judged adequate; (3) physiologic measurements of cardiopulmonary reserve appear compatible with spontaneous ventilation; and (4) general clinical examination and laboratory measurements present no contraindications to maintaining both adequate spontaneous ventilation and cardiopulmonary homeostasis.

Reversal of the Underlying Disease Process

This is solely a medical judgment. The pathology is often obvious (e.g., pneumonia, heart failure) and readily identifiable; often the working diagnosis is tenuous or unknown. Augmented modes of ventilation are helpful in the latter patient, since the ability to tolerate decreasing ventilator rates is helpful in evaluation of the over-all process.

Mechanical Measurements

These have been discussed in detail in Chapter 19. Some useful guidelines are as follows: (1) Vital capacity greater than 15 ml/kg is encouraging; however, vital capacity often dramatically improves over several hours of spontaneous breathing. *Do not* rule out a trial at discontinuance for a vital capacity between 10 and 15 ml/kg. Chronically diseased patients (e.g., chronic obstructive pulmonary disease, quadriplegics) can breathe spontaneously with extremely limited vital capacities. (2) Tidal volumes are difficult to evaluate prior to breathing spontaneously for a period of time. Immediate tidal volumes of greater than 2 ml/kg are encouraging. (3) Spontaneous ventilatory rates of less than 25 per minute are encouraging; greater than this calls for reevaluation. (4) Significant tachycardia on the ventilator is discouraging since the work of breathing will place an additional stress on the heart. Again, augmented modes may prove helpful in these patients. (5) Hypotension on the ventilator is discouraging; hypertension must be carefully evaluated. (6) Cardiac arrhythmia must be evaluated. (7) Hemoglobin content should be optimized.

Physiologic Measurements

These will be discussed in detail in Chapters 27 and 28. Some general guidelines: (1) arterial blood gas measurements must be acceptable on the ventilator; (2) no evidence of acute increased deadspace ventilation should be present; (3) intrapulmonary shunt measurement should be less than 30% and preferably less than 20%; and (4) hemodynamics should be stable on the ventilator.

Seven Steps of Ventilator Discontinuance

Following is a general outline for taking a patient off the ventilator. By no means is this intended to be inflexible; however, any method should include the precautions and evaluations presented.

Step #1.—Psychologic preparation

A conscious patient requires careful explanation of the procedure so that the activity will not be alarming! The patient must understand that, when he is asked to breathe on his own, the initial sensations of difficulty in breathing and shortness of breath are expected and not unusual. Forewarning the patient of the expected sequence of events results in less apprehension when they occur and reassures him that the clinician supervising the program is competent.

The patient must never be "guaranteed" that he will not need the ventilator once again. It should be explained that this is an "initial" attempt and you must express your confidence in his ability to breathe. Do not express disappointment if he is unsuccessful; simply explain that it was an attempt and there will be others. The patient must not become depressed if the initial attempt fails.

Step #2.—Manual ventilation

The initial spontaneous breathing efforts should be manually augmented, providing a smooth transition from the ventilator to spontaneous ventilation. The patient will see that you have things well in control and that you can "breathe for him" at any time.

Step #3.—Oxygen therapy apparatus

There must be appropriate operational equipment at the bedside for oxygen and humidity therapy. Do not discontinue oxygen therapy simultaneously with discontinuance of mechanical support of ventilation! It is unwise and counterproductive to expect a patient to assume the work of breathing and simultaneously to meet the increased cardiovascular demands of diminished inspired oxygen concentrations. The patient should be administered *at least* the same oxygen therapy as he received on the ventilator; some physicians advise a 10% increase in F_{IO_2}.

Step #4.—Discontinuance of manual ventilation

The patient is allowed to assume his own work of breathing while the ECG and blood pressure are closely monitored. The first several minutes of breathing spontaneously are critical and demand the bedside attention of the respiratory care practitioner. Clinical evaluation of the ventilatory pattern, the ventilatory effort, and the cardiovascular system must be continuously accomplished. Any patient stress must evoke immediate and obvious recognition on your part, and that recognition must be obvious to the patient. He must be convinced you are aware and in control!

Several short periods of manually augmented ventilation may be indicated for reassurance. The main criterion and responsibility of the respiratory care practitioner during these first attempts at ventilator discontinuance are to decide whether or not observed distress is a physiologic or psychologic problem.

Step #5.—Assessment of vital sign changes

There are vital sign changes that should be anticipated when a patient assumes spontaneous ventilation: (1) The ventilator has been providing a slower and deeper ventilatory pattern than the patient's natural, spontaneous pattern. When the patient assumes his spontaneous ventilatory pattern, it should not cause concern as long as the pattern is acceptable and remains consistent with cardiopulmonary homeostasis. (2) The ventilator supports the cardiovascular system significantly, so that when the work of breathing is assumed by the patient, it often requires some increase in blood pressure and cardiac rate. (3) Mild diaphoresis (sweating) is a common feature and should not cause concern unless accompanied by other signs of increased sympathetic discharge or physiologic stress.

As long as the vital signs and clinical changes are within acceptable limits, they should not cause concern on the part of the respiratory care practitioner. Far more important than the immediate vital sign changes is their *stability* over the next 15 minutes.

Step #6. — 15-Minute evaluation

During the first 15 minutes of spontaneous ventilation, it is essential that the respiratory care practitioner remain at the bedside and closely monitor the patient. It may be appropriate to intermittently give some deep ("sigh") breaths by manual ventilator, e.g., every 3 or 4 minutes, to augment the patient's ventilatory efforts (as well as for psychologic reassurance). If suctioning is necessary, there must be appropriate support before and after the suctioning process so that the patient is not allowed to become hypoxemic or frightened.

Following 15 minutes of reasonable clinical stability, vital signs, blood gases, and general clinical status must be reevaluated. It is important to assess what has happened to the vital capacity and the ventilatory pattern over these 15 minutes. The blood gases will reveal the net result of cardiopulmonary homeostasis and must be compared with the mechanical work of the cardiopulmonary system so that an evaluation of system efficiency and reserve can be accomplished (see Chapter 19).

Step #7. — Support of the spontaneously breathing patient

If the patient reveals a reasonable clinical status and a stable cardiopulmonary state, his trial of spontaneous breathing should be continued. At this point, it is important for the respiratory care practitioner to recognize the need for adequate bronchial hygiene, as well as for continuance of oxygen and humidity therapy. Appropriate deep breathing and suctioning must be accomplished over the next several hours according to the needs of the patient and his tolerance. The patient will realize that he is now breathing on his own and will interpret this as a very dramatic sign that he is getting better. There should be attempts to make the patient more comfortable, and it must be explained that the artificial airway is still needed (for some period of time) to keep the lungs clear.

While the patient continues to breathe spontaneously over the next several hours, the cardiopulmonary status is closely monitored and evaluated. It has been our experience that if the previously described patient is maintaining adequate cardiopulmonary homeostasis and manifesting adequate reserves at the end of several hours, he will usually remain off the ventilator. It is at this juncture that decisions concerning the airway and other nonventilator support of the patient must be clearly delineated.

Failure to Accomplish Ventilator Discontinuance

Failure of the patient to maintain an adequate cardiopulmonary status with spontaneous breathing must be carefully evaluated — *we must be certain there is no iatrogenic reason for the failure*. The mechanical device through which the patient is breathing must be examined and it must be ascertained that narcotics, sedatives, and muscle ralaxants have been completely reversed. When these factors have been ruled out and the physiologic parameters of cardiopulmonary reserve still indicate that the patient should be able to breathe on his own, the assumption must be made that the patient is either unable to come off the ventilator because the disease is not adequately reversed for his general body reserves, or that psychologic dependence exists. Obviously an unconscious patient cannot manifest psychologic dependence. In our experience, most weaning problems are due to either (1) attempting to discontinue ventilation too early in the disease course; (2) improper ventilator maintenance; or (3) pre-existing chronic disease or malnutrition that severely limits reserves. In the absence of these, the next most common problem is psychologic dependence.

A few patients may have to be placed back on the ventilator at night because they are afraid to fall asleep breathing on their own. This may be a reasonable approach for several days.

Psychologic dependence is a difficult problem and one that demands a great deal of understanding and patience. These individuals are in need of a weaning process in the traditional sense, i.e., the process of taking the patient off the ventilator for short periods of time and trying to lengthen the periods progressively. The problem of having to wean a patient slowly from mechanical support of ventilation for either physiologic or psychologic reasons is a time-consuming and frustrating process.

Augmented Ventilation and Weaning

For the patient who does not assume ventilator independence readily, the techniques of intermittent mandatory ventilation (IMV) or intermittent demand ventilation (IDV) are clinically useful. These techniques hold the advantage of allowing the patient to gradually assume more work of breathing without the constant attention of the respiratory care practitioner. This makes it far more practical (and far less frustrating) to accomplish a weaning process without being limited by the availability of bedside personnel. There still must be appropriate intensive care monitoring, but the process of decreasing the rate of the intermittent ventilation has proved quite beneficial and has shortened the weaning process of many patients.

As useful as augmented techniques have proved for the patient truly in need of a weaning process, these techniques have been misused for ventilator discontinuance. Many physicians "routinely" decrease IMV rates over 24 to 48 hours, a process that unnecessarily prolongs the ventilator course. Since the vast majority of patients do *not* need a weaning process, they do not need several days of tapering with IMV prior to breathing spontaneously. When the disease process has reversed, they will come off the ventilator. IMV/IDV are useful weaning techniques for those patients in need of a weaning process; they should not be misused to prolong unnecessarily the time on the ventilator.

23 • PRINCIPLES OF VENTILATOR MAINTENANCE

THE MAINTENANCE of mechanical ventilation is a multidisciplinary challenge. The respiratory therapist is the cornerstone of this care, since proper use, control, and maintenance of the ventilator and artificial airway are essential. The respiratory intensive care nurse plays an equally vital role in being responsible for bedside monitoring, physical care, and delivery of medications. The chest physical therapist augments the efforts of the respiratory therapist and nurse in maintaining bronchial hygiene.

Respiratory intensive care demands moment-to-moment monitoring and therapy 24 hours a day. The routine change-over of personnel every 8 hours requires established procedures and an excellent system of communication. There are numerous ways to accomplish good care. The essential fact is that the critical care unit must have "a way"—a specific standard operating procedure that is understood by all who participate in patient care. This assures smooth continuation of care from shift to shift and day to day. Unfortunately, inherent in this approach is the necessity for an established program; therefore, the individual preferences of specific physicians, nurses, and therapists cannot always be catered to!

It is not our intention to put forth specific operating procedures of ventilator care. Rather, the purpose is to discuss the *principles* necessary for development of a clinically sound procedural program. The following discussion must not be interpreted as espousing "the way" to accomplish ventilator maintenance. Instead it should be considered a discussion of the physiologic and medical principles that must be satisfied by an acceptable procedure. Discussion of specific procedural methods is avoided where possible; however, in some circumstances it is necessary to describe specific procedures to clarify the discussion. The reader must understand that when such circumstances exist, our standard procedure is presented as an example—not as the only way the goals can be accomplished.

Eucapneic Ventilation

Eucapneic ventilation is the maintenance of an arterial P_{CO_2} within a "normal" range—defined classically as a P_{CO_2} between 35 and 45 mm Hg. The concept of normal ventilation should incorporate the principle of supporting the ventilatory state in the range normally maintained by that patient. A patient who normally carries an arterial P_{CO_2} of 70 mm Hg should be ventilated at an arterial P_{CO_2} close to 70 mm Hg.

Acid-Base Abnormalities

The reasons for maintaining normal ventilation are primarily acid-base and electrolyte considerations. If an individual is maintained at an arterial P_{CO_2} significantly different from his normal range, acute alkalemia or acidemia will result. The kidneys will appropriately respond by holding onto or getting rid of base (HCO_3^-). Normal kidneys will metabolically compensate for a ventilatory pH change in 24 to 36 hours.[298] For example, an individual who normally carries an arterial P_{CO_2} of 70 mm Hg and a pH of 7.40 is in a state of compensated respiratory acidosis (chronic ventilatory failure); an increased amount of base (HCO_3^-) is present. If this individual is suddenly ventilated to and maintained at P_{CO_2} of 40 mm Hg for several days, the kidneys will excrete the "excess" base to correct the sudden "respiratory alkalemia."

The previously described process causes two major problems:

1. The cardiovascular, hepatorenal, and central nervous systems will be challenged to function adequately in an alkalemic milieu and its associated electrolyte environment for several days.[333] Not only is cellular membrane function compromised, but sensitivities and reactivities to various drugs are less predictable. *The goal must be acid-base stability from the moment the patient is placed on the ventilator.*

2. When the ventilator is removed from the patient and he assumes total spontaneous ventilation, he will be required to breathe at an alveolar ventilation far greater than his pre-existent base-line state. If he assumes his previous base-line arterial P_{CO_2} of 70 mm Hg, he will become acidemic secondary to the acute CO_2 rise and the inability of the kidneys to immediately reaccumulate bicarbonate ion. The acute acidemia acts as an additional challenge to his limited cardiopulmonary reserves. Not uncommonly, the patient will end up in severe respiratory and cardiovascular distress because of his inability to maintain ventilation above his "normal" base-line state. This generally results in the patient being placed back on the ventilator and considered a weaning problem. Note that the "problem" is strictly a result of the improper ventilator maintenance.

Cerebral Flood Flow

In addition to the acid-base problem, acute alveolar hyperventilation will result in cerebral vasoconstriction in response to the decreased arterial P_{CO_2}. In most circumstances this leads to a decreased cerebral blood flow. This may be desirable for short periods of time in acute head trauma (see Chapter 34); however, in the critically ill patient without brain damage this decreased blood flow to the brain may be disastrous. There has been much speculation that C.N.S. embarrassment may be the key to major complications confronted in ventilator care. It is theoretically detrimental to routinely maintain ventilator support at arterial P_{CO_2} levels below a patient's pre-existent base line.

Deadspace Tubing Technique

Many patients in the early part of their ventilator course will require control mode ventilation (CMV), some patients for a significant period of time. The optimal IPPV pattern in control mode may result in undesirably low arterial P_{CO_2}'s. In this circumstance, it is necessary to have a means of manipulating the arterial P_{CO_2} so that eucapnia may be maintained in conjunction with the appropriate ventilatory pattern.

The addition of *deadspace tubing* is the process of placing a volume of tubing between the artificial airway and the Y-piece of the ventilator. This "extension of the trachea" results in rebreathing of expired gas and therefore increases the inspired carbon dioxide concentration. The respiratory care practitioner must remember that deadspace tubing will both increase carbon dioxide-inspired concentrations and decrease oxygen concentrations reaching the alveoli. The latter effect is minimized with proper oxygen therapy.

Nomograms are available for estimating the degree of deadspace tubing required; however, we have found that simply "titrating" additions of 50 to 100 ml volumes of tubing is the fastest and most reliable method. In some patients, 300–500 ml of deadspace tubing may be necessary. It is not unusual to add several hundred milliliters of deadspace tubing with only minimal increases in $PaCO_2$ and then to have a marked increase with the addition of another 50 ml of tubing.

Deadspace tubing is reliable and predictable *only* with a control mode of ventilation. *Deadspace tubing is contraindicated with augmented ventilation!* If the clinical decision is made to augment ventilation in a patient with acutely decreased arterial P_{CO_2}, this should be considered a reason for further adjustment in the pattern (rate) of augmentation. In our experience, it is seldom necessary to abandon augmented ventilation because of the patient's desire to maintain a low arterial P_{CO_2}. However, it is also our experience that primarily central nervous system-diseased patients are usually best supported with CMV.

Pharmacology for Ventilator Maintenance

Pharmacologic intervention is indicated when CMV is desired and the patient fights the ventilator. The ideal drug to control ventilation would possess a minimum of eight factors: (1) have a potent central respiratory depressant effect; (2) have minimal cardiovascular side-effects; (3) have a potent euphoric effect, making consciousness tolerable during the ventilator course; (4) have an analgesic effect, since it is not uncommon for these individuals to experience pain; (5) be totally reversible by a pharmacologic agent without dangerous effects of its own; (6) be inexpensive; (7) be clinically familiar to nursing and physician personnel; and (8) have a long, stable shelf life. There are drugs available that come close to meeting these eight criteria; the best example is morphine sulfate.

Morphine Sulfate

Morphine sulfate, the prototype narcotic drug, is a very potent respiratory depressant. It has few clinically significant cardiovascular side-effects when the patient is well ventilated, well oxygenated, and in acid-base balance.[334, 335] The only significant *direct* cardiovascular effect of morphine sulfate is on the venous system where it causes a decrease in the state of venous tone.[336]

Much misunderstanding exists concerning morphine sulfate because the classic pharmacologic effects are related to the spontaneously breathing patient. It has been well documented that large doses of morphine may be extremely dangerous to the cardiovascular system in the spontaneously breathing patient.[207] However, these adverse effects of cardiac arrhythmias and hypotension are secondary to ventilatory depression (hypercarbia, hypoxemia, and acidemia). In the well-ventilated, well-oxygenated, acid-base balanced patient (the patient on CMV), the only *documented* cardiovascular effect of large intravenous doses of morphine is increased venous capacitance.[337, 338] This can be readily compensated by appropriate attention to hemodynamic monitoring and fluid therapy (see Chapter 27).

Morphine sulfate is a good euphoric agent and an excellent analgesic. It is completely reversed by naloxone hydrochloride (Narcan).[339] Morphine sulfate is inexpensive, is familiar in clinical medicine, and has a long shelf life.

Morphine sulfate provides the respiratory care clinician with the almost perfect drug for sedation and control of ventilation. Of course, the patient must have reasonable blood gases and the airway established prior to administration of large doses of morphine. In adults, up to 80 mg has been administered intravenously in the first hour, and up to 20 mg each hour for maintenance without untoward effects. If the guidelines are followed, the only problem with administration of morphine is an increase in the vascular space, which is readily corrected with proper fluid loading. Our usual doses for cardiovascularly stable patients are 10–20 mg (0.2–0.3 mg/kg) the first hour with 3–6 mg (0.05–0.1 mg/kg) every hour for maintenance.

The decision to sedate a patient to accomplish CMV requires an increased responsibility to evaluate the cardiopulmonary system and tissue oxygenation status. Patients often fight the ventilator because of improper ventilation or C.N.S. hypoxia. It must be understood that *sedation is given only after a careful evaluation of the adequacy of ventilatory and oxygenation support.*

Heroin has proved itself superior to morphine in Great Britain. This is probably because of its superiority as a euphoric. The agent is not clinically available in the United States. *Meperidine hydrochloride* (Demerol) may be used, but it is not as good a euphoric as morphine and, therefore, does not work as well in conscious or semicomatose patients. In our experience, none of the narcotics available in the United States have any advantage over morphine sulfate.

Tranquilizing Agents

There are many experts in respiratory care who prefer the use of tranquilizing agents to that of morphine for CMV; others use combinations of morphine and tranquilizers. *Thiazide* agents (e.g., chlorpromazine HCl [Thorazine]) gained popularity for a time. The problem is that these drugs are vasodilators (perhaps by virtue of their alpha blockade effects) and may cause significant hypotension.[207] Droperidol (Inapsine) is a long-acting tranquilizer that may be used in conjunction with narcotics. This is popular in anesthesia and, as a mixture with fentanyl citrate (Sublimaze), is marketed as Innovar. *Diazepam* (Valium) has gained great popularity, especially as an adjunct to augmented ventilation. The greatest objection to the tranquilizing agents is that they are not predictable central respiratory depressants and they are *not reversible.*

Paralyzing Agents

The nicotinic portion of the parasympathetic nervous system includes the motor nerves to skeletal (voluntary) muscles, including the muscles of ventilation. An impulse travels down the motor nerve to the nerve ending, which lies in close proximity to but does not touch the muscle cell membrane. The space between the end of the motor nerve and muscle cell is called the synaptic cleft, and the entire area is known as the *myoneural junction*. The electric impulse travels to the end of the nerve and causes the release of *acetylcholine*, which travels across the myoneural junction and attaches to receptors located on the muscle sole plate, a portion of the muscle cell wall. The attachment of the acetylcholine molecule to the receptor causes depolarization of the cell wall, which leads to an intracellular biochemical process that results in contraction of the muscle fiber. An enzyme (cholinesterase) present in the extravascular fluid metabolizes the acetycholine, allowing the muscle cell wall to repolarize.

The circuit of electric impulse-chemical release-receptor depolarization-chemical metabolism-repolarization occurs very rapidly and allows normal skeletal muscle actions to occur in response to motor nerve stimuli. Pharmacologic intervention at the myoneural junction can lead to muscle paralysis.

Non-Depolarizing Muscle Relaxants

A non-depolarizing muscle relaxant has its effect via the pharmacologic principle of "competition" among substances for the same receptor sites. When the myoneural junction concentration of the competing drug is higher than acetylcholine, the receptor sites will be mostly occupied by the competing drug, and depolarization of the muscle cell by acetylcholine will be blocked. As the relative concentrations of acetylcholine and competing drug change, the degree of muscle blockaid also changes.

d-Tubocurarine has been the traditional non-depolarizing drug of choice for maintenance of controlled ventilation. The initial "curarizing" dose is often up to 30 mg and must be given only by a physician familiar with the drug, since it is a mild ganglionic blocker and may cause hypotension.[206] Although reported to be associated with histamine release, this appears to be of little clinical significance. Maintenance doses of curare are 3–9 mg and seldom cause hypotension. Therefore, it is reasonable to have intensive care nurses administer the maintenance doses of curare, provided appropriate physiologic monitoring is available.

Pancuronium bromide (Pavulon) is widely used in anesthesia as an improved non-depolarizing muscle relaxant and has gained great popularity in the field of respiratory care. The drug has a steroid base and is claimed to have certain advantages over curare in that it is more rapid acting and does not have the ganglionic blocking side-effects. However, tachycardia has been reported as a common side-effect. The usual initial paralyzing dose of Pavulon is approximately 5 mg in the average adult. Again, this must be given only by a physician familiar with the drug. Maintenance doses are 0.5 – 1 mg and it is usually administered by the intensive care nurse. Pavulon is very similar in its clinical uses and clinical actions to that of curare and has become the most commonly used non-depolarizing muscle relaxant.

The non-depolarizing agents are reversible with "anticholinesterase" drugs such as edrophonium chloride (Tensilon) or neostigmine (Prostigmin). Reversal should be attempted only by physicians familiar with the process. Atropine sulfate is usually administered with the neostigmine to block its muscarinic effects. It is generally believed that Pavulon is somewhat more difficult to reverse after long-standing paralysis than is curare. In any case, the non-depolarizing agents are widely favored as the agents of choice for maintenance of muscle paralysis in ventilator care.

Depolarizing Muscle Relaxants

A depolarizing muscle relaxant is a pharmacologic agent whose molecular structure is similar to that of acetylcholine but which is not metabolized by true cholinesterase and which will attach to the muscle cell wall receptor and cause depolarization. This depolarization is seen as muscle twitching or fasciculation shortly after injection. It takes approximately 3 – 10 minutes for an enzyme called *pseudocholinesterase* to metabolize the drug and allow the muscle to repolarize. Such a depolarizing muscle relaxant is succinylcholine chloride (Anectine). Its onset is rapid (within 10 seconds); it is short acting and non-reversible. It is used primarily for facilitating the intubation process and is seldom used for prolonged maintenance of ventilator care.

Combinations of sedation and paralyzation are frequently needed and desirable. Certainly, a conscious patient who must be paralyzed must also be sedated – to do otherwise would be inhumane.

Maintaining Bronchial Hygiene

Maintenance of a clear airway and removal of secretions from the tracheobronchial tree are essential in the care of all patients with tracheal intubations, especially the ventilator patient. The artificial airway results in the loss of an effective cough mechanism and ciliary function, potentially leading to pooling of secretions, atelectasis, and pneumonia. The three main techniques of assuring adequate bronchial hygiene are (1) proper humidification of the airway, (2) positional rotation and aggressive chest physical therapy (CPT) to prevent pooling of secretions, and (3) proper suctioning of secretions from the airway. These techniques have been discussed in Section III. Acute segmental atelectasis is common during ventilator support and is best re-expanded by CPT techniques as previously described (see Chapter 12).

The Fiberoptic Bronchoscope

Bronchoscopy was considered the treatment of choice for atelectasis in acutely ill patients in the United States after World War II. By 1960 the advancement of respiratory therapy had incorporated the techniques of chest physical therapy, aerosol therapy, and IPPB therapy to re-expand atelectasis secondary to retained secretions in the ICU. These techniques proved far more efficient and less traumatic than "rigid" bronchoscopy and, thus, respiratory care abandoned the use of bronchoscopy for bronchial hygiene in acutely ill patients.

The *fiberoptic bronchoscope* became readily available in intensive care in the early 1970s.[340] This new technology allows visualization of the tracheobronchial tree without interruption of ventilation and with minimal risk to the critically ill patient.[341] This new availability and relative safety of fiberoptic bronchoscopy necessitates reevaluation of the role bronchoscopy should play in maintaining bronchial hygiene in ventilator care.

Diagnostic bronchoscopy is indicated when there is bleeding in the tracheobronchial tree or when there is question of tumor, secretions, obstruction, or foreign body. General therapeutic uses of bronchoscopy are suctioning, removal of foreign body, biopsy, and selective lavage.[340] Some physicians prefer routine aggressive suctioning and lavage with the fiberoptic bronchoscope rather than respiratory therapy techniques. Although it will take a period of years for the relative merits of fiberoptic bronchoscopy versus chest physical therapy techniques to be documented, our impression is that the techniques of respiratory therapy (aerosol, IPPB, and CPT) remain the first line of defense in the treatment of atelectasis from pooled secretions.

Essential Ventilator Monitors

The prime concern of intensive care personnel administering ventilatory support must be to eliminate any possibility of death due to mechanical failure or human error. Although there is no replacement for vigilant personnel, monitors to alert the respiratory care practitioner of possible mechanical failure or malfunction are essential.

Exhaled Tidal Volume Monitor

All ventilators should have a mechanism for measuring exhaled tidal volumes. The gas volume exhaled into a spirometer is the best readily available reflection of the volume that has been delivered to the patient. It is not adequate to monitor only the volume of gas being delivered by the machine, since there is no guarantee that all of that gas will be delivered to the patient's pulmonary system. Measurement of exhaled tidal volume (ETV) is usually a reliable reflection of the patient's ventilation.

Ideally, the exhaled tidal volume spirometer should be readily visible. Visual and audial alarms should respond to disconnection as well as to a significant decrease in exhaled tidal volumes. The monitor should have a reasonable delay mechanism (15–20 seconds) so that it is not necessary to turn off the alarm for the suctioning process. *An alarm system that must be routinely turned off is unacceptable since the human tendency is to forget to turn alarms back on.* The audial alarm system should have its own battery power source so that it will be independent of electric power failure.

Oxygen Alarm

All ventilators must have a monitor to assure proper functioning of the oxygen delivery system. This does not delete the responsibility of the respiratory therapist to monitor oxygen concentrations of inspired gas on a routine basis.

Pressure-Relief Mechanisms

The popularity of volume- and time-cycled machines makes it necessary to guarantee that excessive pressures will not be transmitted to the patient's airway. All such machines must have a safety pressure-relief mechanism that will limit the pressure in the inspiratory line. This "pop-off" mechanism should be accompanied by an audial alarm to notify personnel that excessive pressure is being encountered.

Inspiratory Line Thermometer

A thermometer should be placed in the inspiratory line as close to the patient as possible to ensure that the gas is at or near body temperature. Superheated gas can cause hyperthermia, and gas below body temperature will require heat and moisture from the patient's pulmonary system, resulting in drying of the airways and crusting of the artificial airway.

Summary

A detailed discussion of all ventilator monitoring devices is beyond the scope of this text. It is incumbent upon the respiratory therapist to assure that the equipment is maintained in optimal working order and that all reasonable monitors are applied and functioning.

The diligence of all personnel is required to assure patient safety. Some method of periodic, systematic ventilator assessment is mandatory. It is of great assistance to establish some form of "flow sheet" system that requires the therapist to undergo a systematic check of the ventilator at least every 2 hours.

End-Inspiratory Pause (Inflation Hold)

The normal spontaneous inspiratory flow pattern has two characteristics believed to be significant in ensuring optimal peripheral distribution of gas: (1) a *gradual* increase to peak flow; and (2) nearly all of the inspiratory volume being delivered in the first half of inspiration.

The gradual flow increase is believed to minimize turbulence and, thereby, enhances flow through the airways. Although there is much theoretic debate concerning inspiratory flow patterns of ventilators (e.g., sine wave vs. square wave), there is little evidence that it makes a significant difference.[342] The majority of modern ventilators begin inspiration with a square wave flow, a technical convenience that appears to be clinically acceptable.

The delivery of volume in early inspiration is a matter that has received a great deal of attention in the past few years.[315, 342, 343] With time-cycled ventilators, it is relatively simple to deliver the inspiratory volume and then hold inspiration (delay expiration) for an additional period. This *end-inspiratory pause* or *inflation hold* (Fig 23–1) capability appears to have significant clinical application. In simple terms, the longer the time from gas delivery to end inspiration, (1) the greater will be the peripheral distribution of gas (see time constants, Chapter 3), and (2) the better will be distribution of gas to areas of low V/Q due to regional airway resistance variance.[315, 344, 345]

"Manual" inflation hold has been utilized by anesthetists for fifty years to re-expand the retracted lung at the end of chest procedures. This principle was first applied in respiratory care following suctioning procedures to assure expansion of collapsed lung. Whether or not the naturally occurring yawn has a similar function is still being debated; however, many investigators believe that the constant volume hypoventilation of the sleep state leads to miliary atelectasis that is re-

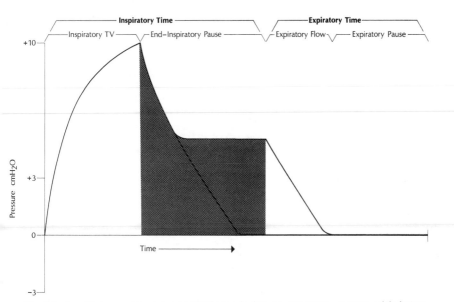

Fig 23–1.—Schematic representation of airway pressure curve with intermittent positive-pressure ventilation and end-inspiratory pause. The shaded area represents the inspiratory time following delivery of tidal volume (VT) to the airway. The rapid initial decrease in airway pressure is the result of significant flow from the upper airway to the lung. Note the pressure plateau that is maintained until expiration begins. This represents a significant period of time between the delivery of inspiratory gas and beginning of expiration (see text).

expanded upon awakening by the "natural inflation hold"—the yawn.[179]

End-inspiratory pause (inflation hold) is a useful and available airway pressure maneuver to provide optimal inspiratory alveolar distribution of gas with positive-pressure ventilation. Tidal volumes between 10 and 20 ml/kg delivered at flow rates allowing complete delivery in not less than 0.5 second and not more than 1.5 seconds, will result in almost identical mean airway pressures.[325] With a ventilator rate of 10 per minute (6-second frequency) and an inspiratory delivery time of 1 second, a 1-second inflation hold may be given and still maintain a 1:2 I:E ratio (2 sec:4 sec). Many clinicians prefer routine use of this airway maneuver. Inflation hold has its greatest potential clinical application in patients with significant airway resistance,[314] although occasionally it may prove helpful in severe compliance disease.

Expiratory Retard

Increased airway resistance is seldom the primary cause for acute respiratory failure requiring ventilator support.[347] However, increased airway resistance is common in patients in need of ventilatory support for other reasons. This increased airway resistance is most commonly due to bronchospasm, pulmonary mucosal edema, bronchiolar inflammation, or combinations of these.

Increased airway resistance results in an obstructive abnormality; i.e., the major problem is exhaling. *Air trapping is common and may be accentuated on the ventilator since inspiratory gas delivery is greater than with spontaneous breathing.* Thus, alveolar gas delivery during inspiration is enhanced, whereas expiratory flow may be impeded.

The airway dynamics of a *forced expiration* in a normal individual is illustrated in Figure 23-2, A. When exhalation begins, the intrapleural pressures increase due to abdominal pressure forcing the diaphragm upward. The alveolar gas is compressed by the positive intrapleural pressure and the elastic recoil forces of the lung, thus creating an alveolar pressure greater than the positive intrapleural pressure. Assuming (1) that the airways are subjected to the intrapleural pressures, and (2) that a gradual pressure decrease occurs from alveolus to mouth, somewhere in the bronchial system the intraluminal and extraluminal pressures will be equal. This theoretic point is called the *equal pressure point* (EPP).[62] Note that airways on the tracheal side of the EPP have extraluminal pressures greater than intraluminal pressures, which would theoretically tend to compress the airways. The normal EPP is believed to be located somewhere above the small bronchi where the airways possess reasonable skeletal rigidity and are not readily compressed or collapsed by increased extraluminal pressures.

In our model (see Fig 23-2), any phenomenon that decreases lung elastic recoil (e.g., acute alveolar distention or emphysema) will decrease the difference between alveolar pressure and intrapleural pressure. During forced exhalation (see Fig 23-2, B) this would tend to move the EPP toward the alveolus, i.e., toward bronchioles that are potentially compressible and perhaps collapsible. Theoretically, this would tend to impede alveolar emptying during exhalation.

The phenomenon illustrated in Figure 23-2, A and B, may occur in the *absence* of forced exhalation with positive-pressure ventilation because the intrapleural pressure may be above atmospheric during exhalation.

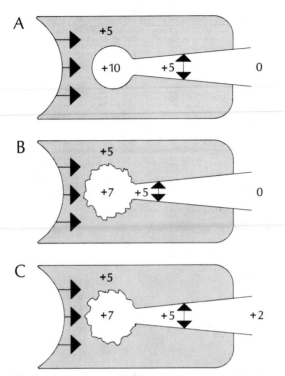

Fig 23–2.—Schematic representation of forced exhalation (the shaded area represents the intrapleural space). **A** represents a normal lung. Note that intrapleural pressure is positive (+5) and intra-alveolar pressure is +10. The airway pressure drop from alveolus to mouth (+10→0) is gradual. The *intraluminal arrows* represent the equal pressure point (EPP). **B** represents forced exhalation with obstructive disease; **C** represents obstructive disease with "retard." See text for full explanation.

Technique of Expiratory Retard

The pressure drop resulting from a gas flowing through a tube with a fixed orifice will be related to the flow, the size of the tube, and the size of the orifice. If a restricted orifice is placed in the extrathoracic airway during exhalation, pressure along the airway will *decrease less* because the restriction acts to diminish the flow. This results in the maintenance of expiratory flow for a longer period of time. Thus, by placing a restricted orifice in the expiratory line of a breathing circuit (Fig 23–3), intraluminal airway pressures will be maintained at a higher level as long as expiratory flow is significant. This type of device is *not* used in patients with normal lung function, as it would needlessly retard flow during exhalation.

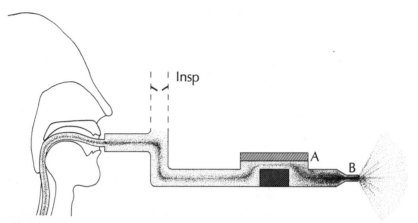

Fig 23–3.—Schematic representation of the expiratory limb of a breathing circuit. *A* represents the exhalation valve in the open position; *B* represents a restricted orifice. The restricted orifice will "retard" expiratory flow (see text).

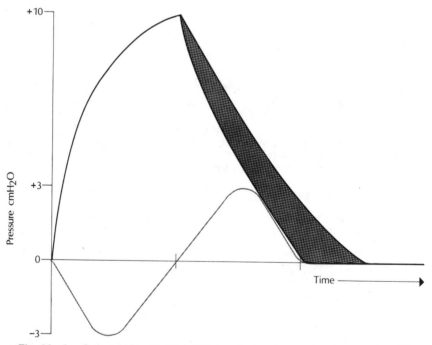

Fig 23–4.—Schematic representation of airway pressure curve resulting from positive-pressure ventilation plus retard. The shaded area represents the increased airway pressure resulting from the "retard."

Paradoxically, the function of the retard in severe obstructive disease is to improve expiratory flow by moving the equal pressure point. Since "expiratory retard" will maintain higher expiratory airway pressures while flow is present, by increasing airway pressure in the trachea, the pressure difference from alveolus to trachea is less (see Fig 23-2, C). Since intrapleural pressures have not been affected, the EPP is *moved away* from the alveolus.

In most cases of severe obstruction, expiratory flow will be markedly improved when retard is appropriately applied. This principle is primarily applicable to patients with air trapping secondary to small airway resistance. It will *not* improve exhalation in a normal lung and may embarrass venous return by increasing mean airway pressure (Fig 23-4).

Pursed lip breathing is believed to be a form of retard exhalation. "Expiratory resistance" or "retard" on the ventilator may prove most beneficial when patients are undergoing acute air trapping secondary to small airways resistance.

24 • PRINCIPLES
OF PEEP THERAPY

OF THE NUMEROUS CLINICAL advances that have evolved in acute respiratory care over the past decade, it appears that positive end-expiratory pressure (PEEP) therapy has made the greatest impact on mortality and morbidity. Routine application of PEEP therapy developed in less than three years. This rapid acceptance has resulted in many clinicians accepting "half-truths" and undocumented concepts, leading to the present day overuse, misuse, and misapplication of PEEP therapy.

Although there is much to be learned, certain facts are obvious: (1) PEEP is *not* the answer to all hypoxemia; (2) PEEP has *not* negated the need for ventilators; and (3) PEEP is *not* harmless. This chapter is designed to aid the respiratory care practitioner in placing PEEP therapy on as solid a physiologic and clinical basis as present knowledge allows while providing a sound foundation with which future knowledge may be properly integrated.

Defining PEEP Therapy

Alveolar Distending Pressure and FRC

Inhalation is an active event in which contraction of ventilatory muscles results in increased thoracic volume. Exhalation is normally a passive event in which relaxation of the ventilatory muscles allows the elastic properties of the lung to create increased alveolar pressures. The resultant alveolar-to-mouth "driving pressure" causes gas to flow until alveolar pressures equal mouth pressure. The volume of gas remaining in the lungs at end exhalation is defined as the functional residual capacity (FRC) and is primarily determined by *elastic properties of the chest wall and elastic properties of the lung* (see Fig 3–1).

At the end of exhalation, the force opposing the lung elasticity is the *alveolar distending pressure* (alveolar pressure minus intrapleural pressure) (see Fig 21–1, C). Since transairway pressure must equal zero at FRC, transpulmonary pressure must equal the alveolar distending pressure at FRC.

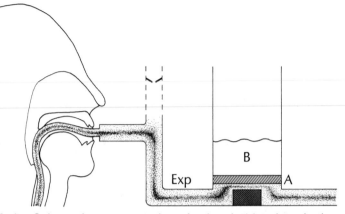

Fig 24–1.—Schematic representation of a threshold resistor in the expiratory limb of a breathing circuit; expiratory *(Exp)* flow is illustrated and is unimpeded. *A* represents a diaphragm that functions as an exhalation valve. When in the "up" position (as shown), flow is unimpeded; when in a "down" position, flow is completely occluded. *B* represents a water column atop the diaphragm. When expiratory pressure falls below the weight (or pressure exerted) by the water column, the diaphragm will shut and flow will cease. Thus, a 10-cm column of water will maintain +10 cm H_2O pressure in the expiratory limb.

Threshold Resistor

A *threshold resistor* is a device that does not interfere with flow as long as the system pressure remains above a predetermined value; when the system pressure falls below that value, the flow completely stops. When a threshold resistor is placed on the exhalation limb of a breathing circuit (Fig 24–1), flow is unimpeded until the pressure falls below the predetermined threshold; when that occurs, the flow completely stops and the pressure is maintained within the system. Thus, it is possible to maintain expiratory airway pressure above atmospheric at the end of exhalation while inspiratory and expiratory flows are unaffected by the system. In this manner it is technically possible to increase the end-expiratory airway pressure to predetermined levels above ambient while leaving inspiratory and expiratory flows essentially unimpeded. This is termed Positive End-Expiratory Pressure (PEEP).

Terminology of PEEP Therapy

As illustrated in Figure 24–2, when PEEP is administered to a patient receiving intermittent positive-pressure ventilation (IPPV), it

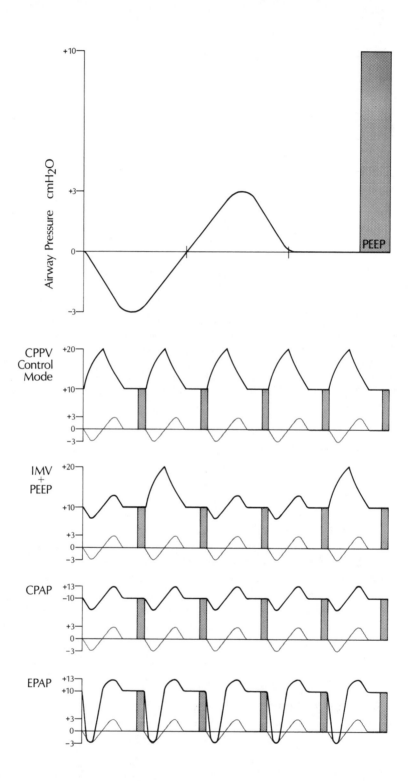

may be referred to as continuous positive-pressure ventilation (CPPV) or "the ventilator with PEEP"; when applied to a patient receiving intermittent mandatory ventilation, it may be referred to as "IMV plus PEEP"; when applied in conjunction with spontaneous ventilation and the inspiratory pressures remain above atmospheric, it is referred to as continuous positive airway pressure (CPAP); when applied to a spontaneously breathing patient whose inspiratory pressure must fall below atmospheric, it is referred to as expiratory positive airway pressure (EPAP). The following discussion concerns the physiologic effects of PEEP alone, i.e., independent of the mechanisms providing the inspiratory flow.

Physiology of PEEP Therapy

Under circumstances in which the intrinsic elastic properties of the lung and chest wall remain reasonably constant, PEEP will increase end-expiratory lung volume (functional residual capacity [FRC]) (Table 24–1). This is purely a *qualitative* relationship! For any increment of PEEP, the "degree" of FRC expansion varies with com-

TABLE 24–1–THEORETIC RELATIONSHIP OF PEEP AND FRC UNDER USUAL CLINICAL CONDITIONS

I. The ideal gas law: $-PV = nRT$
   P = pressure, V = volume, n = number of molecules,
   R = gas constant, T = temperature
II. Since R and T are maintained constant:
   $$\frac{P_1 V_1}{n_1} = \frac{P_2 V_2}{n_2} \quad (1)$$
   Rearranging equation 1:
   $$\frac{P_1}{P_2} = \frac{n_1/V_1}{n_2/V_2} \quad (2)$$
III. Assuming at FRC:
   (a) P_1 represents intra-alveolar pressure ambient
   (b) The ratio n_1/V_1 represents the ambient FRC measurement
   (c) P_2 represents intra-alveolar pressure with PEEP (P_2 is increased without compressing chest wall or lung; i.e., V_2 is *not* less than V_1)
IV. When $P_2 > P_1$; then $n_2/V_2 > n_1/V_1$
   Therefore, **PEEP increases FRC.**

PEEP = positive end-expiratory pressure; FRC = functional residual capacity.

Fig 24–2.—Airway pressure curves of various modes of positive end-expiratory pressure *(PEEP)* superimposed on the normal airway pressure curve. *CPPV* = continuous positive-pressure ventilation; *CPAP* = continuous positive airway pressure; *EPAP* = expiratory positive airway pressure; *IMV* = intermittent mandatory ventilation.

pliance, e.g., the lesser the compliance, the lesser the FRC expansion for any increment of PEEP. The *distribution* of that increased lung volume will depend on several factors that are best illustrated by developing a theoretic lung model based on well-documented pulmonary physiology.

In the normal erect lung at FRC: (1) the majority of blood flow is to the bases (see Fig 4–2); (2) intrapleural pressures are more subatmospheric at the apex than at the base (see Fig 4–3); and (3) intra-alveolar pressures are equal throughout the lung (see Fig 4–3). As discussed in Chapter 4 and illustrated in Figure 24–3, transpulmonary pressure (alveolar distending pressure) at FRC is greater at the apex than the base and results in larger alveoli at the apex. In addition, the normal FRC includes approximately one-half the total lung capacity (TLC), which (1) favors the distribution of inspired gases toward the bases, and (2) renders the lung compliance optimal for inspiration.

As discussed in Chapter 20, any acute decrease in FRC will (1) affect the ventilation-perfusion relationship adversely, and (2) provide a less than optimal compliance for inspiration. In addition, acute decreases in FRC *may* decrease alveolar volumes to the degree that the smaller alveoli collapse.

Normal airways and normal chest wall properties are assumed in our model (see Fig 24–3), upon which a *homogeneous* disease process that acutely decreases lung compliance is imposed (Fig 24–4). Thus, the TLC and FRC are significantly diminished. The increased lung elasticity results in greater negative intrapleural pressure (at FRC the intrapleural pressure is -14 cm H_2O at the apex and -6 cm H_2O at the

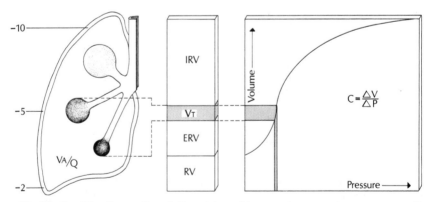

Fig 24–3.—The theoretic relationships of lung volume, pulmonary compliance, and ventilation-perfusion (see text). IRV = inspiratory reserve volume; VT = tidal volume; ERV = expiratory reserve volume; RV = residual volume.

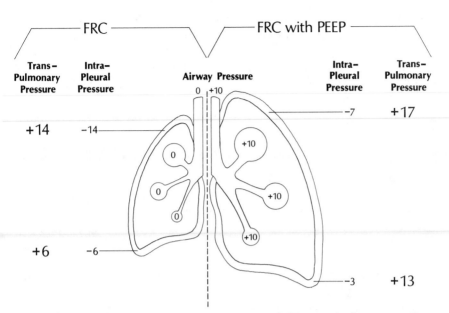

Fig 24–4.—Acute restrictive disease without PEEP results in greater than normal negative intrapleural pressures at FRC. All alveolar pressures are equal and equal to mouth pressure (see text). With 10 cm H_2O PEEP, more pressure is transmitted to the pleural space at the apex (7 cm H_2O transmitted) than at the base (3 cm H_2O transmitted). Thus, transpulmonary pressure is increased 7 cm H_2O at the base and only 3 cm H_2O at the apex. *PEEP =* positive end-expiratory pressure; *FRC* = functional residual capacity.

base). These values are for illustrative purposes only and are not known to represent actual measurements. It should be recalled that at FRC, transpulmonary pressures (TPP) are equal to alveolar distending pressures. Therefore, the apical TPP in our model is zero minus a minus fourteen $[0-(-14)]$ and equals a plus fourteen. The basilar TPP equals a plus six.

Let us now apply a PEEP of 10 cm H_2O, which results in alveolar pressures of $+10$ at FRC. Some degree of FRC expansion must occur (see Table 24–1). A portion of that increased alveolar pressure will be dissipated in enlarging the lung, whereas the remainder will be transmitted to the pleural space. In general, the poorer the initial alveolar compliance, the greater portion of the pressure that must be dissipated to increase alveolar size. Since the basilar alveoli are less compliant than the apical alveoli, a greater portion of the increased alveolar pressure will be dissipated at the bases than at the apex. In other words, more of the increased alveolar pressure will be *transmitted* to the apical intrapleural space than to the basilar intrapleural space. As exemplified in Figure 24 – 4, 7 of the 10 cm H_2O are transmitted at the apex while 3 of the 10 cm H_2O are transmitted at the base. This results in an apical TPP increase of 3 cm H_2O and a basilar TPP increase of 7 cm H_2O. Thus, *a RELATIVELY greater portion of the increased FRC per unit lung will be distributed to the basilar areas.*

This discussion has assumed a *homogeneous* lung disease causing an acute and significant decrease in lung compliance. Indeed the model closely resembles the adult respiratory distress syndrome (ARDS) (see Chapter 30). Remember that the model refers to the lung in an erect human being. All relationships apply in any position; the basilar alveoli would be the gravity-dependent alveoli.

In our theoretic model, a logical argument may be made to support the statement that the closer the FRC is restored toward normal, the less effective PEEP will be in favoring expansion of the less compliant basilar alveoli. A similar argument could be made for regionally isolated disease in that the increased FRC from PEEP may tend to go to the undiseased lung. From a clinical viewpoint, *PEEP therapy is primarily effective in reasonably nonregional lung disease that causes significant acute decreases in lung compliance.*

Closing Volumes and PEEP

The closing volume pulmonary function test has been discussed in Chapter 3. It is believed to represent the point in the exhaled vital capacity at which flow ceases through the small airways of the gravity-dependent areas of lung. Teleologically, this concept is very attractive, since it would assure the maintenance of a minimum gas volume within these dependent alveoli and help prevent their collapse.

Interest in this pulmonary function test increased when it was noted that patients with chronic obstructive pulmonary disease (COPD) had significantly increased closing volumes.[348] It was theorized that early changes in closing volume may signify early small airway disease, a theory that is seriously questioned at present.[349, 350] It was also hypothesized that COPD patients with closing volumes greater than FRC may suffer significant hypoxemia because a portion of the tidal volume cannot be distributed to basilar alveoli.

It must be understood that although the existence of closing volumes is generally accepted,[351] their measurement and physiologic significance are highly questionable.[352] What few data are available concerning PEEP and closing volumes do not justify the sweeping assumptions made by some investigators and authors. *There is no direct evidence to support the hypothesis that PEEP directly affects closing volumes.* The observation that PEEP may alter the relationship of FRC to the closing volume is attractive;[201, 311, 328, 353] however, to assume that this is *the* mechanism by which PEEP improves arterial oxygenation is misleading.

The direct effects of PEEP on airway patency, inspiratory flow through small airways, and closing volumes are undocumented at present, whereas the direct effects of PEEP on FRC are well documented.[327, 354-359, 367] We strongly urge that PEEP therapy be clinically conceptualized and rationalized primarily in terms of its effects on FRC. Although the future may reveal the existence of a significant relationship between PEEP and closing volumes, at present the relationship is speculative and presumptive.

Common Pathophysiology Requiring PEEP Therapy

The major therapeutic application of PEEP is with acute restrictive disease processes in which the FRC has been very significantly decreased (see Fig 20 – 1, type C). This type of pulmonary pathology presents two major physiologic abnormalities that are potentially life threatening: (1) increased intrapulmonary shunting (Qs/Qt), and (2) decreased lung compliance.

The *increased intrapulmonary shunting* is mainly due to collapsed alveoli, with perfusion through the adjacent pulmonary capillaries. Inevitably this occurs primarily in the gravity-dependent portions of lung. Since pulmonary artery blood (mixed venous blood) is passing through the lung and entering the left heart without the opportunity to oxygenate, the administration of increased oxygen to open alveoli will have little affect on the oxygen content of the blood in the left heart. Thus, a *refractory hypoxemia* exists, i.e., an arterial hypoxemia that is essentially unaffected by breathing increased oxygen concentrations.

The *decreased lung compliance* is primarily due to the disease process and secondarily due to the acute lung volume loss. Not only is the significant drop in FRC responsible for inspiration occurring on a less advantageous portion of the compliance curve, but often the disease process is responsible for "shifting" the curve to a yet more disadvantageous slope.

It is essential to realize that both of these pathophysiologic factors result from a particular type of acute lung volume loss, i.e., an acutely decreased FRC with significant decrease in residual volume (see Chapter 20). These patients often have very adequate ventilatory reserves, expend a great deal of energy to spontaneously ventilate, and manifest significant alveolar hyperventilation (decreased arterial PCO_2). This significantly increased work of breathing is accompanied by a significant arterial Po_2 deficit that is relatively unresponsive to oxygen administration.

Clinical Goals of PEEP Therapy

PEEP therapy is capable of accomplishing three primary clinical goals when appropriately applied: (1) improvement in arterial oxygenation, (2) decrease in work of breathing, and (3) improvement in V/Q inequality.

Improvement in Arterial Oxygenation

When a refractory hypoxemia is caused by intrapulmonary shunting secondary to a diffusely decreased FRC, the application of PEEP usually results in *dramatic* improvement of arterial Po_2. The distribution of the increased lung volume will tend to favor the collapsed or nearly collapsed alveoli. Once these alveoli are adquately re-expanded, concentrations of inspired oxygen below 40% will result in adequate arterial oxygenation.[357]

Decrease in Work of Breathing

When acute restrictive disease exists, if the FRC can be increased toward normal, inspiration will begin from a more advantageous point on the compliance curve. This improved compliance results in less energy required to move the same tidal volume or minute volume.[360]

Improvement in V/Q Inequality

Increasing FRC toward normal will improve the ventilation-perfusion relationship.[361] Not only will "shunt effect" be diminished, but deadspace ventilation will be decreased in most instances (see Fig 30 – 1).

Summary

When applied to an acutely decreased FRC secondary to reasonably homogeneous lung disease, PEEP will dramatically improve compliance, decrease true shunting, decrease deadspace ventilation, and decrease shunt effect. Adequate arterial oxygenation (Po_2 of 60 mm Hg or better, with normal hemoglobin) may be accomplished with 40% inspired oxygen concentrations or less. In a spontaneously breathing patient the PEEP will result in much less work of breathing, while any necessary positive-pressure ventilation will be accomplished at significantly lower airway pressures.

In our experience, *therapeutic levels of PEEP in the adult are usu-*

ally between 10 and 30 cm H_2O. Generally, higher PEEP levels are required with CPAP or low IMV rates than with control mode IPPV. The over-all clinical goal of PEEP therapy must be to assure adequate *tissue* oxygenation; thus, the pulmonary advantages must never be evaluated separately from the cardiovascular effects and other potential detriments of PEEP.

Undesirable Cardiopulmonary Effects of PEEP Therapy

When applied improperly or when not indicated, PEEP may manifest three undesirable cardiopulmonary effects: (1) decreased cardiac output; (2) increased intrapulmonary shunting; and (3) decreased lung compliance.

Decreased Cardiac Output

It has been previously stated that PEEP increases mean airway pressure and thereby may increase intrapleural pressure. This increase in intrapleural pressure may *potentially* decrease venous return to the heart and thus decrease cardiac output (see Chapters 26 and 27). No matter how strong the heart may be, it cannot pump more blood than comes to it! Tissue oxygenation cannot be maintained or improved by decreasing cardiac output; therefore, *if PEEP is to be of physiologic benefit, it must not cause significant decreases in cardiac output.*

The decreased venous return secondary to PEEP can usually be reversed by appropriate fluid therapy (see Chapter 27); however, in some circumstances the cardiac output may be improved pharmacologically.[362] These are medical judgments and must be made individually for each patient. However, if PEEP therapy is causing decreased cardiac output that cannot be reasonably reestablished, that level of PEEP therapy is contraindicated.

It is our experience that almost all patients in whom PEEP therapy is clearly indicated have few problems with decreased cardiac output that cannot be readily overcome with proper fluid therapy. This is probably because such patients have a significant portion of the increased airway pressure dissipated in providing the necessary distending pressure to improve FRC. Therefore, a relatively small portion of the increased airway pressure is apparently transmitted to the pleural space.

When PEEP therapy causes a significant decrease in cardiac output, two questions should be answered: (1) Is the pathologic process one that should benefit from PEEP? and (2) Is too much PEEP being applied?

Increased Intrapulmonary Shunting

Since a primary goal of PEEP therapy is to decrease shunting, there can be no argument that if PEEP causes increased shunting it is contraindicated. PEEP most likely results in increased shunting when overdistention of reasonably undiseased alveoli results in decreased perfusion to those alveoli. Such a process may favor pulmonary blood flow to diseased areas of lung unaffected by the PEEP. This is believed to occur most frequently when PEEP is applied to lung disease with fluid-filled alveoli or airway obstruction (e.g., bacterial pneumonitis; multiple lung abscesses; non-re-expanding segmental or lobar atelectasis). It may also be hypothesized to occur when too much PEEP is applied or when PEEP is applied to a normal lung.

No matter what the etiology or how controversial the theory, one clinical statement remains irrefutable: *PEEP therapy that results in increased intrapulmonary shunting is contraindicated!*

Decreased Lung Compliance

Overdistention of alveoli results in decreasing lung compliance (see Chapter 3) as well as decreasing chest wall compliance. Therefore, too much PEEP may result in decreasing pulmonary compliance.[360] In most circumstances a decreasing compliance resulting from an increased PEEP is an indication to decrease PEEP therapy.

Monitoring PEEP Therapy

All patients with refractory hypoxemia and increased work of breathing will *not* favorably respond to PEEP therapy. In addition, PEEP therapy may cause harm when inappropriately applied. These statements lead to the inevitable conclusion that *PEEP therapy must not be applied without appropriate monitoring.* The term "appropriate" is a clinical judgment and varies widely for different patient populations and different health care institutions. The following discussion is designed as an organized and objective discussion of monitoring techniques from the simplest to the most complex. They are presented so that the respiratory care practitioner may be familiar with their *potential* application; their *actual* applications must be based on clinical judgment and availability.

There are three general areas of monitoring that are applicable to PEEP therapy: (1) airway pressure and gases, (2) hemodynamics, and (3) oxygenation.

Airway Monitoring

The minimum requirement is to monitor the degree of PEEP being applied. Simply applying a PEEP device is *not* adequate; there must exist a manometer within the system that reflects the existing airway pressures. The closer the manometer is to the patient's airway, the more reliable the measurements. In addition to monitoring PEEP levels, this manometer may be used to help reflect compliance changes of the system.

Effective Static Compliance

Compliance is an important *concept* in the application of PEEP therapy. A simple method of grossly reflecting changes in pulmonary compliance would be an obviously desirable clinical tool. When appropriately measured and interpreted, the *effective static compliance* (ESC) measurement is such a tool.

Figure 24–5 illustrates a typical tracing of a positive-pressure inspiration with an end-inspiratory pause. The *peak pressure* is the result of the system's impedance to flow (see Chapter 3). This impedance includes both compliance and resistance factors within the pulmonary system and breathing circuit. If expiration is delayed for a period following delivery of the inspiratory volume, a significant portion of gas

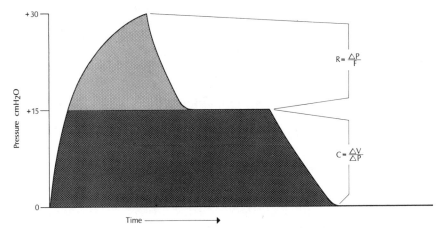

Fig 24–5.—Positive-pressure ventilation with end-inspiratory pause (see text). The lightly shaded area represents the pressure change related to resistance phenomena. R = resistance; ΔP = pressure change; F = flow. The darkly shaded area represents the pressure change related to compliance factors. C = compliance; ΔV = change in volume.

in the upper airways will be distributed toward the alveolar level (see time constants, Chapter 3, and end-inspiratory pause, Chapter 23). The rapidly diminishing transairway pressure gradient results in rapidly diminishing flows. Since the pressure resulting from resistance factors is flow related, *as flow significantly decreases, the pressure related to resistance will significantly decrease.*

It is reasonable to assume that the pressure change represented between the inspiratory plateau and peak pressure in Figure 24–5 is attributable to resistance factors. Thus, *the pressure differential between inspiratory plateau and base line is essentially attributable to compliance factors.*

Compliance (C = Δ V/Δ P) is a static measurement; i.e., it can only be measured in the absence of flow. However, a reasonable *estimate* of the system compliance can be calculated by dividing the exhaled tidal volume (ΔV) by the pressure differential between base-line and inspiratory plateau (ΔP). This measurement is termed the effective static compliance to denote that, although flow is greatly diminished, it is not entirely absent.

To avoid confusion, it is necessary to explain the term *effective dynamic compliance* (EDC). Historically, initial clinical attempts to estimate system compliance utilized the base line to peak pressure as ΔP. Obviously this was misleading, especially if significant resistance factors were present. Even though it was later "understood" that EDC was to be measured with inspiratory plateau pressures, many clinicians were confused and various texts were unclear. The term EDC should be relegated to history and the confusion avoided.

Inspired Oxygen Concentration (FI_{O_2})

Appropriate monitoring of ventilation-perfusion relationships demands accurate measurement of FI_{O_2}. In addition, optimizing arterial oxygenation while minimizing FI_{O_2} is a prime goal of PEEP therapy. The respiratory care practitioner must assure accurate and frequent measurement of inspired oxygen concentrations.

Mass Spectrometry

This technology promises the clinical ability to accurately monitor all airway gases, including trace amounts of inert gases, in combination with flow measurement. When combined with recent computer technology, the mass spectrometer becomes a noninvasive bedside monitor of the critically ill patient with exciting potential. For example, it is possible that oxygen consumption, compliance, and resistance may be routine bedside measurements in the near future. Even more exciting is the probability that routine FRC measurements will be available.[299, 300] It appears that the ideal PEEP monitor may well be the serial FRC measurement.

Hemodynamic Monitoring

Circulation of blood is an essential prerequisite for tissue oxygenation. Measurements reflecting blood circlulation are termed *hemodynamics*, which is discussed in depth in Chapters 26 and 27. Hemodynamic monitoring in some form is indicated when PEEP therapy is instituted. Minimal hemodynamic monitoring includes measurements of arterial blood pressure and pulse and the clinical estimation of peripheral perfusion, none of which require invasive measures. In some cases a central venous pressure measurement may suffice, although the most satisfactory technique of invasive hemodynamic monitoring is the *pulmonary artery catheter*, which allows ventricular preload and afterload measurement as well as actual cardiac output measurement. These are all discussed in Section VII.

Oxygenation Monitoring

Since a major clinical goal of PEEP therapy is to improve arterial oxygenation, serial measurement of *arterial blood gases* is a requisite. In most circumstances placement of an indwelling arterial catheter is appropriate.[35]

Pulmonary artery blood gases (see Chapter 28) are valuable in that serial measurement of arterial-venous oxygen content differences $(A-V_{O_2})$ reflects the adequacy of cardiac output in relation to oxygen consumption. Mixed venous oxygen tension $(P\bar{v}_{O_2})$ is helpful in estimating the adequacy of tissue oxygenation. Serial calculation of intrapulmonary shunt (Qs/Qt) is of great aid in monitoring PEEP therapy.

Summary

The need for some form of airway, hemodynamic, and oxygenation monitoring during PEEP therapy is beyond question. The degree and sophistication of monitoring techniques will vary from patient to patient.

Base-line measurements are always necessary since it is the physiologic *changes* resulting from PEEP that are paramount. As a general rule, we do not increase or decrease PEEP in increments greater than 5 cm H_2O and repeat all measurements within 15 minutes of any change. Development of a flow chart in which the necessary information is shown sequentially is invaluable.

Airway Suctioning and PEEP Therapy

When arterial oxygen tensions are in excess of 200 mm Hg, airway suctioning may result in PO_2 decreases greater than 100 mm Hg. This has been widely interpreted as meaning that PEEP *must* be maintained during suctioning—a technique that is cumbersome, expensive, and time consuming. When airway suctioning is properly accomplished, as described in Chapter 16, it is our experience that arterial oxygenation does not fall below the maintenance level even though PEEP is transiently discontinued. Thus, we have not found it clinically necessary to change our routine suctioning technique for patients on 30 cm H_2O PEEP or less.

Physiologic PEEP

A widely observed clinical phenomenon is that spontaneously breathing, intubated patients often have gradually decreasing arterial PO_2's despite consistent oxygen therapy and adequate bronchial hygiene. This oxygenation deficit is usually reversed when 3–5 cm H_2O PEEP is applied.[363, 364] In our experience, this observation is valid primarily in patients with pre-existing chronic pulmonary disease or neuromuscular deficits.

Pulmonary physiologists have hypothesized the existence of a "glottic mechanism" that plays a role in maintaining "normal FRC." This mechanism does not appear to be a simple resistance factor at the glottic level but more likely an indirect effect on small airway caliber. In any case this has been a proposed explanation for decreased FRC's in intubated patients.

The glottic mechanism hypothesis seems to have been combined with the above-documented findings and has resulted in a concept known as *physiologic PEEP*. In essence, this concept states that 5 cm H_2O PEEP in the intubated patient will replace the glottic mechanism and help to maintain a normal FRC. It should be emphasized that there are no conclusive data available upon which any definite statements may be based. One recent study in postoperative patients showed no effect of 5 cm H_2O on FRC;[365] other studies indicate the opposite.[366]

It is our opinion that *routine* use of physiologic PEEP is unwarranted. It is very expensive to set up PEEP systems on *every* intubated patient when the benefits are questionable. On the other hand, we believe *selective* use of physiologic PEEP is justified. Our present criteria for applying physiologic PEEP to spontaneously breathing, intubated patients apply to (1) those who have demonstrated a drop in PO_2

attributable to the removal of 5 cm H_2O PEEP; (2) those with significant pre-existent chronic lung disease; and (3) those on augmented modes of ventilation at rates of less than 4 per minute.

Physiologic PEEP in conjunction with augmented ventilation should not be considered significant PEEP therapy. Seldom are PEEP levels of 5 cm H_2O or less critical to the supportive therapy of adults. It is perfectly appropriate to extubate from 5 cm H_2O PEEP.

25 • APPLICATION AND COMPLICATIONS OF AIRWAY PRESSURE THERAPY

THE PHYSICS, physiology, and pathology pertinent to the development of clinical rationale for applying airway pressure therapy have been presented in the previous seven chapters. No simple rules such as "all hypoxemia requires PEEP" or "all tachypnea calls for a ventilator" are applicable. Therefore, a prerequisite to applying airway pressure therapy is an over-all evaluation of the patient's status by a qualified and conscientious physician. The respiratory care practitioner must be capable of functioning knowledgeably and effectively within that over-all clinical evaluation.

The clinical goal of airway pressure therapy may be simply stated: *To optimize respiration at the pulmonary level while minimizing physiologic stress to the cardiovascular and pulmonary systems.* Since patients requiring airway pressure therapy are usually subjected to significant cardiopulmonary stress, any additional stress from the therapy itself must be minimized. Thus, it is imperative to comprehend not only when and how to apply airway pressure therapy, but when and how the therapy may be detrimental or contraindicated. One purpose of this chapter is to combine previously presented information, concepts, and rationale into *guidelines* we believe germane to safe and effective application of airway pressure therapy.

Guidelines for Application of Airway Pressure Therapy

Control Mode IPPV

Capabilities: (1) To provide the total power necessary for maintenance of ventilatory homeostasis; (2) to determine ventilatory pattern; and (3) to manipulate inspiratory pressure and flow patterns.

Direct V/Q effect: Increases deadspace ventilation (V_D/V_T) and shunt effect by favoring distribution of ventilation to non-gravity-dependent portions of lung.

Clinical indications: (1) Apnea; (2) acute ventilatory failure (acute respiratory acidosis) in the absence of corrective therapy expected to be immediately beneficial; (3) impending acute ventilatory failure;

380

and (4) oxygenation deficit due to (a) increased work of breathing or (b) a cardiovascular system unable to maintain adequate circulation because of the added stress of the work of breathing.

Monitors: (1) Ventilator and airway (appropriate monitors) (see Chapter 23); (2) arterial blood gases (indwelling arterial line preferable); (3) blood pressure and ECG; and (4) CVP or pulmonary artery catheter when there is question of adequacy of cardiovascular reserves.

Suggested application: (1) Tidal volumes of 10–20 ml/kg (not applicable in patients with *chronic* restrictive disease in which smaller tidal volumes and more rapid rates are indicated); (2) rate of 8–12 per minute; (3) inspiratory flow time of 0.5–1.5 seconds; (4) I:E ratio of greater than 1:2; (5) sedation and/or paralyzation as needed to avoid "fighting ventilator" and to ensure patient comfort; (6) eucapneic maintenance; and (7) a change to augmented mode if (and as soon as) patient status permits.

In our experience, control mode is most commonly applied (1) in the first 12 hours following ventilator commitment to accomplish (a) clinical stabilization, (b) evaluation, and (c) placement of required monitors and therapeutic catheters; (2) in primary C.N.S. disease or malfunction; and (3) in *severe* primary cardiac disease.

Augmented Mode IPPV (IMV/IDV)

Capabilities: (1) To provide a spontaneously breathing patient with the *additional* ventilatory energy necessary to maintain ventilatory homeostasis without excessive or detrimental cardiopulmonary work; (2) to allow spontaneous inspiration of desired gas mixtures during IPPV; and (3) to provide intermittent deep lung inflations to optimize V/Q and minimize atelectasis.

Direct V/Q effects: (1) Minimizes increased deadspace ventilation and shunt effect of IPPV and (2) optimizes favorable V/Q effects of spontaneous ventilation.

Clinical indications: Same as for control mode with the exception of apnea.

Monitors: Same as for control mode.

Suggested application: (1) Tidal volumes of 10–20 ml/kg; (2) rate of 2–7 per minute; (3) inspiratory flow time of 0.5–1.5 seconds; (4) sedation and/or analgesia as required for patient comfort; (5) fighting the ventilator must not be tolerated for long periods; (6) more than 50 ml of deadspace tubing is contraindicated; (7) consider adding PEEP of 5 cm H_2O when rate is less than 4 per minute; and (8) consider utilizing end-inspiratory pause with rates less than 4 per minute.

Maintain the minimal ventilator rate consistent with acceptable vital signs, arterial blood gases, and general condition. Do not *misuse* augmented modes by unnecessarily prolonging the ventilator course for weaning. In the vast majority of cases, ventilator discontinuance does *not* require prolonged stepwise decreases in ventilator rate.

End-Inspiratory Pause (Inflation Hold)

Capabilities: To increase the time available for peripheral distribution of inspired gases.

Direct V/Q effect: Improves distribution of ventilation to alveoli, particularly to low V/Q alveoli when increased airway resistance or decreased compliance is present.

Clinical indications: (1) Unacceptably high $PaCO_2$ despite adequate minute ventilation and adequate pulmonary perfusion; and (2) the maintenance of eucapnia with minimal minute ventilation in the presence of significant airway resistance.

Monitors: Same as for control mode plus accurate I:E ratio calculation.

Suggested application: (1) Assure the presence of an adequate time for volume delivery (0.5 – 1.5 seconds) before applying inflation hold; (2) maintain I:E ratios of at least 1:2 in adults; (3) add inflation hold in increments of 0.25 – 0.5 second; (4) *not* a substitute for PEEP or retard; and (5) may be applied fairly routinely with square wave generators.

Expiratory Retard (Expiratory Resistance)

Capabilities: To facilitate expiratory gas flow in the presence of increased small airway resistance.

Direct V/Q effects: Controversial.

Clinical indications: Evidence of significant expiratory wheezing and/or air trapping.

Monitors: (1) Clinical examination of chest (auscultation); (2) arterial blood gases; and (3) blood pressure and ECG.

Suggested application: (1) Increase incrementally; (2) adjust independent of other airway pressure maneuvers (i.e., do not change two factors at once); (3) frequently reevaluate need for continuing the retard; and (4) is compatible with any other airway pressure therapy.

PEEP

Capabilities: (1) To increase functional residual capacity (FRC); (2) to improve lung compliance when decrease is secondary to acute and reasonably diffuse pulmonary pathology; and (3) to improve arterial oxygenation by decreasing true shunting created by acute and reasonably diffuse pulmonary pathology.

Direct V/Q effects: (1) When reasonably diffuse pulmonary pathology results in a significantly diminished FRC, PEEP should (a) reverse true shunting by reestablishing and maintaining ventilation of perfused alveoli and (b) preferentially increase end-expiratory volume of smaller alveoli; (2) when FRC decrease is due to *non-diffuse* disease, PEEP (a) may hyperexpand the more compliant lung and potentially increase deadspace ventilation and (b) may promote pulmonary blood flow to diseased portions of lung, thereby increasing intrapulmonary shunting.

Clinical indications: (1) Presence of refractory hypoxemia and increased work of breathing when *not* attributable to lobar or segmental lung disease; and (2) intubated spontaneously ventilating patients who manifest gradually decreasing PaO_2 in spite of adequate cardiopulmonary function and adequate bronchial hygiene.

Monitors: (1) Arterial blood gases; (2) FIO_2; (3) blood pressure and ECG; (4) effective static compliance; (5) work of breathing and perfusion status (clinical evaluation); and (6) pulmonary artery catheter if cardiac status (reserve) is not otherwise assessable.

Suggested application: (1) In therapeutic ranges (10–30 cm H_2O): (a) PEEP levels should be increased or decreased by 5 cm H_2O increments, repeating measurements and evaluation before next change; (b) adequate fluid status must be assured since proper ventricular filling (preload) is essential to effective PEEP therapy; (c) evidence of decreased cardiac output (hypotension, increased A-VO_2), in spite of adequate preload and pharmacologic manipulation of myocardium, requires that PEEP be appropriately readjusted downward; and (d) FIO_2 changes must be accomplished independent of PEEP level changes. (2) Criteria for "enough" PEEP are when (a) "adequate arterial oxygenation" is provided while acceptable cardiac output is maintained at an FIO_2 of 0.40 or less, (b) serial measurements of effective static compliance show optimal improvement in patients with excellent cardiovascular reserve,[381] (c) measured QS/QT decreases to 15%,[380] (d) cardiac output decreases (as reflected in direct measurement or indirectly as increased A-VO_2 difference); or (e) QS/QT increases from a previously lower level.

"Super PEEP" (levels above 30 cm H_2O) is not routinely required and is associated with an increased incidence of barotrauma.[368] These levels are almost never applied in conjunction with control mode IPPV. In spite of the dismal patient prognosis, PEEP levels of greater than 30 cm H_2O should be attempted if clinically indicated.

Control Mode CPPV (IPPV + PEEP)

Capabilities: Same as for control mode IPPV and PEEP.
Direct V/Q effects: Same as for control mode IPPV and PEEP.
Clinical indications: Same as for control mode IPPV and PEEP.
Monitors: Same as for control mode IPPV and PEEP.
Suggested application: (1) Stabilize IPPV as best as possible, then titrate PEEP; (2) always reevaluate necessity for control mode once adequate PEEP level is reached. Control mode is frequently unnecessary *unless* there is C.N.S. or severe cardiac malfunction. Frequently a higher level of PEEP is required once the augmented mode is established.

Augmented Mode CPPV (IMV/IDV + PEEP)

This is the most physiologically advantageous mode of PEEP therapy in critically ill adults!
Capabilities: Same as for augmented mode IPPV and PEEP.
Direct V/Q effects: Same as for augmented mode IPPV and PEEP.
Clinical indications: Same as for augmented mode IPPV and PEEP.
Monitors: Same as for augmented mode IPPV and PEEP.
Suggested application: Priorities for decreasing therapy: (1) decrease FI_{O_2} to 0.4; then (2) decrease ventilator rate to the lowest reasonable level (even if some increase in PEEP level is necessitated); and then (3) decrease PEEP levels.

CPAP

This is PEEP therapy applied to the patient who is capable of assuming all the work of breathing.

EPAP

Capabilities: Same as for PEEP.
Direct V/Q effects: Same as for PEEP. Compared to CPAP, EPAP may improve cardiovascular function in patients in whom an increased work of breathing is not detrimental.
Clinical indications: (1) Same as for PEEP but only when the patient's ventilatory reserve is excellent, and (2) when intermittent PEEP therapy is desired in non-intubated patients.[369]
Monitors: Same as for PEEP.
Suggested application: (1) In patients with excellent ventilatory reserve but limited cardiovascular reserve; and (2) since the equipment is less expensive and simpler than CPAP equipment, EPAP appears a cost effective technique if the patient can tolerate the increased work of breathing.

Non-Cardiovascular Complications
of Airway Pressure Therapy

The critically ill patient succumbs to either (1) the primary disease process becoming overwhelming; (2) the primary process causing malfunction of originally uninvolved organ systems; or (3) iatrogenic (doctor-caused) physiologic stress from diagnostic, therapeutic, and "supportive" interventions. These three factors are often difficult or impossible to delineate clinically. For example, a 50-year-old previously healthy man contracts a severe bilateral gram-negative pneumonia and experiences septic shock. Thirty-six hours after septic shock the kidneys stop functioning. Is the renal failure a result of (1) the initial septic insult; (2) the sustained hypotension that followed; (3) a renal toxic effect of the antibiotics administered; or, as most often occurs, (4) a combination of all these factors?

In order for the respiratory care practitioner, nurse, and physician to intelligently evaluate such matters, it is essential to understand the *potential* insult of airway pressure therapy on various organ systems. Following is a discussion of the potential non-cardiovascular complications of airway pressure support. The cardiovascular effects (e.g., decreased cardiac output, hypotension, vascular volume-space relationships) are discussed in detail in Section VII.

Mechanical Malfunction

This is probably the most common *preventable* and *reversible* complication of airway pressure therapy. The myriad of interconnected tubes, valves, gas sources, alarms, monitors, and gauges create the milieu for malfunction. The probability of less than optimal functioning of some component of the system is significant, even when the equipment is excellently maintained and monitored. The possibility of catastrophe is ever present! A well-organized, well-trained, and dedicated respiratory therapy department is essential to safe and optimal respiratory intensive care. The question is not how little can one get away with but, rather, how much is needed to provide optimal therapy at the least patient risk and cost?

A basic rule must never be violated: *treat patients, not machines!* Any questionable machine or circuitry malfunction must be addressed *after* the patient is assured adequate ventilation and oxygenation. A properly functioning self-inflating hand ventilator that can be easily connected to an oxygen source *must* be at each bedside. An appropriate PEEP attachment should be readily available when the patient is receiving greater than 10 cm H_2O PEEP. Whenever equipment malfunction is suspected, the patient should be disconnected from the apparatus and hand ventilated. Patient evaluation to assure adequacy must be immediately undertaken. Only after the *patient's safety* is assured should the equipment be examined!

Airway Malfunction

Obstruction, cuff malfunction, displacement (extubation or bronchial intubation), and disconnection are probably the second most common preventable and reversible complications of airway pressure therapy. These have been discussed in Chapter 16. Appropriate alarms and the appropriate personnel response to these signals are paramount in preventing catastrophe.

Pulmonary Barotrauma

Barotrauma generally refers to lung rupture secondary to airway pressure phenomena. In relation to airway pressure therapy, *barotrauma refers to an alveolar gas leak to extraparenchymal structures.* Pulmonary barotrauma includes interstitial emphysema, pneumomediastinum, subcutaneous emphysema, pneumoperitoneum, and pneumothorax.

INTERSTITIAL EMPHYSEMA. — A chest x-ray diagnosis. It is usually the result of a surface bleb or alveolus that ruptures but does *not* disturb the visceral pleura. Gas dissects along blood vessel connective tissue sheaths toward the hilus. The clinical significance of interstitial emphysema is that the gas must decompress and, therefore, poses a constant threat of dissection that will tear the pleura and result in pneumothorax.

PNEUMOMEDIASTINUM. — A chest x-ray diagnosis. Seldom will "tension" become a problem since decompression readily occurs via dissection either to (1) the cervical fascial planes; (2) the retroperitoneal space via the esophageal diaphragmatic hiatus; or (3) pleural rupture at the hilus. Although pneumopericardium is rare, it is potentially life threatening and must be immediately evaluated for decompression.

SUBCUTANEOUS EMPHYSEMA. — Most commonly the result of mediastinal gas decompressing via the contiguous cervical fascial planes. Neck crepitus (palpation of subcutaneous air) is often the first observed clinical indication of barotrauma in patients on airway pressure therapy. Although not harmful in and of itself, full-blown subcutaneous emphysema makes the patient appear grotesque. Pneumothorax must constantly be ruled out. Subcutaneous emphysema of mild degree may result from tracheostomy or chest tube wounds.

PNEUMOPERITONEUM. — Most commonly encountered following closed chest cardiac massage; however, it does occur in other circumstances. This usually represents mediastinal decompression via the retroperitoneal space.

PNEUMOTHORAX. — The most dangerous type of barotrauma that commonly occurs in patients receiving airway pressure therapy. The pleural air compresses lung and creates hypoxemia. *When pneumothorax is present in conjunction with airway pressure therapy, a chest tube must be placed!* This will almost always relieve the lung compression and will usually avoid tension pneumothorax.

Tension Pneumothorax

Tension pneumothorax is air in the pleural space under greater than atmospheric pressure. When untreated in conjunction with airway pressure therapy, it will collapse lung, compress the mediastinum, and compress the great veins and atria contained therein. *Tension pneumothorax in conjunction with IPPV or PEEP may rapidly result in total inability to ventilate and total circulatory collapse.* Without immediate thoracic cavity decompression, death will ensue.

Decompression

A needle inserted into the chest in adults will usually confirm the diagnosis, but most often will not adequately decompress the gas under tension for any significant period of time. *The chest must be opened!* A small skin incision is made over the second or third rib between the midclavicular and anterior axillary line. This is followed by placement of a closed hemostat through the incision and insertion into the chest cavity immediately *above* the rib (intercostal vessels run below the rib). Once the hemostat is inserted and opened, adequate decompression will occur and the immediate emergency is over. Positive-pressure ventilation does not require a closed chest; therefore, the insertion of a chest tube is not immediately necessary and should be accomplished under more sterile conditions by skilled personnel.

PEEP Therapy and Barotrauma

In a review of over 600 consecutive patients receiving airway pressure therapy in our institution, 7% had pulmonary barotrauma. A majority of patients with barotrauma had either pre-existing chronic obstructive pulmonary disease (COPD) or had experienced pulmonary trauma (including surgery, closed chest massage, and subclavian vein needle punctures). Of the patients *not* included in the above categories, all but two received PEEP therapy of 10 cm H_2O or greater. Thus, it appears that pulmonary barotrauma seldom occurs with airway pressure therapy in the absence of pre-existing lung abnormality or chest wall trauma. It is not unexpected that a significant incidence of barotrauma with airway pressure therapy exists in patients with COPD (in which blebs and air trapping are common) or with decreased lung compliance.

PEEP therapy of 10 cm H₂O or greater is associated with a significant incidence of barotrauma. However, this is usually attributable to the pulmonary disease process requiring therapy and must not be interpreted as a contraindication for the therapy. *If the patient requires PEEP therapy, the risk of barotrauma is inherent!* A 14% incidence of barotrauma has been reported in patients requiring PEEP therapy above 25 cm H_2O;[368] however, there are no data to support the assumption that barotrauma incidence increases in tandem with the PEEP level. It is our impression that PEEP levels between 10 and 30 cm H_2O have the *same* incidence of barotrauma. Appropriate PEEP therapy should not be withheld due to fear of initiating barotrauma.

Pulmonary Atelectasis and Infection

Lobar and segmental atelectasis are common complications of airway pressure therapy. The diagnosis should be made within several hours to allow complete re-expansion by chest physical therapy techniques and/or fiberoptic bronchoscopy. The diagnosis is most commonly made by observing vital signs and/or arterial blood gas changes, and confirmed by chest x-ray. *Pulmonary infection* is a common complication of intubated patients in general. This has been discussed in Chapter 16. The most effective means of decreasing the incidence of these complications appears to be meticulous airway care and aggressive bronchial hygiene therapy.

Gastrointestinal Malfunction

Gastrointestinal bleeding is common in all critically ill patients. It has been estimated that without prophylactic therapy, as high as 40% of patients requiring IPPV for more than 3 days will have gastrointestinal bleeding; half of these patients will have severe enough bleeding to require blood transfusion.[44] Gastrointestinal bleeding is greatly increased in incidence and severity by the pre-existence of gastrointestinal ulcer and long-term steroid therapy.[373]

It appears that the great majority of gastrointestinal bleeding in conjunction with airway pressure support is due to *acute* ulceration of gastric and bowel mucosa.[370] Antacid regimens aimed at maintaining gastric fluid pH above 5.0, as well as early and frequent nasogastric feedings, have almost completely abolished major gastrointestinal bleeding (4 units of blood or more) caused by *acute* gastrointestinal ulceration in conjunction with airway pressure therapy.[371, 372]

Cimetidine is a new drug that decreases the acidity of gastric secretion. Although used frequently at present, its effects on the incidence of gastrointestinal bleeding in patients receiving airway pressure therapy have yet to be established.

The *direct* effects of airway pressure therapy on splanchnic blood flow are not presently known; however, some presumptive evidence exists that mesenteric blood flow may be decreased.[374]

Renal Malfunction

Acute renal failure is a grave prognostic sign in all critically ill patients. Airway pressure therapy has been directly related to changes in renal function, CPPV to a greater degree than IPPV. In general, positive airway pressure results in (1) decreased urine output, (2) sodium retention, and (3) water retention.[375] This may be partly attributable to increased levels of antidiuretic hormone,[376, 377] but more recent studies have revealed changes in the distribution of intrarenal blood flow directly attributable to positive airway pressure.[378] Although total renal blood flow may remain unchanged, renal function may be significantly impaired by airway pressure therapy in critically ill patients.[371]

C.N.S. Malfunction

The effects of acute changes in P_{CO_2}, pH, and P_{O_2} on cerebral blood flow are discussed in Chapter 34. With the exception of the effect on cerebral blood flow,[379] there are no known *direct* effects of airway pressure therapy on C.N.S. function. On the other hand, C.N.S. malfunction is believed to have profound effects on pulmonary function and lung metabolic functions.

Psychologic Trauma

Intensive care patients are exposed to significant emotional stress, especially patients on mechanical devices (e.g., ventilators, dialysis machines). The realization that one cannot "breathe" without the aid of a machine is frightening. Appropriate action of the intensive care staff is a necessity for the emotional well-being of the patient. Communicating with the patient, explaining procedures, and showing concern are the most obvious ways of meeting the patient's needs for emotional support.

SECTION VII
CARDIOVASCULAR MONITORING AND SUPPORTIVE THERAPY

26 • THE PHYSIOLOGY
OF CIRCULATION
AND PERFUSION

GAS EXCHANGE at the pulmonary level (external respiration) demands the presence of adequate pulmonary blood flow. However, external respiration is of little value to the organism unless adequate internal respiration (gas exchange between blood and tissue) is assured. In other words, respiratory homeostasis demands adequate functioning of the lungs, heart, and circulatory system. The process incorporating all these factors is referred to as *cardiopulmonary function.*

Airway pressure therapy is designed to support pulmonary function and external respiration. Unfortunately, its application can threaten the maintenance of adequate circulation and perfusion. For this reason, the principles of monitoring and maintaining adequate *cardiovascular* function (circulation and perfusion) must be appreciated by the respiratory care practitioner. The physics and physiology of circulation and perfusion must be mastered if one is to comprehend the clinical assessment and support of cardiovascular function.

Defining Circulation

A simple example of circulation mechanics is a system in which a pump forces fluid through a rigid tubular system that eventually empties the fluid back into the inlet of the pump (Fig 26 – 1). The flow is determined by a basic relationship known as the "law of flow": Flow = $\frac{\Delta P}{R}$. The term ΔP (mm Hg) represents the drop in pressure from the output of the pump to the input. R represents the resistance in the circuit. In this simplified model the conduits are rigid and, therefore, resistance remains constant. The pump must supply adequate force (energy) to the fluid to overcome all the factors tending to impede the flow. Thus, flow (or circulation) through the system will be directly related to the capabilities of the pump. Note that a prerequisite for adequate circulation is the presence of enough fluid to fill the system.

A schema of the human cardiopulmonary system (Fig 26 – 2) is composed of two pumps in series (ventricles), each of which supply the

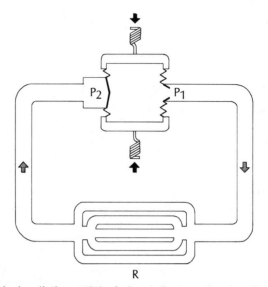

Fig 26–1.—A simplistic model of circulation mechanics. The pump forces fluid to flow out and circulate through the conduits. P_1 represents the pressure at the pump outlet; P_2 represents the pressure at the pump inlet; R represents the resistance to flow in the conduits (see text).

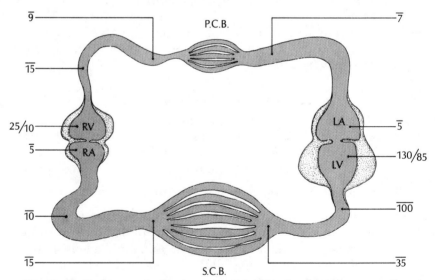

Fig 26–2.—Schema of circulatory mechanics in the human cardiopulmonary system. *LA* = left atrium; *RA* = right atrium; *LV* = left ventricle; *RV* = right ventricle; *S.C.B.* = systemic capillary bed; *P.C.B.* = pulmonary capillary bed. The numbers represent *mean* pressures except in the ventricles where systolic and diastolic pressures are noted (see text).

394

necessary energy to propel the fluid (blood) through the respective vascular conduits (systemic and pulmonary). In general, cardiac output depends upon the pump capacities of the ventricles and the adequacy with which blood is returned to the ventricles. Resistance varies with the geometry of the vascular components, contractile alterations of vascular smooth muscle, changes in blood viscosity, and presence of valvular heart disease. Since the systemic circulation nourishes the vast majority of body tissues, it consists of a more extensive vasculature than the pulmonary circulation. This normally results in a systemic resistance six times greater than pulmonary resistance (see Fig 26-2). Therefore, with each contraction the left ventricle must work approximately six times more than the right ventricle to accomplish the same flow.

Myocardial Function

Circulation in the human cardiopulmonary system may be considered as the flow of blood through a series of conduits resulting from the energy imparted to the blood by the ventricles. Therefore, ventricular output *(cardiac output)* depends on (1) pump capability of the ventricle *(myocardial contractility)*; (2) return of blood to the ventricle *(preload);* and (3) presence or absence of factors impeding outflow from the ventricle *(afterload)*.

Myocardial Contractility

Myocardial contractility may be conceptualized as the force developed while the ventricular muscles shorten. At present, a true measurement of contractility in the clinical setting is not feasible. However, *changes* in the contractile status may be inferred through careful clinical evaluation and serial hemodynamic measurements.

An improvement in myocardial contractility is referred to as *positive inotropism* and is usually associated with an improved physiologic milieu (e.g., improved oxygenation status or normalization of pH) or the administration of positive inotropic drugs (e.g., isoproterenol, dopamine). A decrease in myocardial contractility is referred to as *negative inotropism* and is usually associated with a deteriorating physiologic milieu or negative inotropic drugs, as well as certain toxins and anesthetics.

Ventricular Preload

In an isolated myocardial muscle, preload can be thought of as the degree of "stretch" imposed prior to contraction. Such stretching in the

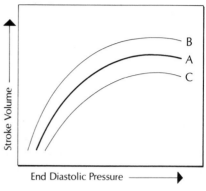

Fig 26–3. — The Frank-Starling relationship. *A* represents a normal heart, *B,* a heart with increased contractility (positive inotropism), and *C,* a heart with decreased contractility (negative inotropism).

intact heart results in an enlarged end-diastolic volume (EDV). In general, then, increased EDV is correlated with an increase in ventricular preload. Under normal conditions the end-diastolic pressure (EDP) will vary with the EDV.

Early studies on isolated heart revealed a relationship between EDP and cardiac output (stroke volume), known as the Frank-Starling relationship (Fig 26–3).[32] This relationship demonstrates that *within limits,* increasing the EDP (preload) results in an increased stroke volume; however, beyond a given point there is no longer improvement in cardiac output as end-diastolic pressures are increased. This relationship exists on an infinite family of curves in which changes are determined by such factors as circulating hormones, autonomic stimulation, and the general physiologic milieu.

In the adequately functioning heart, pressure dynamics are such that (in the absence of atrioventricular valvular abnormality) the mean atrial pressure will provide reasonable reflections of ventricular end-diastolic pressures. Thus, *measurement of atrial pressure provides a clinically reliable reflection of ventricular preload.*

Ventricular Afterload

Ventricular afterload refers to the force against which the ventricle must work to eject blood. The primary afterload component is the resistance within the vascular system; however, valvular disease and increased blood viscosity also will result in increased impedance to the ejection of blood. Generally, an increase in vascular resistance leads to an increase in arterial blood pressure. Therefore, *changes* in mean arterial pressure may be used to clinically reflect *changes* in ventricular afterload.

Body Water Compartments

The human vascular system is composed of "dynamic" conduits capable of contraction and expansion. Thereby, vascular resistance and *blood volume* are variable. The multiple factors affecting intravascular volume are essential to comprehend before the factors involved in venous return can be understood.

The adult human body is composed of 40–60% water by weight. Fatty tissue contains less water than other tissue; thus, total body water by weight varies inversely with obesity. Males have approximately 60% of normal body weight as water, females about 50%.

Figure 26–4 illustrates that total body water (TBW) is distributed between two major compartments—*intracellular* and *extracellular*. The extracellular compartment is in turn divided into two subcompartments—*interstitial* (extravascular) and *intravascular*. Since water can move across cellular membranes and capillaries, all body compartments maintain an equilibrium with reference to water.

The intracellular compartment contains about two thirds of the TBW in the adult; distribution of the remaining one third is normally 75% in the interstitial compartment and 25% intravascular (blood). The RBC mass, although intravascular, is considered part of the intracellular fluid compartment.

The larger protein molecules are primarily contained within the intravascular compartment. The small amount of protein that enters the interstitial space is removed by the lymphatics and returned to the

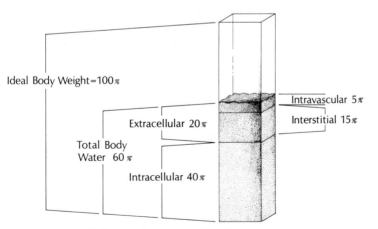

Fig 26–4.—Normal distribution of total body water expressed as percentage of total body weight (see text).

TABLE 26-1.—BLOOD VOLUME

| | % NORMAL BODY WEIGHT | | |
	Range	Mean	ml/kg
Males	7.5–9.0	7.5	75
Females	6.0–7.5	6.5	65

blood. The *colloid osmotic pressure* (COP) exerted by proteins (see Chapter 29) plays an important role in maintaining intravascular volume at the capillary level. Representative values for blood volumes are listed in Table 26–1.

Absolute Hypovolemia

Absolute hypovolemia is defined as a decrease in blood volume from the patient's "normal" volume. The most common clinical causes for absolute hypovolemia are (1) acute hemorrhage, (2) dehydration, and (3) third space fluid losses.

ACUTE HEMORRHAGE.—This commonly occurs secondary to trauma, gastrointestinal bleeding, or surgical manipulation and is a common clinical cause of absolute hypovolemia in adults. Most patients can sustain a 10% loss in blood volume (e.g., donating a unit of blood) without significant effects. Up to 20% of the blood volume can be acutely lost with minimal effects as long as the patient remains supine and inactive. However, upon assuming an upright position, that individual will usually experience postural hypotension and tachycardia. Most patients who acutely lose 30–50% of their blood volume will show clinical evidence of a severe "low flow state" and require rapid reestablishment of their blood volume. Patients acutely losing more than 50% of their blood volume frequently develop what is termed "irreversible shock" in spite of rapid and aggressive blood volume replacement. The degree of acute blood loss cannot be accurately quantitated by measuring the hematocrit or hemoglobin content because 24–72 hours is required for equilibration of total body water between intracellular and extracellular compartments.

DEHYDRATION.—This blood volume depletion results from a loss of total body water. Initially several mechanisms allow water to shift from the interstitial to intravascular compartment in response to dehydration (e.g., protein mobilized from lymphatics to blood). Such mechanisms are effective for only *limited* periods of time. Chronically ill patients and those at bed rest for prolonged periods have lower blood volumes than would be predicted. Ultimately, all water shifts must be proportional in all compartments. *Maintenance of total body water is essential to maintenance of adequate blood volume.*

THIRD SPACE FLUID LOSS. — This refers to fluid lost from normal functioning compartments but still remaining within the body. The most common examples are found with abdominal surgery, where fluid is sequestered in the bowel peritoneal surfaces, or with bowel obstruction or paralytic ileus, which often results in retention of large amounts of fluid within the lumen of the gastrointestinal tract. This type of problem can be very difficult to deal with: the exact amount of fluid lost is difficult to quantitate since it remains within the body.

Absolute Hypervolemia

Absolute hypervolemia is defined as an increase in blood volume from the patient's normal volume. This is most commonly seen in patients with congestive heart failure, with severe oliguric renal disease, and after administration of *excessive* intravenous fluid.

Venous Return

Cardiac output equals the stroke volume times the rate (CO = SV × rate). Ventricular preload (and therefore stroke volume) is greatly dependent upon the venous return of blood to the heart, since *the heart cannot pump out more blood than it receives!* Thus, a thorough understanding of venous flow capabilities becomes paramount in understanding venous return.

The anatomy and general physiology of the vascular system have been discussed in Chapter 2. It should be recalled that 65–70% of the intravascular volume is contained within the venous system. The arterial system is relatively fixed in its ability to alter volume compared to the venous system, which has a relatively great ability to alter volume.

Venous Driving Pressure

For blood to flow through the venous system to the atrium requires a pressure gradient (ΔP). Flow in the large veins can be affected by abdominal and intrathoracic pressure changes. However, flow through the smaller (peripheral) veins and venules is primarily a reflection of local organ system demands and the pressure gradient developed by smooth muscle activity varying the vessel caliber.

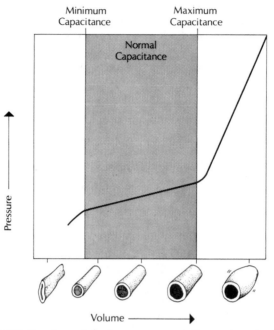

Fig 26–5.—A model of venous capacitance (see text).

Venous Capacitance

Figure 26–5 represents a model in which the venous capacitance may be conceived as an ability to store blood. Whenever the venous system contains a blood volume below its upper limit of storage capability, *maximum capacitance,* variations in volume result in relatively small pressure changes. When the venous system contains a blood volume above its maximum storage capacity, addition of further volume results in relatively large increases in pressure.

Although this model is *not* identical to lung compliance, similarities between lung compliance and venous capacitance are found in terms of pressure-volume interrelationships. In general, at any moment in time the venous capacitance is determined in part by venous tone. Volumes below this storage capacity may be varied, with resultant small pressure changes; volume variation above storage capacity results in large pressure changes (see Fig 26–5).

VENOTONE.—This may be defined as the state of contraction of smooth muscle within the venous walls. This is primarily under the

$$\text{CONDUCTANCE} = \frac{F}{\triangle P}$$

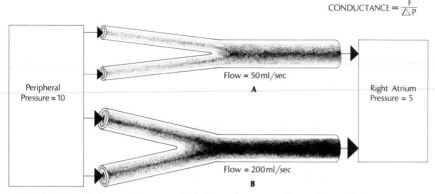

Flow = 50 ml/sec
A

Peripheral
Pressure = 10

Right Atrium
Pressure = 5

Flow = 200 ml/sec
B

Fig 26–6. – Schematic representation of venous flow when driving pressure remains constant while conductance increases. *A* represents constricted veins with a driving pressure (peripheral pressure minus atrial pressure) of 5 and a flow of 50. Conductance equals 10 (50 ÷ 5). *B* represents dilated veins with a driving pressure of 5 and flow of 200. Conductance equals 40.

Increasing conductance will result in increased flows if the driving pressure is kept constant (see text). F = flow; ΔP = pressure change.

control of the sympathetic nervous system. *Venotone and venous capacitance are inversely related;* i.e., as venotone increases, venous capacitance decreases. When venotone is maximum, a state of *minimum capacitance* may be defined. When a state of minimum capacitance exists, any reduction in venous fluid volume will result in a marked decrease in pressure (see Fig 26–5).

VENOUS CONDUCTANCE. – This is the capability to convey flow easily. Since the concept of resistance is generally well understood by the respiratory care practitioner, it is easier to approach the concept of conductance by first considering resistance. The smaller a caliber of a vessel, the greater the resistance to flow $\left(R = \frac{\Delta P}{F} \right)$. This relationship is as valid from the opposite viewpoint, i.e., the less the resistance, the greater the ability to convey flow. Thus, conductance may be defined as the reciprocal of resistance* $\left(\text{conductance} = \frac{F}{\Delta P} \right)$. The greater the conductance (the less the resistance), the greater the ability to convey flow. From yet another viewpoint, the greater the conductance, the greater the flow resulting from a given driving pressure (Fig 26–6).

*The reciprocal of resistance equals $\frac{1}{R}$.

Vascular Volume-to-Vascular Space Relationship

Venous flow may be theoretically improved by two mechanisms: (1) increasing driving pressure and (2) improving conductance. Venous driving pressures may be increased by either decreasing atrial pressure† or increasing venotone in the more peripheral portions of the venous system. Venous conductance may be enhanced by increasing vessel caliber. Clinically, an increased venous volume is most often accompanied by decreasing venotone. It is this mechanism which usually allows intravenous fluid therapy to increase conductance and maintain venous driving pressure.

Increasing driving pressure (venoconstriction) is the most common mechanism increasing venous return that the *body* invokes in response to acute physiologic stress. Improving conductance (intravenous fluid administration) is the most common mechanism accomplished in acute supportive care. In other words, *optimizing the relationship of vascular volume to vascular space is the primary means for medically optimizing venous return and thereby ventricular preload.*

Perfusion

Circulation and perfusion of blood are responsible for supplying all nutrients to living cells and removing their metabolic waste products. To accomplish this task, there must be adequate blood flow through the capillary beds that pervade all tissue. These capillary beds are referred to as the *microcirculation;* their anatomy and general physiology have been discussed previously (see Chapter 2).

Perfusion is defined as blood flow through the microcirculation of organ systems. It is imperative to appreciate that *circulation* and *perfusion* are not synonymous. Inadequate circulation is almost always accompanied by inadequate perfusion; however, adequate circulation does not necessarily assure adequate perfusion. Thus, perfusion depends not only on adequate circulation, but also on appropriate arteriolar and microcirculatory function.

Distribution of Circulation

The primary role of arteries is to rapidly transport blood from the heart to the microcirculation. *Arterioles* have the ability to significantly

---

†Note that an increased atrial pressure is directly produced when airway pressure therapy is instituted. It is often this increased intrathoracic pressure that directly causes decreased venous return.

alter their resistance and thereby determine the distribution of blood to various organs as well as to tissue beds within those organ systems. This crucial function is under the control of numerous mechanisms (e.g., autonomic nervous system, hormonal systems). The combination of these mechanisms acting on both the arterioles and the microcirculation is referred to as *autoregulation*.

Under normal circumstances the distribution of blood flow to organ systems correlates with oxygen requirements. In other words, organ systems generally receive portions of the total cardiac output that are proportional to that organ's metabolic demand. In a simplified fashion then, metabolic demands may be equated with organ system oxygen consumption *except* in three organ systems: (1) kidneys, (2) skin, and (3) heart. The *kidneys* normally receive about 25% of the cardiac output while utilizing only 10% of the body's total oxygen consumption. This disparity is in response to the kidney's role in filtering metabolic waste products from the blood. The *skin* normally receives about 10% of the cardiac output while using only 5% of the body's total oxygen consumption. This is secondary to the role of cutaneous circulation as a temperature regulator. The *heart* normally receives about 5% of the cardiac output while utilizing 10% of the body's total oxygen consumption. This necessitates a large extraction of oxygen from the coronary blood supply and results in extremely desaturated coronary sinus blood. The clinical implication is that, since there is normally very little available oxygen remaining in coronary sinus (venous) blood, oxygen supply to the heart is vitally dependent upon maintenance of adequate coronary blood flow.

Assessment of Perfusion

The capillary beds of various organ systems function as indigenous units. The functions of true capillaries, postcapillary sphincters, and metarterioles (see Chapter 2) are mediated by numerous local vasoactive mediators and metabolites that reflect local metabolic phenomena. This "local" autoregulation or "vasomotion" is in addition to "regional" and "central" regulatory mechanisms.

The autoregulatory capabilities of various capillary beds vary dramatically, e.g., the autoregulatory capabilities of the pulmonary capillaries are relatively limited compared to those of the C.N.S. However, when confronted with significant physiologic stress, vital organ perfusion will generally be favored over musculoskeletal perfusion.

The next chapter is devoted to the clinical assessment of *circulation*. Presently available measurements and techniques allow quantitative and objective assessment of the circulation but, unfortunately, the same is not true of clinical assessment of perfusion. We must still depend on routine clinical observations to assess perfusion status.

A decrease in *peripheral skin temperature* is an early clinical indication of perfusion deficit. The skin normally receives a significant portion of the cardiac output, and this can be readily decreased with minimal detriment to the organism. "Cold and clammy" extremities are early signs of perfusion deficit.

The fingernail beds are readily available for clinical observation of the microcirculation. After compressing and following release of the nail, the resultant "blanching" should readily disappear if microcirculatory blood flow is adequate. Good nail bed *capillary fill* is reassuring, since extremity perfusion is usually diminished early in a perfusion crisis.

Sensorium is a useful basis for assessment. C.N.S. perfusion is usually favored in stress. Conscious cerebral function is very sensitive to oxygen lack, and therefore changes in sensorium (agitation, obtundation, confusion) will occur when perfusion to the brain is diminished. An alert and oriented patient has adequate perfusion of the brain.

Assessment of *urine output* is a very useful reflection of kidney perfusion status. In physiologic stress the urine output is initially somewhat diminished because of increased fluid reabsorption. However, in prolonged, severe physiologic stress renal blood flow is significantly decreased and therefore urine output approaches zero. Placement of a urinary catheter allows serial observations of urine output. A major limitation to this evaluation process is the difficulty in separating pre-existent renal disease from the acute process.

Summary

Circulation has been defined as blood flow through the heart and vascular system, *perfusion* as blood flow through the microcirculation of organ systems. Perfusion is dependent on an adequate circulation and on numerous autoregulatory mechanisms.

Circulation is dependent on adequate myocardial function and venous return. Myocardial performance is affected by the state of contractility as well as by adequate ventricular preload and acceptable ventricular afterload.

Venous return is primarily a function of the vascular volume-to-vascular space relationship, which is determined by the interrelationships of venous capacitance, conductance, and blood volume.

Clinical assessment and support of the circulatory and perfusion states demand comprehension of the physics and physiology presented in this chapter.

27 • CLINICAL ASSESSMENT OF VENOUS RETURN

HEMODYNAMIC MEASUREMENTS were originally utilized to aid in the care of patients with myocardial disease. Their primary application in respiratory care is to aid in optimizing venous return and cardiac output in patients requiring airway pressure therapy.[383] The following discussion is *not* intended as a complete presentation of clinical hemodynamic monitoring; rather, it presents reasonable rationale and guidelines for hemodynamic measurements in most patients receiving airway pressure therapy.

Atrial Pressure Measurement

The atria are chambers with thin muscle walls and relatively low pressure. Atrial contraction has an insignificant effect on the mean pressure measurement; thus, for clinical purposes the atrial pressure may be considered the result of two major variants: (1) blood volume within the chamber and (2) intrathoracic pressure compressing that volume. *Assuming that intrathoracic pressure is normal and consistent, the major factor altering atrial pressure is atrial blood volume.*

Pressure-Volume Relationship

The atria function as capacitance chambers and are continuous with the large capacitance veins within the thorax. Thus, pressure-volume relationships in the atria are similar to those of the venous system; i.e., volume changes below maximum capacitance result in relatively small pressure change; volume changes approaching maximum capacitance result in relatively large pressure change (see Fig 26–5). *Atrial pressure changes are not linearly related to atrial volume changes.*

Volume-Flow Relationship

Atrial volume will be determined by the relationship of blood flow into and out of the chamber. When inflow exceeds outflow, atrial volume increases; when outflow exceeds inflow, atrial volume decreases. Of course, such imbalances of flow are transient. A new inflow-outflow equilibrium state is rapidly achieved, but a *changed atrial volume constitutes part of the new steady state.*

405

Pressure-Flow Relationship

Since atrial pressure is directly related to intra-atrial blood volume, low atrial pressure reflects decreased inflow potential in relation to outflow potential; however, high atrial pressure reflects increased inflow potential in relation to outflow potential.

Myocardial inotropy (ventricular contractility status) will be the main determinant of atrial outflow in the absence of atrioventricular valvular disease. For example, an acute *negative inotropic state* will result in increased ventricular end-diastolic pressures, which will result in a transiently decreased atrial outflow. The new equilibrium state requires an increased intra-atrial volume and a higher atrial pressure.

Obtaining Atrial Pressure Measurements

Central Venous Pressure (CVP) Monitor

Central venous pressure is classically obtained from a catheter placed at the junction of the superior vena cava and right atrium and traditionally attached to a vertical water column device. Therefore, the common unit of measurement is cm H_2O. The "normal" range for CVP is 5–15 cm H_2O; however, the delta (Δ) factor (i.e., ΔP_{AT} with volume loading) is the most significant measurement.

A CVP measures right atrial pressures and, therefore, reflects the systemic venous return and right ventricular preload. In patients in whom it is reasonable to suspect that function of the left heart is as capable as the right heart, the CVP is a useful and valuable monitor.[383] However, often in the very critically ill patient the left heart is incapable of functioning similarly to the right heart.[384, 385] Such circumstances require the placement of a pulmonary artery catheter to properly monitor left ventricular preload.[386]

Pulmonary Artery Catheter

Development of the Swan-Ganz (pulmonary artery, balloon-tipped) catheter has made catheterization of the right heart and pulmonary artery technically feasible and relatively safe to perform at the bedside of the patient in intensive care.[387, 388] The basic double-channel catheter has a fluid channel, which opens at the distal tip, and a second air channel connected to a balloon located close to the end of the catheter. The balloon may be repeatedly inflated and deflated with small amounts of air.

Placement

The catheter can be introduced into the systemic venous system either by a surgical cut down over the antecubital fossa or percutaneously via the subclavian, external, or internal jugular veins. Occasionally the femoral vein may be used. The catheter is advanced with the balloon deflated until it lies within the chest cavity. The balloon is then appropriately inflated and further advanced, allowing the blood flow to carry the balloon tip in a manner similar to an embolus.[387] In essence, the blood flow "carries" the tip of the catheter through the right ventricle and pulmonic valve into the pulmonary artery. Prior to introduction of the catheter, the fluid channel is filled with heparinized saline and connected to a pressure transducer, allowing instantaneous display of the various pressure patterns on an oscilloscope (cathode ray tube projection on a phosphorescent screen). A continuous ECG recording is essential for careful monitoring during advancement of the catheter. It is not unusual for the catheter tip to cause a few ventricular premature contractions as it passes through the right ventricle. Occasionally a severe ventricular arrhythmia will occur, necessitating immediate removal of the catheter from the right ventricle. The balloon should not be deflated with the tip of the catheter in the right ventricle.

Pressure Patterns

Figure 27–1 illustrates the classic pressure patterns displayed as the catheter tip traverses the right atrium, right ventricle, and main pulmonary artery and eventually lodges in a pulmonary artery branch in a wedge position.

Wedge Position

The catheter tip is positioned so that the inflated balloon completely occludes proximal blood flow through a branch of the pulmonary artery. When the balloon is deflated, there must be free flow of pulmonary artery blood around the tip of the catheter, and the pressure reading will represent the phasic (systolic/diastolic) pulmonary artery pressures. Inflation of the balloon should be kept to a minimum, since blood flow to a significant portion of lung is obstructed while the balloon is occluding the vessel. It is also possible for the tip of the catheter to advance (migrate outward) after being initially positioned. In some circumstances this can result in an occlusion of the arterial branch even with the balloon deflated. This complication can be

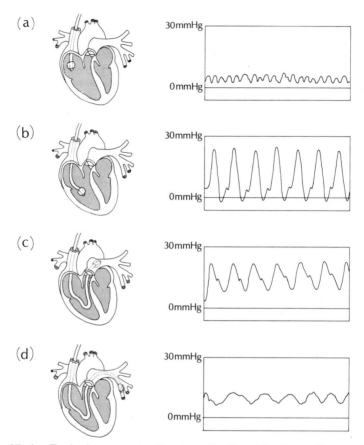

Fig 27–1.—Typical pressure patterns as the tip of the Swan-Ganz catheter traverses the right heart and pulmonary artery. **a,** right atrial pressure; **b,** right ventricular pressure—note that diastolic pressure is zero base line or below; **c,** pulmonary artery pressure—note that diastolic pressure is signifi-cantly above zero baseline; **d,** pulmonary wedge pressure—catheter tip senses only pulmonary capillary back pressure since balloon obstructs ar-terial flow. Deflation of the balloon should result in immediate return of the pulmonary artery pressure pattern (see text). (From Shapiro, B. A., Harrison, R. A., and Walton, J. R.: *Clinical Application of Blood Gases* [2d ed.; Chicago: Year Book Medical Publishers, Inc., 1977].)

avoided by careful, continuous monitoring of the phasic pulmonary artery pressure pattern. When a dampened pressure reading is ob-served, the catheter channel should be vigorously irrigated and the integrity of the pressure transducers thoroughly evaluated. If the trac-ing is still dampened, the catheter must be retracted and repositioned

until a satisfactory pulmonary artery pressure pattern is obtained.[389]
With the balloon properly inflated, the pressure reading just beyond the catheter tip will reflect back pressure through the pulmonary circulation. These "wedge" pressure readings (PWP) relate to the filling pressure of the left ventricle in a manner similar to the way central venous pressure readings relate to right ventricular filling pressures.[390]

With the balloon deflated and the catheter in proper position, pulmonary artery blood will be flowing past the tip of the catheter. Under these circumstances a blood sample properly drawn through the fluid channel[391] will have a true mixed venous oxygen tension and content.

Pulmonary Wedge Pressure (PWP)

This is *not* a direct left atrial pressure measurement; however, when the catheter tip is properly positioned, the pressures are very close approximations of left atrial pressures, and "delta factors" correlate reliably.[390] The "normal" range of PWP is 4–12 mm Hg; however, pressures up to 18 mm Hg are acceptable in critically ill patients.

Optimizing Venous Return—the Fluid Challenge Principle

A finite volume of fluid added to the vascular space in a given time period is referred to as a *volume load*. The difference between atrial pressures measured before and after a volume load is referred to as ΔP_{AT}.

Relative hypovolemia exists whenever the vascular volume is insufficient to fill the existing vascular space. A model system has already been constructed (see Fig 26–5) in which the minimum and maximum venous capacitances are predetermined. In Figure 27–2, the model is modified to show the relationship between ΔP_{AT} and flow. In this schema a state of relative hypovolemia exists below the point of minimum capacitance. This results in a low peripheral venous pressure, which leads to an inadequate venous driving pressure: venous return is significantly diminished.

In the circumstances depicted in Figure 27–2, repeated volume loads will result in insignificant changes in atrial pressure (ΔP_{AT}) in *area A*. As the vascular volume is increased, the relative hypovolemia is essentially reversed so that an additional volume load in *area B* should produce a small change in ΔP_{AT}. Further volume loading now results in measurable atrial pressure changes with corresponding improvement in flow *(area C)*. At this time, increases in vascular volume are also resulting in increasing venous caliber, thereby improving

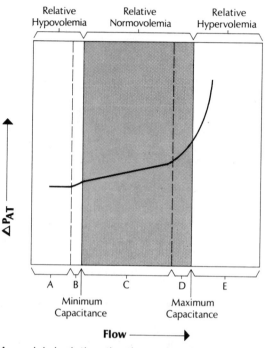

Fig 27–2.—A model depicting the theoretic relationship between venous flow and the change in atrial pressure resulting from a specific fluid load (ΔP_{AT}). See text for details.

conductance. As the point of maximum capacitance is approached (*area D*), larger changes in atrial pressure are observed with continued volume loading. When the maximum capacitance of the venous system is exceeded (*area E* — a state of relative *hyper*volemia), further volume loading will result in extremely large atrial pressure changes with minimal improvement in flow.

In other words, at the point represented by *area D*, atrial venous return has been theoretically optimized. Therefore, continued inadequacies in cardiac output must be secondary to factors interfering either with atrial or ventricular outflow or to primary myocardial dysfunction. When atrial-ventricular valvular disease exists, changes in atrial pressure measurements cannot be assumed to reliably indicate changes in outflow. Furthermore, in patients with chronic myocardial dysfunction, much higher than "normal" atrial pressures may be needed to optimize outflow.

In most clinical circumstances, when a state of relative hypovolemia exists, the vascular space is significantly contracted (i.e., approaching minimal capacitance). However, a state of relative hypovolemia can exist *without* increased venous tone. In general, early "septic shock" usually represents a state of relative hypovolemia in which venous volume was initially normal but becomes inadequate secondary to an abnormal reduction in venous tone.

The fluid challenge principle is a clinical means of assessing the adequacy of venous return and its interface with ventricular (preload) function, as schematized in Figure 27–2. Since pressure measurements are taken at only one point in the system (the atria), understanding the physiologic phenomena causing pressure *changes* is paramount to their proper clinical application.

Base-Line Assessment of Circulation and Perfusion

The unstable cardiopulmonary system requires serial evaluations for assessment of improvement or deterioration. A simple observation or measurement (unless extremely abnormal) is often misleading. The delta factors that occur with time and/or therapy are more meaningful and easier to assess in terms of clinical significance.

A general clinical evaluation of the circulatory and perfusion status is essential as a base line, since even the most sophisticated of monitoring systems are of little value unless evaluated in conjunction with the general clinical status. Such an evaluation in critically ill patients must include at least the following: (1) *Blood pressure*—mean arterial pressures below 60 mm Hg and above 110 mm Hg are disturbing; however, even "normal" blood pressure does not assure adequate flow. The *changes* that occur or do not occur are more significant. In critically ill patients, routine *cuff* blood pressure measurements are extremely inaccurate. More accurate and reliable values can be achieved by direct monitoring using an arterial catheter.[35] (2) *ECG monitoring,* which allows evaluation of myocardial rate and electric patterns; rates below 60 per minute or greater than 140 per minute in adults are disturbing since reserves for increasing cardiac output are limited. The presence of arrhythmias must be observed and evaluated. (3) *Peripheral perfusion*—skin temperature and color, sensorium, and urine output. (4) *Arterial blood gases.*

Guidelines for Fluid Challenge

The following is a guideline that we find useful for a "fluid challenge principle" with pulmonary artery wedge pressures. It is called the *3–7 mm Hg rule* and is correlated with the schema in Figure 27–2.

Step #1.—Obtain general clinical and laboratory base lines and measure PWP.

Step #2.—Give 50–200 ml of appropriate solution within 10 minutes. (Exact volume depends on the clinician's appraisal of the patient's condition.)

Step #3.—Observe the systemic circulation for improvement in blood pressure, peripheral perfusion, and urine output. Reexamine the chest for presence of rales, wheezes, or other adventitious sounds.

Step #4. — Evaluate change in PWP (ΔP_{pwp}):

- If less than 3 mm Hg (*areas A* and *B*, Fig 27–2)—repeat process until there is either (a) improvement in systemic circulatory function, or (b) emergence of adverse chest physical findings.
- If more than 7 mm Hg (*area E*, Fig 27–2)—continued volume expansion is not likely to improve venous return; administer more fluid only if the clinical situation dictates the need for further increase in ventricular preload.
- If between 3 and 7 mm Hg (*areas C* and *D*, Fig 27–2)—wait 10 minutes and again measure PWP to compare with "base-line" measurement:
- If increase is now less than 3 mm Hg—repeat entire process.
- If increase remains between 3 and 7 mm Hg—repeat entire process but reduce quantity of fluid challenge.

The same guideline may be used with a CVP catheter. It is then the *2–5 cm H₂O* rule; i.e., ΔP_{cvp} of 2 cm H_2O and 5 cm H_2O are used in step #4.

The controversy concerning *colloid* (blood, plasma, albumin, dextran) versus *crystalloid* (saline, lactated Ringer's, 5% dextrose in water) administration is beyond the scope of this text. Suffice it to say that the principle of fluid challenge is appropriate irrespective of what solution is deemed advisable for volume expansion.

Improving Ventricular Function

When negative inotropy exists after proper assessment of vascular volume-to-space relationship, pharmacologic manipulation of the cardiovascular system may be indicated. Such manipulation generally consists of positive inotropic drugs and/or diuretic therapy.

Positive Inotropic Agents

Isoproterenol

Drugs that will immediately improve myocardial contractility (beta-1 adrenergic stimulators) are titrated in appropriate intravenous solution. The classic beta drug with excellent inotropic and chronotropic (increased heart rate) effects is *isoproterenol*. This drug displays a significant incidence of arrhythmia when administered to patients with limited ventricular function. Often the accompanying peripheral vasodilatation results in a drop in systemic blood pressure. Since patients with significant heart disease frequently have partial obstruction of the coronary arteries, this hypotension may further compromise coronary blood flow. Thus, isoproterenol may have an over-all detrimental effect on myocardial metabolism, causing a significant increase in oxygen demand while tending to decrease oxygen delivery to the myocardium.

Dopamine

Dopamine is a naturally occurring catecholamine and precursor of norepinephrine and epinephrine. It has most of the beneficial properties of isoproterenol while possessing fewer of the disadvantages. At lower infusion rates (1–2 μg/kg/minute), a direct "dopaminergic" effect results in renal and splanchnic vasodilatation. This may increase renal blood flow. At infusion rates of 3–10 μg/kg/min, adrenergic effects of positive chronotropism and positive inotropism are added. However, the increase in heart rate is generally not as excessive as with isoproterenol, and the tendency toward arrhythmias is not as prominent as with isoproterenol. Continued increases in dopamine dosage (greater than 10–15 μg/kg/minute) cause the alpha-adrenergic effects to become predominant. The resulting vasoconstriction will frequently lead to a decrease in cardiac and renal output. Thus, the general advantages of dopamine compared to isoproterenol are (1) less significant tachycardia, (2) less oxygen demand on the heart, and (3) decreased potential for development of arrhythmias.

Diuretic Therapy

The decrease in cardiac output that accompanies heart failure causes renal hypoperfusion, which results in sodium and water retention. This salt and water retention leads to increased venous pressure and causes transudation of water and salt to the interstitial space. Thus, total body water and sodium are increased.

The aim of diuretic therapy is to achieve a net loss of sodium and its associated water. A potent diuretic such as furosemide (Lasix) is a very effective agent in this circumstance because of its (1) prompt onset of action; (2) inhibition of sodium and chloride transport back into the circulation; and (3) effectiveness irrespective of the acid-base status. Furosemide is also a direct venous dilator.[412]

An initial dose of 5–20 mg given intravenously is followed by waiting an appropriate time interval (approximately 30 minutes to 1 hour) for assessment of its effects. Increasing doses are administered when indicated. Often the patient will recover a significant amount of cardiovascular function as fluid is lost, and the preload is adjusted downward to a more appropriate range. However, many patients require a positive inotropic agent to be incorporated into the regimen either primarily or as an adjunct to diuretic therapy.

Airway Dynamics and Atrial Pressures

Transmural atrial pressure (intra-atrial pressure minus intrapleural pressure) is a function of intra-atrial blood volume. When intrapleural pressure is normal and consistent, changes in atrial pressure are directly reflective of changes in venous return following fluid administration. However, *when intrapleural pressures are manipulated, atrial pressures must be considered in relation to intrapleural pressure.*[392] For example, when intrapleural pressures are significantly increased, any increase in atrial pressure is *not* directly reflective of changes in venous return.[393] In fact, under these circumstances the venous return is often greatly diminished, leading to inadequate ventricular filling. Since reliable intrapleural pressure measurements are not readily available at present,[394] estimations of the effects of airway pressure therapy on pleural pressures must be applied.

Airway Pressure-to-Intrapleural Pressure Relationship

With *spontaneous ventilation* (see Fig 21–2), the intrapleural pressure during inspiration must be less than airway pressure. Normally the transpulmonary pressure gradient is small (2–10 cm H_2O). As airway resistance increases, or lung compliance decreases, the transpulmonary pressure (TPP) gradient must increase in order for the patient to achieve the same tidal volume.[395] When severe pulmonary pathology exists, the inspiratory TPP gradient may be as high as 50–60 cm H_2O. During passive expiration the intrapleural pressure returns to resting values. Therefore, in most circumstances when lung pathology is present, spontaneous ventilation results in mean intrapleural pressures being more subatmospheric than normal—an obvious advantage for venous return.

Airway pressure therapy always results in increased mean airway pressures that must be transmitted to the intrapleural space to some degree. The degree of transmission varies primarily with lung compliance and secondarily with pulmonary resistance.

Control Mode IPPV (see Fig 22-1)

With normal lungs, IPPV control mode increases the mean airway pressure 5-10 cm H_2O. The major variant affecting mean airway pressure is the expiratory time. Mean intrapleural pressures are believed to be affected to the same degree as mean airway pressures.[395, 401]

When increased airway resistance is present, greater positive pressure is required to deliver the same tidal volume. Some of this increased airway pressure is believed transmitted to the pleural space. When lung compliance is acutely decreased, much greater airway pressures are required for tidal volume delivery, but relatively little of this increased airway pressure is believed transmitted to the pleural space. However, when chest wall compliance is decreased, higher airway pressures are required to deliver the tidal volume, and most of this will be transmitted to the pleural space. This occurs clinically every time a patient fights the ventilator.

An advantage to having an IMV circuit in line with control mode ventilation is that any attempts to breathe "around" or "between" ventilator breaths will result in lower intrapleural pressures. Theoretically this is a cardiovascular advantage as long as the energy expenditure involved is not detrimental and the efforts do not result in fighting the ventilator or decreasing chest wall distensibility.

Augmented Mode IPPV

The less IPPV required, the lower are the mean airway and intrapleural pressures.

Inspiratory Hold

With normal lungs, the mean airway and intrapleural pressures are increased. When airway resistance is increased, the mean intrapleural pressure will be increased to a lesser degree than mean airway pressure.[400]

Retard with IPPV

Intrapleural pressures are minimally affected when retard is appropriately applied for airway resistance.

PEEP

Of all positive airway pressure maneuvers, PEEP has the greatest effect on mean airway pressure. With normal lungs there will be a significant transmission of increased pressure to the pleural space[396, 397, 400]—as great as 90% of the increased airway pressure. With acutely decreased lung compliance, transmission of increased airway pressures appears proportional to the degree of decreased lung compliance. When PEEP is appropriately applied in usual therapeutic ranges (10–30 cm H_2O) to such lungs, it is doubtful that more than 40% of the increased mean airway pressure is transmitted to the pleural space.

Suggestions for Interpretation of Atrial Pressures in Conjunction with Airway Pressure Therapy

1. *Attempt to estimate mean intrapleural pressure.*—The normal mean intrapleural pressure in spontaneous breathing is estimated to be minus 5 cm H_2O[395]: (a) appropriate control mode IPPV is estimated to increase mean intrapleural pressure 5 cm H_2O; (b) one third of appropriate PEEP therapy is estimated to be transmitted to the pleural space.

2. *Transform atrial pressure readings to estimated atrial transmural pressures.*—For example, if normal CVP is 10 cm H_2O, normal right atrial transmural pressure is 15 cm H_2O [10−(−5) = + 15]: (a) with IPPV control mode, a CVP of 15 cm H_2O probably represents an atrial transmural pressure of 15 cm H_2O, since mean intrapleural pressure is close to zero. In other words, a CVP of 15 cm H_2O on control mode probably represents the same transmural pressure as a CVP of 10 cm H_2O in a spontaneously breathing patient; (2) with CPAP of 20 cm H_2O, a CVP of 17–18 cm H_2O is estimated to reflect an atrial transmural pressure of about 15 cm H_2O [17 − (+2) = 15], since a third of the PEEP (about 7 cm H_2O) is transmitted and increases mean intrapleural pressure from minus 5 to plus 2.

Remember, these are only *suggestions* to help interpret absolute values and to make comparisons when airway pressures are changed. The delta factors remain paramount!

For PWP measurements, 1 mm Hg equals 0.75 cm H_2O. Assuming that normal intrapleural pressure is a mean of minus 3 mm Hg and that a normal PWP is 10 mm Hg, normal atrial transmural pressure is 13 mm Hg (16 cm H_2O): (1) with control mode IPPV, a PWP of 13 mm Hg would represent a normal atrial transmural pressure; (2) with 20 cm H_2O PEEP (15 mm Hg), a PWP of approximately 15 mm Hg would reflect an atrial transmural pressure of 10 mm Hg.

3. *Take measurements at end of exhalation regardless of ventilatory pattern or types of airway pressure support.*[399]

4. *Do not remove the airway pressure therapy from the patient to measure atrial pressure.*—(a) Proper venous return and ventricular

preload must be maintained *with* airway pressure therapy; therefore, measurement must be made *with* airway pressure therapy;[400] (b) in general, when IPPV and PEEP therapy are appropriately applied, changes in atrial pressure readings are not significant when therapy is removed;[398] and (c) unless adequate time (more than 30–45 seconds) is allowed for new steady state equilibration, atrial pressure readings are unreliable off airway pressure support.[398]

Summary

The patient with pulmonary decompensation is generally manifesting an increased cardiac output. When airway pressure therapy is instituted to prevent or reverse pulmonary decompensation, the cardiovascular system is placed at a potential disadvantage. The increased mean intrapleural pressures frequently result in increased atrial pressures but not necessarily in decreased venous return. To increase venous return, the venous system must respond by increasing its venotone. This can be minimized by proper assessment and support of the vascular volume-to-vascular space relationship.

Many critically ill patients are "overloaded" in terms of total body fluid but have inadequate intravascular volumes and compensate by decreasing the vascular space. In these circumstances, airway pressure therapy may cause profound decreases in venous return capability. For example, the initiation of ventilator therapy usually results in an elevation of mean intrapleural pressure, which tends to impede venous return and ventricular preload. Agents frequently used to allow appropriate application of airway pressure therapy (such as morphine, sedatives, and tranquilizers) may alter the venous tone and contribute to relative hypovolemia. Furthermore, normalization of arterial blood gases (improved arterial oxygen tension, diminished carbon dioxide tension, improved acid-base status) may lead to a significant reduction in endogenous catecholamines which results in decreased venous tone.

The respiratory care practitioner, nurse specialist, and physician must properly evaluate vascular volume-to-vascular space relationships when instituting and maintaining airway pressure support. The patient's well-being depends on the ability of "the team" to function smoothly.

Ventricular Afterload

Ventricular afterload is defined as the forces impeding flow out of the ventricle. The greater the impedance, the greater the energy required to achieve a given stroke volume. If the ventricle is unable to eject blood adequately because it cannot generate the required energy, decreasing the afterload will reduce the energy required to eject the blood and therefore ventricular output can be increased. In the absence of anatomic outflow tract abnormality (valvular disease, muscle hypertrophy), the major impedance to flow is the peripheral vascular resistance.

The use of peripheral vasodilating agents has recently become significant in the armamentarium of pharmacologic support for the patient with limited cardiovascular reserves. The basic premise is to reduce systemic arterial blood pressure (reduce afterload) so that cardiac output may be maintained while reducing the work of the left ventricle. This technique is particularly effective in patients with limited cardiovascular reserves who manifest hypertension.

Sodium nitroprusside (Nipride) is a direct, fast-acting, and potent vascular smooth muscle dilator. Its rapid onset of action and metabolism allow excellent moment-to-moment control with intravenous infusion. The primary disadvantage of sodium nitroprusside is that large amounts of the drug may result in toxic blood levels of cyanide.

A major disadvantage to the pharmacologic reduction of afterload is that coronary blood flow is decreased because diastolic pressure is lowered. The *counterpulsating aortic balloon device* is designed to overcome this disadvantage, since it allows reduction in ventricular afterload while augmenting aortic root diastolic pressure. The success of this device, except in cardiac surgical candidates or early postoperative cardiac surgical patients, has been disappointing.

28 • CLINICAL ASSESSMENT OF INTRAPULMONARY SHUNT, OXYGENATION, AND CARDIAC OUTPUT

THE PLACEMENT OF PULMONARY artery catheters for monitoring left ventricular hemodynamic function in critically ill patients has become accepted clinical practice. Although the initial purpose for developing such catheters was primarily to monitor left heart filling pressures their contribution to acute respiratory care has been notable, since the critically ill patient with a significant hypoxemia often presents a diagnostic challenge to ascertain the extent to which the cardiac and pulmonary systems are implicated. The exact pathophysiology is often in doubt despite careful clinical evaluation, including a detailed history and physical examination, routine laboratory studies, chest x-ray, and routine blood testing. Since a diagnosis determines the emphasis of treatment, differentiation of a large primary intrapulmonary shunt from a primary myocardial dysfunction is often of critical importance.

The Fick Equation

Approximately one hundred years ago, Adolph Fick described a procedure whereby the concentration of a dissolved substance in the blood could be used as an indicator for determining blood flow.[402] This concept became known as the Fick principle. When oxygen is used as the dissolved substance, the determination is known as the Fick equation.

The quantity of oxygen potentially available for tissue consumption in a given unit of time is expressed as the arterial oxygen content (C_{aO_2}) multiplied by the quantity of arterial blood presented to the tissues per unit time ($\dot{Q}T$).

$$\text{Oxygen availability} = (\dot{Q}_T)(C_{aO_2}) \tag{1}$$

The quantity of oxygen returned to the lungs is expressed as the total cardiac output multiplied by the mixed venous oxygen content ($C\bar{v}_{O_2}$), obtained from pulmonary artery blood.

$$\text{Oxygen returned} = (\dot{Q}_T)(C\bar{v}_{O_2}) \qquad (2)$$

Therefore, the tissue oxygen consumption in a given time interval ($\dot{V}_{O_2}$) equals the oxygen that has been extracted from the blood, i.e., the difference between the oxygen available (Equation #1) and oxygen returned (Equation #2).

$$\dot{V}_{O_2} = (\dot{Q}_T)(C_{aO_2}) - (\dot{Q}_T)(C\bar{v}_{O_2}) \qquad (3)$$

Equation #3 can be simplified and rewritten as follows:

$$\dot{V}_{O_2} = (\dot{Q}_T)(C_{aO_2} - C\bar{v}_{O_2}) \qquad (4)$$

Equation #4 is the Fick equation, which states simply that the oxygen consumed per unit time equals the oxygen extracted from the blood per unit time.

Deriving the Shunt Equation

Rather than expressing the Fick equation as Equation #4, it is more commonly written as

$$\dot{Q}_T = \frac{\dot{V}_{O_2}}{[C_{aO_2} - C\bar{v}_{O_2}]} \qquad (5)$$

$\dot{Q}_T$ is cardiac output per unit time (L/min); $\dot{V}_{O_2}$ is oxygen consumption per unit time (cc/minute); and $[C_{aO_2} - C\bar{v}_{O_2}]$ is the oxygen content difference between arterial and mixed venous blood (vol%).

As illustrated in Figure 28-1, the total cardiac output ($\dot{Q}_T$) is arbitrarily divided into two major components:

$$\dot{Q}_T = \dot{Q}_c + \dot{Q}_s \qquad (6)$$

$\dot{Q}_c$ is the portion of cardiac output that exchanges perfectly with alveolar air. $\dot{Q}_s$ is the portion of cardiac output that does not exchange at all with alveolar air. $\dot{Q}_s$ may be considered equivalent to absolute shunting. Where shunt effect (decreased $\dot{V}/\dot{Q}$) exists, the blood will be incompletely oxygenated. Shunt effect is mathematically divided as though a portion of that blood exchanged perfectly ($\dot{Q}_c$) and the remainder did not exchange at all ($\dot{Q}_s$).

$\dot{Q}_c$ mathematically represents all the blood to which oxygen is being ideally added as it traverses the lung. The blood leaving these perfectly exchanging alveolar-capillary (A-C) units may theoretically be said to contain an end-pulmonary capillary oxygen content (Cc_{O_2}). This value is based on the assumption that complete equilibration between an alveolar gas tension and an end-pulmonary capillary gas tension can exist. In those A-C units with capillary transit times within normal ranges (0.3–0.7 second) and alveolar oxygen tensions (PA_{O_2}) greater than 100 mm Hg, the assumption is clinically valid.[403] The calculated alveolar oxygen tension does not represent any real tension in the various alveoli but, rather, an average value that is dependent on the physical laws of gas exchange and the respiratory exchange ratio.

The mixed venous oxygen content ($C\bar{v}_{O_2}$) represents the blood oxygen content being returned to the lungs. It can be measured *only* in pulmonary artery blood. The oxygen content of shunted blood ($\dot{Q}s$) is unchanged from the mixed venous oxygen content. Therefore, instead of Equation #4, the organism's oxygen consumption may be derived from an expression written as Equation #7:

$$\dot{V}_{O_2} = \dot{Q}c[Cc_{O_2} - C\bar{v}_{O_2}] \tag{7}$$

Therefore,

$$\dot{Q}T[C_aO_2 - C\bar{v}_{O_2}] = \dot{Q}c[CcO_2 - C\bar{v}_{O_2}] \tag{8}$$

The physiologic shunt equation expresses the relationship between total cardiac output and shunted cardiac output. Therefore, Equation #6 is solved in terms of $\dot{Q}_C$:

$$\dot{Q}_C = [\dot{Q}T - \dot{Q}s] \tag{9}$$

Substituting Equation #9 for $\dot{Q}_C$ in Equation #8 results in the following equation:

$$\dot{Q}T[C_aO_2 - C\bar{v}_{O_2}] = [\dot{Q}T - \dot{Q}s][Cc_{O_2} - C\bar{v}_{O_2}] \tag{10}$$

Expanding Equation #10 algebraically:

$$\dot{Q}TC_{aO_2} - \dot{Q}TC\bar{v}_{O_2} = \dot{Q}TCc_{O_2} - \dot{Q}TC\bar{v}_{O_2} - \dot{Q}sCc_{O_2} + \dot{Q}sC\bar{v}_{O_2} \tag{11}$$

Note that two of the six terms ($\dot{Q}TC\bar{v}_{O_2}$) are identical and common to both sides of the equation and, therefore, may be removed from the equation. The collection and factoring of all $\dot{Q}s$ terms on the left side and all $\dot{Q}T$ terms on the right side of the equation results in

$$\dot{Q}s[Cc_{O_2} - C\bar{v}_{O_2}] = \dot{Q}T[Cc_{O_2} - C_{aO_2}] \tag{12}$$

This relationship can now be written as a ratio of shunted cardiac output to total cardiac output:

$$\frac{\dot{Q}s}{\dot{Q}T} = \frac{[CcO_2 - C_{aO_2}]}{[Cc_{O_2} - C\bar{v}_{O_2}]} \tag{13}$$

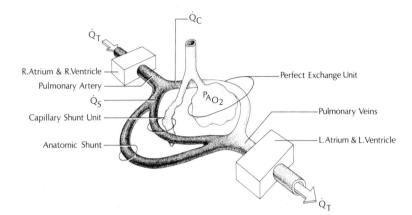

Fig 28–1.—Mathematical concept of physiologic shunting (see text). $\dot{Q}T$ is cardiac output per unit time; $\dot{Q}c$ is the portion of the cardiac output that exchanges perfectly with alveolar air; $\dot{Q}s$ is the portion of the cardiac output that does not exchange with alveolar air; PA_{O_2} is the alveolar oxygen tension. (From Shapiro, B. A., Harrison, R. A., and Walton, J. R.: *Clinical Application of Blood Gases* [2d ed.; Chicago: Year Book Medical Publishers, Inc., 1977].)

Equation #13 is the classic shunt equation.[404] It has the advantage of being derived as a ratio so that no absolute measurement of cardiac output is required. In this form the equation very clearly demonstrates that as the shunted cardiac output ($\dot{Q}s$) approaches zero, the arterial oxygen content must approach the theoretic value of the end-pulmonary capillary oxygen content. As long as a portion of the cardiac output exists as shunted blood, the arterial oxygen content will always be less than the end-pulmonary capillary oxygen content. In other words, since shunted blood has the same oxygen content as mixed venous blood ($C\bar{v}_{O_2}$), when this blood mixes with the perfectly exchanging cardiac output ($\dot{Q}c$), a lowered oxygen content equilibrium (Ca_{O_2}) must be established. This may be conceptualized as oxygen leaving the $\dot{Q}c$ hemoglobin and attaching to previously desaturated $\dot{Q}s$ hemoglobin. The end result is always an arterial oxygen content somewhere between the end-pulmonary capillary oxygen content and the mixed venous oxygen content.

Clinical Shunt Measurement

The intrapulmonary shunt can be calculated whenever both systemic arterial and pulmonary arterial blood gases are performed. The Cc_{O_2} is calculated by assuming that the end-pulmonary capillary hemoglobin content is the same as arterial and by calculating the alveolar P_{O_2} by the alveolar gas equation.

Clinical intrapulmonary shunt measurements should be done at the patient's *maintenance* $F_{I_{O_2}}$. It is not necessary to place the patient on 100% oxygen for the measurement; in fact, 100% oxygen inspired often increases the shunt.[110-112]

Total Oxygen Consumption

Oxygen consumption can be readily measured in cooperative patients breathing room air; however, it is not readily measurable in the critically ill patient. Although the mass spectrometer shows promise of being able to provide serial oxygen consumption measurements in the critically ill patient, at present the technique is not widely available. However, when cardiac output and the arterial-venous oxygen content difference are measured, the oxygen consumption can be *calculated* from the Fick equation.

In most clinical situations the following general statement is valid: in a patient who is adequately perfused, normothermic, and not shivering or seizing, the metabolic oxygen demands are reasonably normal and can be represented by a value of *3.5 ml O_2/kg of normal body weight.* If any of the criteria are not met, this manner of approximating oxygen consumption cannot be reliably assumed.

Arterial-Venous Oxygen Content Difference

The arterial oxygen content minus the mixed venous oxygen content difference $[C_{a_{O_2}} - C\bar{v}_{O_2}]$ represents an assessment of the cardiac output in relation to the metabolic rate. This becomes obvious when the arterial-mixed venous oxygen content difference is considered in the context of the Fick equation (Equation #4). Under conditions in which the oxygen consumption ($\dot{V}_{O_2}$) remains constant, changes in cardiac output ($\dot{Q}_T$) can be related to changes in arterial-mixed venous oxygen content difference ($C_{a_{O_2}} - C\bar{v}_{O_2}$). In other words, as cardiac output increases under these circumstances, oxygen extraction per unit volume of blood decreases (Table 28-1). Although normal A-V content difference is 4.5-6 vol%, in the critically ill patient with a competent cardiac reserve, the A-V content difference is approximately 3.5 vol%.[532]

Table 28-2 lists reference values relating to pulmonary artery blood gas samples and the derived values. As stated previously, clinical application of these values also requires simultaneous measurement of an arterial blood gas. These values should be considered only as guidelines, and they assume a normal oxygen-carrying capacity, clinical evidence of adequate peripheral perfusion, adequate alveolar ventilation, and normal acid-base status with the patient either

TABLE 28-1.—RELATIONSHIP OF CARDIAC OUTPUT
TO OXYGEN EXTRACTION

CONDITION	OXYGEN CONSUMPTION (cc/min)	CARDIAC OUTPUT ($\dot{Q}T$) (L/min)	OXYGEN EXTRACTION $(Ca_{O_2} - C\bar{v}_{O_2})$ [vol% (cc/L)]
Normal cardiac output	250	5	5 (50)
Increased cardiac output	250	10	2.5 (25)
Decreased cardiac output	250	2.5	10 (100)

breathing spontaneously or being supported on the ventilator.[405] When factors such as severe anemia, lack of peripheral perfusion, severe hypercarbia, and acidemia are superimposed, these guidelines begin to lose their clinical usefulness.

These physiologic measurements should be used as early warning indicators of impending or early cardiovascular decompensation. Their clinical value lies in the fact that changes in pulmonary artery blood gases secondary to cardiopulmonary stress often occur earlier than changes in systemic arterial blood gases. This allows for initiation of corrective therapeutic maneuvers, reversing the pathophysiology at an earlier stage.

In patients who meet the criteria for assuming that oxygen utilization is consistent, changes in A-V content difference may be interpreted as correlating with changes in cardiac output.

Thermodilution Cardiac Output Measurements

A triple-channel pulmonary artery catheter contains a second fluid-filled channel that ends approximately 30 cm from the tip of the cathe-

TABLE 28-2.—PREDICTED BLOOD GAS VALUES IN HEALTH
AND DISEASE FOR PULMONARY ARTERY BLOOD

CONDITION	$P\bar{v}_{O_2}$ RANGE	$P\bar{v}_{O_2}$ AVERAGE	% Hb SAT. RANGE	% Hb SAT. AVERAGE	$[Ca_{O_2} - C\bar{v}_{O_2}]$ (vol%) RANGE	$[Ca_{O_2} - C\bar{v}_{O_2}]$ (vol%) AVERAGE
Healthy resting human volunteer	37-43	40	70-76	75	4.5-6.0	5.0
Critically ill patient, cardiovascular reserves excellent	35-40	37	68-75	70	2.5-4.5	3.5
Critically ill patient, cardiovascular stable, limited cardiovascular reserves	30-35	32	56-68	60	4.5-6.0	5.0
Critically ill patient, cardiovascular decompensation	< 30	< 30	< 56	< 56	> 6.0	> 6.0

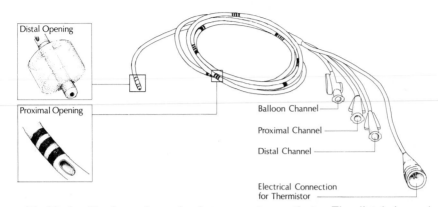

Distal Opening

Proximal Opening

Balloon Channel

Proximal Channel

Distal Channel

Electrical Connection
for Thermistor

Fig 28–2. — The four-channel pulmonary artery catheter. The distal channel and balloon channel comprise the basic two-channel catheter. Addition of the proximal channel that opens in the right atrium results in the triple-channel catheter, usually 7 French in diameter. Addition of the thermistor channel results in the four-channel catheter used for thermodilution cardiac output measurements, usually 7 French in diameter. (From Shapiro, B. A., Harrison, R. A., and Walton, J. R.: *Clinical Application of Blood Gases* [2d ed.; Chicago: Year Book Medical Publishers, Inc., 1977].)

ter. This opening is designed to lie in the right atrium or superior vena cava and is used as a CVP monitor.

The four-channel pulmonary artery catheter (Fig 28 – 2) has a thermistor at the end of the catheter.[406] Cardiac output can be calculated by knowing the amount of cold injected and the average temperature change (concentration of cold) during the time required for total ejection of the cold solution from the right ventricle.[407, 408] In reality, this technique represents an application of the basic Fick principle.[409] The quantity of cold injected, representing the solute, replaces the term oxygen consumption ($\dot{V}O_2$), and the average measured temperature change in the pulmonary artery blood replaces the arterial-mixed venous oxygen content difference ($C_{aO_2} - C\bar{v}_{O_2}$) in the Fick equation.

Tissue Oxygenation

The diffusion of oxygen from the blood to tissue depends primarily on the oxygen pressure gradient between capillary blood and tissue. The lower the capillary oxygen tension, the less the potential for oxygen diffusion.

Hemoglobin-Oxygen Affinity

A factor of paramount importance to tissue oxygenation is the strength with which hemoglobin chemically combines with oxygen.

This chemically bound oxyhemoglobin is intimately related to the P_{O_2} but does not itself exert a partial pressure, since it is not in the dissolved state.[35] Because nearly all oxygen in the blood exists in chemical combination with hemoglobin, almost all of the oxygen molecules that diffuse to tissues must first break their chemical bond with hemoglobin. *Bulk flow of oxygen to tissues requires the dissolution of oxygen binding with hemoglobin.*

The strength with which the hemoglobin chemically binds the oxygen is referred to as *hemoglobin-oxygen affinity.* This affinity is affected by such factors as hydrogen ion concentration, carbon dioxide content, and temperature. An increase in these factors decreases the hemoglobin-oxygen affinity, i.e., "shifts the curve to the right" (see Fig 6–4). Phosphorylase enzyme systems within the red blood cell are also known to affect the affinity. *The theoretic significance of an increased hemoglobin-oxygen affinity is that any pressure gradient will transfer fewer oxygen molecules per unit time.*[35]

Each of the four iron-binding sites in the hemoglobin molecule is affected by the oxygenation status of the other three sites. As each successive heme iron moiety is occupied by oxygen, the distance between them is decreased. These spatial relationships are believed to significantly affect the ability of the unoxygenated heme moieties to combine with oxygen.[410] This physiochemical relationship is probably the basis for the sigmoid shape of the hemoglobin dissociation curve.[35]

When normal blood is 75% saturated, the vast majority of hemoglobin molecules have three oxygenated heme sites and, when 50% saturated, have two oxygenated heme sites. It may be inferred that removal of oxygen from the hemoglobin becomes progressively more difficult as the blood falls below 75% and then 50% saturation. Normal tissue oxygenation demands only oxygen from the fourth heme site, since normal $P\bar{v}_{O_2}$ is 40 mm Hg (75% saturation) (see Fig 6–2).

A venous oxygen tension represents the lowest possible oxygen tension existing in that capillary bed. Therefore, when $P\bar{v}_{O_2}$ falls below 27 mm Hg, it may be inferred that oxygen must leave hemoglobin that is less than 50% saturated in order to meet tissue oxygen demands.

Clinical Assessment of $P\bar{v}_{O_2}$

In the presence of normal hemoglobin values, *the existence of tissue hypoxia must be considered when $P\bar{v}_{O_2}$ falls below 27 mm Hg.* For example, a $P\bar{v}_{O_2}$ of 20 mm Hg can mean either (1) tissue oxygen needs are being met through significant desaturation of hemoglobin, or (2) further desaturation is not possible and tissue oxygen needs are *not* being met. In a patient with normal hemoglobin and adequate perfusion, a $P\bar{v}_{O_2}$ above 30 mm Hg almost always ensures that tissue oxygen needs are being met.

Summary

The development of the balloon-tipped pulmonary artery catheter has made pulmonary artery measurements available at the bedside of the critically ill patient. Besides hemodynamic monitoring, blood gas measurements of true mixed venous blood values, in conjunction with arterial blood gas values, have allowed the clinician to identify more clearly the cardiopulmonary pathophysiology and have further reinforced the interdependence of the two systems.

SECTION VIII

COMMON PULMONARY PATHOLOGY IN ACUTE RESPIRATORY CARE

29 • PULMONARY EDEMA

THE TRACHEOBRONCHIAL TREE, respiratory bronchioles, alveolar ducts, and alveoli must be maintained in a relatively dry state for the lungs to function adequately as a gas exchange organ. Appropriate diffusion and $\dot{V}/\dot{Q}$ relationships require an interstitial space without excessive water content. The "tightness" of alveolar epithelial cell junctions (see Chapter 1) appears to provide an effective barrier to water entering the air spaces until either the epithelial cells are directly damaged or interstitial fluid pressures become excessive.[10] Since capillary endothelial cell junctions are normally permeable to water and small molecules[19] (see Chapter 2), it appears that prevention of interstitial water accumulation is the result of several phenomena in delicate balance: (1) the pulmonary vascular system is normally a low-pressure system; therefore, the *capillary hydrostatic pressure* forcing fluid from blood to interstitium is relatively small; (2) larger intravascular molecules are responsible for a counterforce *(colloid osmotic pressure)* tending to keep fluid within the vascular compartment and completely counterbalancing the hydrostatic pressure under normal conditions; and (3) the pulmonary *lymphatics* normally remove any excess water from the interstitial area.

Pulmonary edema may be broadly defined as the excessive movement of fluid from the vascular space to the interstitial and air spaces of the lung.[411] Numerous pathologic conditions may upset the normal delicate water balance and result in pulmonary edema. For the clinical purposes of this discussion, pulmonary edema will be divided into two major categories — cardiogenic and non-cardiogenic.

Cardiogenic Pulmonary Edema

Pathophysiology

Pulmonary edema as a consequence of increased pulmonary vascular hydrostatic pressure is most often related to left heart failure. Myocardial disease, either acute or chronic (Table 29–1), is the most commonly encountered cause of a negative inotropic state. In other words, inadequate myocardial contractility results in increased end-

431

TABLE 29-1.—CAUSES OF CARDIOGENIC
PULMONARY EDEMA

Acute myocardial infarction
Mitral valvular disease
Excessive fluid administration
Arrhythmias
Rheumatic heart disease (myocarditis)
Pulmonary embolus
Infection—sepsis
Anemia—severe
Thyrotoxicosis
Malnutrition—(beriberi)
Systemic hypertension
Renal failure

NOTE: Most often these physiologic insults are associated with a pre-existent degree of chronic congestive heart failure.

diastolic volumes, which result in increased left atrial pressure (see Chapter 26) and pulmonary vascular engorgement. When the patient is being monitored with a pulmonary artery catheter, elevated pulmonary wedge pressures will be measured.

The increased pulmonary blood volume and elevated hydrostatic pressure result in fluid movement into the interstitial compartment. This increased water content results in significant enlargement of the normally small interstitial space. This process is termed *interstitial pulmonary edema*. The lymphatics initially function to remove the excess fluid but eventually are overwhelmed by the ever-increasing extravasation. As pressures become even higher, the alveolar epithelial barrier is broken and fluid extravasates into the alveolar spaces, ducts, and respiratory bronchioles. This process is now termed *alveolar pulmonary edema*.

Clinical Presentation

In early pulmonary edema (interstitial edema), the main complaint generally is *dyspnea*. The patient tends to manifest tachypnea while maintaining reasonably normal tidal volumes; i.e., an increased minute ventilation is common. Blood pressure remains reasonably normal, with an associated mild tachycardia. Chest auscultatory findings are usually limited to basilar rales and a few expiratory wheezes. The wheezing associated with pulmonary vascular engorgement is referred to as *cardiac asthma*. Chest x-ray remains unremarkable except for evidence of lymphatic engorgement. Arterial blood gases reveal reasonably acceptable Pco_2 and pH values with mild to moderate reduction in Po_2.

A classic finding associated with pulmonary edema is called paroxysmal nocturnal dyspnea (PND). After lying supine for several hours, the patient will suddenly wake up with extreme respiratory distress and paroxysms of coughing and wheezing. Relief is obtained by sitting upright at the side of the bed. These episodes, though usually of short duration, may last for several hours, in which case the patient will also demonstrate diaphoresis and frothy secretions.

As interstitial edema progresses to a more severe stage (alveolar pulmonary edema), the patient becomes more severely stressed; dyspnea, shortness of breath, tachycardia, hypotension, and frequent coughing are present. The cough may produce a frothy blood-tinged sputum. Auscultatory chest findings now consist of bilateral "wet" rales, ronchi, and diffuse expiratory wheezes. The patient refuses to assume the supine position and is often diaphoretic, agitated, and manifests direct evidence of myocardial instability. Chest x-ray reveals vascular engorgement, diffuse haziness throughout the lung fields, and often a classic "butterfly" pattern. Arterial blood gases reveal a marked hypoxemia (even with aggressive oxygen therapy), a normal to slightly elevated P_{CO_2} with corresponding pH change and/or metabolic acidemia.

If untreated, the process may progress to a state of "massive" alveolar pulmonary edema involving all lung fields and associated with cardiac hypoxia, C.N.S. hypoxia, and eventually death. During this terminal phase the patient becomes obtunded or comatose and shows minimal evidence of adequate perfusion (e.g., cold, clammy extremities; absent urine output). If an endotracheal tube is placed, copious and continuous frothy, blood-tinged fluid emanates from the tube. Arterial blood gases will reveal severe hypercarbia, acidemia of both respiratory and metabolic origin, and marked hypoxemia even with maximal oxygen therapy.

Therapy

The symptomatology of cardiogenic pulmonary edema is readily relieved by decreasing pulmonary vascular hydrostatic pressure. Appropriate therapeutic intervention prior to cardiopulmonary collapse is usually dramatic. There are three primary goals of therapy: (1) decrease venous return; (2) increase ventricular inotropy; and (3) improve gas exchange. Although the physician and nurse are primarily involved with the first two regimens, it is essential for the respiratory care practitioner to comprehend the therapy so that he or she may appropriately participate in the over-all care. On the other hand, although the third area of therapy is primarily the involvement of the physician and respiratory therapist, it is essential for the nurse to understand the role and indications for such therapy.

Therapy to Decrease Venous Return

FOWLER'S POSITION (SITTING UP). — Pulmonary vascular intraluminal pressure increases approximately 2 mm Hg for each inch below the heart. Since the root of the pulmonary artery lies in the midportion of the chest, the patient in pulmonary edema accomplishes the following by sitting up: (1) minimizes areas of lung where excessive hydrostatic pressure exists; (2) decreases pulmonary blood volume by decreasing right heart venous return secondary to peripheral pooling; and (3) gains mechanical pulmonary advantages (increased vital capacity) for the work of breathing.

ROTATING TOURNIQUETS. — Placing venous tourniquets on three of four extremities impedes venous flow and promotes pooling of blood, thereby reducing the central or core blood volume. This reduction in vascular volume results in decreased right atrial pressure and, eventually, decreased venous return to the left heart (see Chapters 26 and 27). The tourniquets are rotated every 15 minutes so that no single extremity is continuously obstructed for more than 45 minutes.

MORPHINE SULFATE. — Appropriate administration of morphine sulfate (1 – 2 mg incrementally given intravenously) will accomplish considerable venodilatation and venous pooling. In addition, morphine is a euphoric, and the psychologic effects can reduce anxiety and thereby decrease the release of endogenous catecholamines. However, all of the exact modes by which morphine improves these patients is not clear.[207] Careful monitoring of respiratory function is essential so that the respiratory drive is not adversely affected.

DIURETICS. — Furosemide (Lasix) is rapid acting. Removal of salt and water via the kidneys results in decreased vascular volume. This drug also has an immediate direct vasodilating action.[412]

PHLEBOTOMY. — Removal of 250 – 500 ml of blood may be lifesaving in severe conditions.

Therapy to Increase Inotropy

Diminishing pulmonary vascular volume by decreasing venous return results in decreased ventricular filling. The decreased end-diastolic volume may allow improvement in contractility (see Chapter 26). If this does not occur, therapy aimed specifically at increasing myocardial inotropy may be instituted.

AMINOPHYLLINE. – This has been a popular mode of therapy for many years. The drug has beta-stimulating properties and when effective is believed to improve inotropy as well as vasodilate and bronchodilate. The popularity of this mode of therapy in pulmonary edema does not appear justified in the medical literature.[207, 411]

DOPAMINE/ISOPROTERENOL (ISUPREL). – This may be instituted in severe pulmonary edema that is not responsive to usual therapy.

DIGITALIS (CARDIAC GLYCOSIDES). – This is seldom used in acute pulmonary edema due to the potential problems associated with rapid digitalization.[413]

DECREASE AFTERLOAD. – Nitroprusside infusion is often attempted in very refractory cases or where systemic hypertension is present.[411]

Therapy to Improve Gas Exchange

OXYGEN THERAPY. – Since hypoxemia is present and is caused in large part by shunt effect ($\dot{V}/\dot{Q}$ inequality), the hypoxemia should be reasonably responsive to oxygen therapy. This is especially true with interstitial edema. Initial concentrations of 30–60% are recommended, preferably by high-flow system. Greater than 60% oxygen is usually not of benefit and, indeed, may result in a worsened state of oxygenation (see Chapter 7). The exception to this general statement is the patient with massive pulmonary edema and severe cardiopulmonary instability: 100% oxygen should be administered until the situation improves. Arterial blood gas measurements are required, and in severe cases measurement of pulmonary artery blood gases is extremely helpful. *Appropriate oxygen therapy is indicated in all pulmonary edema.*

IPPB THERAPY. – The use of this modality will result in some patients responding dramatically, whereas in others it causes further deterioration. This can best be explained by identifying the nature of the heart failure. For example, with isolated left heart failure, the left ventricle may be depending on the right ventricular output to maintain a higher preload. If IPPB therapy causes an acute decrease in systemic venous return, the result may be a catastrophic drop in left ventricular output. On the other hand, the patient with both right and left ventricular failure may experience a more moderate decrease in right and left ventricular filling with IPPB therapy. This may result in a beneficial reduction of biventricular preload.[153]

When IPPB therapy is administered, the patient must be carefully monitored and therapy discontinued if detrimental. If tolerated, there are some advantages: (1) work of breathing is transiently diminished; (2) deep tidal volumes may improve alveolar ventilation and oxygenation; and (3) many patients have decreased anxiety because they feel "something is being done" for them. IPPB *therapy* must not be confused with IPPV, whose indications and application have been discussed in Chapters 22 and 23.

INTUBATION. — This therapy is often indicated in severe cases and usually for the purpose of supporting the ventilation by positive-pressure means (IPPV). Often, the foaming and frothing may be so copious that ventilaton is hindered. We have found administration of *20 – 50%* *ethyl alcohol* by aerosol to be dramatic as a defoaming agent. The bubbles and froth disappear and ventilation and oxygenation improve. Do *not* assume that the pathologic process has improved! The alcohol aerosol is only a temporizing maneuver while more definitive therapy is being accomplished.

PEEP THERAPY. — With the patient intubated, application of 5 – 10 cm H_2O PEEP is often beneficial in improving oxygenation until the pathologic process is controlled.

Non-Cardiogenic Pulmonary Edema

These disease processes must be caused by (1) decreased colloid osmotic pressure; (2) altered capillary permeability; (3) altered lymphatic function; (4) damage to the alveolar epithelium; or (5) combinations of these factors.

Colloid Osmotic Pressure (COP)

Osmotic Pressure

A substance dissolved in a solution (a solute) contains a force that can potentially attract water molecules to itself. The magnitude of this force is directly related to the solute concentration and is referred to as *osmotic pressure*. The quantity of osmotically active particles in a solution is referred to as *osmolarity* and is expressed as milliosmoles per liter (mOsm/L). Substances such as sodium chloride (NaCl) dissociate in solution and form two osmotically active particles (Na^+ and Cl^-), whereas substances such as glucose ($C_6H_{12}O_6$) remain undissociated and account for only one active osmotic particle.

Normal serum osmolarity is 285 – 310 mOsm/L. Total osmotic pressure in blood would exceed 5,000 mm Hg if most of these particles could not freely move across membranes separating the fluid subcompartments of the body. The physiologically significant osmotic pres-

TABLE 29-2.—TRANSCAPILLARY
FLUID EXCHANGE

$$J = k(P_{cap} - P_{is}) - (\pi_{pl} - \pi_{is})$$

J = net fluid movement across capillary membrane
k = capillary permeability factor
P = hydrostatic pressure (capillary and interstitial)
π = oncotic pressure (plasma and interstitial)

sure that will determine water distribution among the subcompartments is related to particles that are *limited* to one of the compartments.

COP

Large solute particles cannot normally pass through capillary micropores with ease and thus would essentially be contained within the vascular compartment. Colloid particles such as albumin (approximately 90,000 molecular weight) and globulin (approximately 200,000 molecular weight) are particles present in significant quantities in blood. They do not pass freely through normal capillaries and, thereby, exert a colloid osmotic pressure that will hold water in the vascular compartment. This pressure is often referred to as *oncotic pressure*.

Normal COP (oncotic pressure) is 25–30 mm Hg and comprises approximately 1.6 mOsm/L. The relationship between intra- and extravascular oncotic and hydrostatic pressures was classically expressed by Starling (Table 29-2).[414] Simply stated, distribution of fluid between the intravascular and interstitial compartments will be greatly determined by the balance between oncotic and hydrostatic pressures within those compartments.

Decreased COP

This is seldom the sole cause of pulmonary edema but is probably a contributing factor more often than is realized. To be sure, chronic debilitating diseases result in decreased total body colloid. However, the most common clinical problem is a physiologic insult that affects the capillary permeability and allows abnormal movement of colloid to the interstitium. If the lymphatic system cannot adequately remove the interstitial colloid, the result will be movement of water into the interstitium. It should be noted that this response to physiologic stress is *not* an acute change in total body colloid, but rather an acute change in the *distribution* of colloid from blood to interstitium.[415, 416] Most *acute* decreases in COP are secondary to this type of phenomenon.

Altered Capillary Permeability

Many infectious and inflammatory processes are believed to alter the integrity of pulmonary endothelial cell micropores.[417] These appear to be more vulnerable than most other endothelial complexes. The factors affecting the pulmonary endothelial cells are an active area of research at present (see Chapter 30).

Altered Lymphatic Function

The pulmonary lymphatic system has been described in Chapter 1. Although little specific knowledge is available, it is obvious that alterations in lymphatic function have profound effects on fluid distribution in the lung.[411, 417]

Alveolar Epithelial Damage

Alveolar type I cells form a "watertight" pavement epithelium. Alveolar fluid tends to occur either when interstitial pressure is excessive (cardiogenic edema) or when the epithelium is damaged (lung burn, severe hypoxia, prolonged atelectasis). Little specific information is known concerning the factors that control or affect alveolar epithelial function (see Chapter 30).

Summary

Although well-established pulmonary edema is a reasonably easy clinical diagnosis, the differential between cardiogenic and non-cardiogenic origins is often difficult, especially in the critically ill patient. This is probably because factors causing cardiogenic and non-cardiogenic pulmonary edema often occur simultaneously.

One type of non-cardiogenic pulmonary edema is known as the adult respiratory distress syndrome (ARDS). The following chapter is devoted to discussion of this entity.

30 • THE ADULT RESPIRATORY DISTRESS SYNDROME (ARDS)

Defining ARDS

History

AN ORGAN SYSTEM'S response to physiologic stress is limited to several cellular and/or tissue reactions. For example, *inflammation* is a general type of tissue reaction to stress. Pulmonary inflammation may be caused by bacterial, viral, allergic, traumatic, or chemical stresses. Although there are variations in the inflammatory response, it remains a single type of tissue response to stresses of varying etiology.

The lung may react to stress by becoming "stiff," i.e., poorly compliant. This was first recognized as a common occurrence in World War II and was termed "shock lung." For the following twenty-five years, this type of lung response to stress was referred to by etiology. Table 30 – 1 lists some of the names under which this "stiff lung syndrome" was reported in the medical literature from 1940 to 1970.

This phenomenon was first described as a *syndrome* in 1967[418] and the name adult respiratory distress syndrome (ARDS) suggested. The most distinguishing factor in this description was the suggestion that an acutely decreased functional residual capacity (FRC) was present and common to all ARDS. The following four years saw numerous investigations and documentations of this "new lung syndrome." In 1971, the definitive publication describing and classifying the ARDS appeared.[419] Table 30 – 2 lists only some of the causes that have been described for the ARDS in the past ten years. It appears that almost any severe physiologic stress may result in ARDS.

Pathology

The lungs are "beefy" in appearance and do not readily collapse when removed from the chest cavity. Microscopically, there are three "typical" findings: (1) *Hyaline membranes* covering all alveolar epithelium and unassociated with significant bronchial pneumonia. (2) *Interstitial edema and fibrosis:* thickening of alveolar and intralobular septa, which occurs early and is most probably secondary to accumu-

TABLE 30-1.—CHRONOLOGIC ORDER
OF SOME NAMES APPEARING IN
MEDICAL LITERATURE
REFERRING TO ARDS

Oxygen toxicity
Oxygen pneumonitis
Respirator lung syndrome
Shock lung
Wet lung
Adult hyaline membrane disease
Congestive atelectasis
Hemorrhagic pulmonary edema
Non-cardiac pulmonary edema
Stiff lung syndrome
Post pump lung
Post-traumatic pulmonary insufficiency
Post-nontraumatic pulmonary insufficiency

TABLE 30-2.—CAUSES OF ARDS
COMMONLY FOUND IN RECENT
MEDICAL LITERATURE

Aspiration
Chemical-induced lung injury
Disseminated intravascular coagulation
Drug ingestion
Fat or air emboli
Interstitial viral pneumonitis
Massive blood transfusion
Near drowning
Non-thoracic trauma
Oxygen toxicity
Pancreatitis
Prolonged cardiopulmonary bypass
Radiation-induced lung injury
Sepsis
"Shock"
Thoracic trauma
Uremia

lation of interstitial fluid. This early *exudative phase* progresses to a *proliferative phase* in which fibroblastic proliferation occurs.[420] This later-occurring fibrotic process is believed to be the only irreversible portion of the ARDS.[421] (3) *Pneumocyte hyperplasia* seen on appropriately stained light microscopic preparations as well as with the electron microscope. The hyperplasia is primarily type II cell proliferation and swelling, although type I cells are abnormal.

Electron microscopic findings in ARDS include (1) interstitial edema; (2) proliferation of type I and II cells, with evidence of both nuclear and cytoplasmic abnormalities; and (3) abnormality of cytoplasmic organelles of endothelial cells.[422]

Clinical Pathophysiology

The vast majority of pulmonary abnormalities leading to acute respiratory failure are acute restrictive diseases,[347] i.e., an acute decrease in total lung capacity, vital capacity, and functional residual capacity (see Chapter 20). All available evidence appears to support the statement that the ARDS involves an acute decrease in FRC similar to the third type of acute restrictive disease outlined in Figure 20–1. ARDS appears to involve a greater decrease in FRC than vital capacity, leading to the interpretation that significant loss of residual volume must be involved.[303, 356, 357, 359, 423] Measurement of FRC in critically ill patients is difficult at present and must still be considered a clinical research endeavor.[300, 347] However, application of mass spectrometry at the bedside promises to provide routine serial measurement of FRC in the future.

The first clinical pathophysiologic hallmark of ARDS is the presence of *refractory hypoxemia* (a moderate to severe arterial hypoxemia that is poorly responsive to increased concentrations of inspired oxygen). *Any hypoxemia that dramatically responds to oxygen therapy is probably not the result of ARDS.* This is *not* to intimate that all refractory hypoxemia is ARDS. To the contrary, other causes of refractory hypoxemia must be ruled out (e.g., anatomic shunt, lobar or segmental atelectasis, consolidating pneumonia) prior to diagnosing the existence of ARDS.

The second clinical pathophysiologic hallmark of ARDS is a dramatically *decreased lung compliance.* In a spontaneously breathing patient, this is manifested as a significant increase in the work of breathing required to accomplish a normal minute ventilation; in a patient receiving IPPV, the presence of high inflation pressures or decreased effective static compliance is noted.

Although increased deadspace ventilation is present, *the most clinically significant physiologic abnormalities in ARDS are refractory hypoxemia and decreased lung compliance.*

Radiologic Findings

The chest x-ray typically reveals diffuse alveolar infiltrates in a honeycomb pattern similar to that seen in alveolar proteinosis. The x-ray findings are often quite typical, but unfortunately lag behind the pathophysiologic process by approximately 24 hours. In addition, a significant percentage of patients will not show classic patterns but, rather,

mimic the picture of cardiogenic pulmonary edema or a diffuse pneu-
monitic process. Often, viral and other interstitial pneumonias will
look similar to ARDS. Thus, the chest x-ray should be considered con-
firmatory evidence for the diagnosis of ARDS, but cannot be counted
upon as an independent diagnostic tool.

Clinical Presentation

In the spontaneously breathing patient without obvious acute cardiopulmonary disease (e.g., heart failure, pneumonia, atelectasis),
*respiratory distress that appears disproportionate to the blood gas
and radiologic abnormalities* is the most common early presentation
of ARDS.

It must be remembered that ARDS has a smaller infringement on
vital capacity than most other acute restrictive pulmonary diseases
and, therefore, ventilatory reserves remain surprisingly intact. Thus,
patients maintain a "reasonably stable" clinical status in spite of the
increased work of breathing for a significant period of time. In addition, these patients most often have normal or below normal arterial
Pco_2's in response to the hypoxemia and seldom manifest cyanosis
prior to cardiopulmonary collapse. In other words, the presence of
cyanosis is an extremely late and in extremis event for ARDS.

In the patient being closely monitored in intensive care, ARDS
most commonly presents as decreasing arterial Po_2's that are poorly
responsive to increases in inspired oxygen concentration despite a
clinical absence of obvious cardiopulmonary malfunction.

Clinical Diagnosis

The clinical diagnosis of ARDS is often difficult, especially in the
patient with pre-existing cardiopulmonary disease. The clinician must
consider ARDS a response of the lung to significant physiologic stress,
and therefore any patient who has been subjected to significant physiologic stress is a potential candidate.

The syndrome occurs in all degrees of severity from very mild to
overwhelming. Lesser degrees of ARDS may be of clinical significance in patients with limited cardiopulmonary, hepatorenal, or
C.N.S. reserves. Symptomatology and threat to life are as much related
to cardiopulmonary reserves as to pathologic severity. The clinical
index of suspicion for ARDS must be higher in patients with limited
reserves.

Making an *early* diagnosis is important because *the process is totally reversible in almost all patients in whom appropriate therapy is
applied early in the disease.*[424-426] All patients who have undergone

significant physiologic stress and then manifest refractory hypoxemia in conjunction with an increased work of breathing must be evaluated for ARDS.

Infant Respiratory Distress Syndrome

Much activity in the field of neonatology was devoted to the problem of the infant respiratory distress syndrome (IRDS) in the 1950s and 1960s. This disease, known as "hyaline membrane disease of the newborn," was responsible for a very high mortality (80%) in premature babies. Pathologically and clinically there is little difference between the respiratory distress syndrome of the infant and the adult; in fact, the name *adult* respiratory distress syndrome was coined because of its profound similarity to the *infant* respiratory distress syndrome. The cause of IRDS is most likely "immature" alveolar type II cells rather than "stressed" alveolar type II cells.[427] In spite of similarities, the respiratory care practitioner must *not* consider the discussion of ARDS in this text as generally applicable to the neonate.

ARDS — a Metabolic Malfunction of Lung

The adult respiratory distress syndrome (ARDS) is a confusing subject in the medical literature. Although much of this confusion is due to the short time span that the "syndrome" has been studied (about fifteen years), we believe a significant degree of confusion is secondary to the failure to consider the syndrome as *an intrinsic metabolic malfunction of lung parenchyma.* Prior to 1950 little attention was paid to the existence of intrinsic pulmonary metabolism. The electron microscope has revealed the lung to be a significant metabolic organ. Perhaps the greatest challenge to pulmonary clinicians at present is to apply this recent realization of metabolic lung function to clinical practice. Without question, it is no longer acceptable to consider the lung a "passive" organ.

Parenchymal Metabolic Function

Epithelial Function

Type I alveolar epithelial cells provide 95% of the surface area for gas exchange, but the type II cell is the most numerous.[8] The cytoplasmic junctions between alveolar type I cells are either touching or overlapping; i.e., there are no "micropores," as exist with endothelial cells. Thus, the epithelium normally provides a "watertight" surface.[10] The same appears to be true for the cytoplasmic junctions between alveolar type I and alveolar type II cells; however, there remains some controversy concerning this matter.[9, 10] The type I cells appear to be "oxygen sensitive" in that hypoxia results in cytoplasmic changes that affect cellular junctions and allow interstitial fluid to enter the air spaces.

The normal fluid layer covering the epithelium is produced in type II cells and is secreted via microvilli that extend onto the alveolar surface.[11] This fluid differs from plasma in both electrolyte and protein content. Production and secretion of *surfactant* also take place within the alveolar type II cells (see Chapter 1). It is logical to assume that malfunction of these cells would lead to two phenomena: (1) an aberrance from the normal content of the alveolar fluid lining, and (2) a change in either the quantity or quality of pulmonary surfactant.[429]

The mechanisms responsible for removing the fluid layer from the alveolar surface are not known. One suggestion is that the fluid flows toward the terminal bronchioles and becomes part of the mucous blanket as a result of normal expansion and contraction of the alveoli.[428] Although this is an attractive theory, there are no supportive data at present. Another theory is that the macrophages remove all or part of the fluid—again an attractive theory with little documentation. It can be safely stated that the *fluid lining and its contents are constantly produced and removed from the alveolar surface*. The mechanisms responsible for removal are unknown at present.

Like all metabolically active cells, the alveolar type II cells appear to be easily damaged when severely physiologically stressed.[12] A basic physiologic protective mechanism for prevention of such malfunction is the provision of increased blood and oxygen supply during periods of physiologic stress.[430] In other words, a general body response to stress is to increase the nutrient supply to meet the increased metabolic demand placed on cells and tissues. The alveolar type II cells appear extraordinarily vulnerable, since they are *not* supplied by systemic arterial blood (see Chapter 1).

It must be assumed that oxygenation of alveolar epithelial cells occurs by diffusion of alveolar oxygen or from interstitial fluid when alveolar oxygen is not present. In addition, type II cell *hyperoxia* would result from *alveolar hyperoxia* and not from systemic arterial hyperoxemia.

The profound metabolic activity of type II cells is unquestioned,[9, 12] although specific functions and mechanisms are largely unknown. A generally accepted pathologic observation is that when type II cells are abnormal, aberrant interstitial and endothelial cell function is almost always present.[431] By contrast, pulmonary endothelial cell malfunction commonly occurs independent of type II cell abnormality. This raises the question: Does the type II cell have functions that are essential to the proper functioning of pulmonary endothelial cells? Some indirect evidence has been found that pulmonary sodium ion concentration may be monitored and altered by type II cell mechanisms.[432] At present it appears reasonable to ask: Are normal alveolar type II cell functions required for normal interstitial and endothelial function? Future research will produce definitive answers.

Lymphatic Function

The ultrastructure of the pulmonary interstitial space has been described (see Chapter 1). A constant flow of fluid and electrolytes normally exits from pulmonary blood to interstitium. Likewise, a constant removal by the lymphatics of these substances (along with protein) normally occurs. Since interstitial pressures are less than right atrial pressure, the lymphatic flow must be due to active mechanisms.[13] Although the lymphatic ducts have peristaltic capabilities,[14] the mechanisms by which substances are transported to the ostia of the lymphatic ducts are completely unknown. Reasonable theories include the autonomic nervous system,[14] smooth muscle contractions,[15] and cyclic lung movement.[16] Regardless of specifics, a combination of complex lymphatic mechanisms removes sodium, chloride, proteins, and water from the interstitial space.[17] Thus, the net result of sodium and protein content within the interstitium is at least partly dependent upon lymphatic function.

Generalized failure of lymphatics is seen as *anasarca*, interstitial edema of the entire body that is believed secondary to both endothelial and lymphatic malfunction. However, most non-cardiogenic pulmonary edema occurs *independently* of systemic interstitial edema.[17] *Perhaps* this results from failure of mechanisms responsible for transporting fluid, electrolytes, and proteins to the lymphatic duct ostia rather than from failure of the lymphatics proper. Are such mechanisms influenced by alveolar type II cells? The answers are not known.

Endothelial Function

The metabolic function of pulmonary and systemic endothelial cells has been discussed (see Chapter 1). Pulmonary endothelium is more "porous" than most other organ systems except the kidney and liver.[19] The exact mechanisms involved in determining pulmonary endothelial micropore size and function are not known. Since some endothelial cell functions have been demonstrated to be sodium dependent,[8, 9] perhaps similar mechanisms control cytoplasmic function in terms of pulmonary capillary micropores.

Micropore malfunction (endothelial cell abnormality) occurs in numerous disease states in which type II cells appear normal; however, almost always when type II cells are abnormal, endothelial micropore function is found to be abnormal.[431]

A Clinical Concept of ARDS

The authors' present clinical concept of ARDS (Table 30–3) is based on available information and on the applicability of the schema to clinical practice. By no means should this concept be considered complete or unchangeable. To the contrary, it is presented as an incomplete schema that has undergone, and will continue to undergo, significant change as new information and further experience are gained.

Alveolar type II cells are exceptionally vulnerable to physiologic stress. When significantly stressed or damaged, they attempt to meet

TABLE 30–3.—PROPOSED COMMON PATHWAY OF ARDS

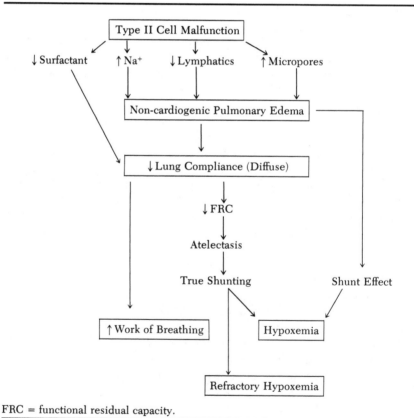

FRC = functional residual capacity.

metabolic demands by proliferation and hypertrophy, inevitably re-sulting in metabolic malfunction. Such malfunction leads to (1) de-creased production or abnormal production of pulmonary surfactant; (2) interstitial sodium (and water) retention; (3) suboptimal interstitial lymphatic function; and (4) endothelial cytoplasmic abnormality, causing micropore enlargement. These factors lead to a diffuse and relatively homogeneous lung abnormality with (1) *decreased lung compliance*, primarily due to surfactant deficiency and secondarily to the interstitial edema; and (2) *non-cardiogenic pulmonary edema*, primarily due to "leaky" capillaries, allowing increased colloid to en-ter the interstitium, and secondarily due to increased sodium reten-tion in the interstitium (a non-diuresible edema secondary to deficient "sodium pump" function of the type II cells)—and both of these com-pounded by a decreased lymphatic function.

The diffuse decrease in lung compliance results in a significantly decreased FRC. Due primarily to the surfactant abnormality, the gravity-dependent alveoli will begin to collapse, resulting in atelec-tatic lung that is relatively well perfused. As this process continues, it results in a *refractory hypoxemia*. The continuing decrease in com-pliance requires greater muscular energy to inflate the lung and there-fore increase the work of breathing. Based on this general schema (Fig 30–1), a rational discussion of the clinical management of oxy-genation supportive care is possible.

Principles of Oxygenation Support in ARDS

ARDS represents a serious oxygenation threat to all tissues. Its management must be aimed at supporting tissue oxygenation through optimization of cardiopulmonary function. In the 1950s and 1960s, such therapy consisted of high inspired oxygen concentrations to sup-port the hypoxemia and of positive-pressure ventilation to support the work of breathing. The results of this therapy were dismal, the patient almost always dying from overwhelming lung pathology.

Alveolar Oxygen Tension

The biochemical sequelae of alveolar epithelial cell hyperoxia have been discussed in Chapter 7. When normal alveolar epithelium is exposed to oxygen tensions greater than 350–400 mm Hg, cellular dysfunction becomes apparent in several days.[433-435] In fact, 100% oxy-gen delivered to normal lungs over several days will directly result in epithelial cell damage.[101, 102, 436] In addition, previously malfunction-ing type II cells may undergo rapid degeneration when exposed to alveolar oxygen tensions as low as 250 mm Hg.[93] Since inspired oxygen concentrations of 40% at sea level will result in alveolar oxygen tensions of about 250 mm Hg, it would appear that an F_{IO_2} of greater than 40% would be potentially detrimental in ARDS.

Superficially it may appear a paradox to discuss minimizing F_{IO_2} in a patient with severe hypoxemia. Remember, these patients have *refractory* hypoxemia and will have essentially the same arterial oxygenation with 50% inspired oxygen as with 100% inspired oxygen. Also, a pulmonary death is virtually guaranteed if high inspired oxygen concentrations are continued.

Positive-Pressure Ventilation

Appropriately administered positive-pressure ventilation to normal lungs may be maintained for prolonged periods without pulmonary damage. However, excessively high pressures within the lung are believed detrimental to type II cells.[436] Thus, positive-pressure ventila-

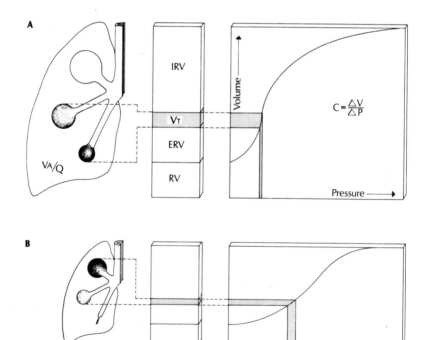

Fig 30–1.—**A** represents the normal relationships between lung volumes, compliance, and V̇A/Q̇. **B** represents the changes that occur in ARDS (see text). *IRV* = inspiratory reserve volume; *V̇T* = tidal volume; *ERV* = expiratory reserve volume; *RV* = residual volume.

tion would be anticipated to be detrimental in ARDS, since the poor compliance usually requires excessive pressures to accomplish ventilation.

A spontaneously breathing patient receiving 40% oxygen or less would not be expected to develop ARDS from the oxygen therapy; a patient on appropriate positive-pressure ventilation receiving less than 40% oxygen would not be expected to develop ARDS from the ventilator; however, a patient on PPV receiving 100% oxygen *would* be expected to develop ARDS within several days![437, 438] This is probably why the therapy of the 1950s and 1960s (PPV + 100% oxygen) was so uniformly unsuccessful.

PEEP Therapy

No single therapeutic intervention is more essential in ARDS than the appropriate application of PEEP therapy.[439] ARDS can be conceived of as an acute restrictive disease in which FRC is greatly diminished owing to a relatively *uniform* metabolic malfunction throughout the lung; therefore, the pathology matches almost perfectly the theoretic principles on which the application of PEEP therapy was discussed in Chapter 24.

In general, ARDS is a relatively homogeneous acute restrictive disease that is exquisitely amenable to reversibility toward more physiologic circumstances with appropriate application of PEEP therapy. Two crucial pathophysiologic processes are apparently reversed with appropriate PEEP therapy: (1) The decreased FRC is increased toward a more favorable position on the lung compliance curve (see Fig 30–1). This results in a decreased work of breathing for the patient or lower inflation pressures on the ventilator. (2) The expansion of FRC favoring those areas of lung previously collapsed (see Chapter 24) will result in a significant reversal of true intrapulmonary shunting. Therefore, the refractory hypoxemia will become responsive to oxygen therapy, which will allow appropriate arterial oxygen levels to be achieved with relatively low inspired oxygen concentrations.

From a pulmonary viewpoint, the application of PEEP therapy is absolutely appropriate and indicated in ARDS; however, we must always consider the *potential* deleterious effects on cardiovascular function. It is clear that any increase in airway pressure may cause some degree of increase in intrapleural pressures. As discussed in Chapters 24 and 27, the degree of transmission of increased airway pressures is dependent upon the severity of the decreased lung compliance. In other words, the less compliant the lung, the less the portion of increased airway pressure that will be transmitted to the pleural space. Thus, the more severe the ARDS, the greater should be the cardiovascular tolerance for high levels of PEEP.

However, PEEP therapy cannot be increased indiscriminately. Once a reasonable effect has been accomplished (i.e., FRC and lung compliance significantly restored toward normal), a greater portion of any additional PEEP will be transmitted to the pleural space. This brings to the fore the questions: How much PEEP is clinically adequate? How does one appropriately monitor PEEP therapy?

Monitoring PEEP Therapy

The effects of PEEP therapy on intrapulmonary shunt, compliance, arterial oxygen tension, and cardiac output in the ARDS have been voluminously studied.[356-360, 363, 380, 381, 410-442] Figure 30–2 combines this information into a schema that assumes that the starting point is severe ARDS. As increasing levels of PEEP are applied: (1) at some point arterial P_{O_2} will begin to improve and continue to do so if $F_{I_{O_2}}$ is kept constant; (2) intrapulmonary shunting ($\dot{Q}s/\dot{Q}T$) will decrease; and (3) effective static compliance (ESC) (see Chapter 24) will improve.

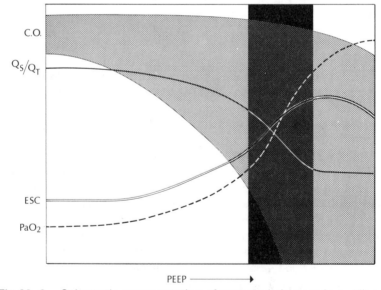

Fig 30–2.—Schematic representation of expected changes in cardiac output *(C.O.)*, intrapulmonary shunting *($\dot{Q}s/\dot{Q}T$)*, effective static compliance *(ESC)*, and arterial P_{O_2} *(Pa_{O_2})* as PEEP is increased. The schema assumes that the starting point represents severe ARDS (see text). *PEEP* = positive end-expiratory pressure. The black area represents the PEEP level of greatest physiologic advantage, assuming cardiac output remains adequate.

However, if PEEP is increased too far, the compliance will begin to decrease.

Note that the significant improvement in arterial P_{O_2}, intrapulmonary shunting, and compliance tends to occur in the same PEEP range. This appears reasonable, since it may be assumed that reversal of the underlying pathophysiology (decreased FRC) is responsible for all these changes.

The effects of any PEEP level on cardiac output are believed dependent upon the cardiac reserves, availability of adequate intravascular volume, and lung compliance. Patients with a healthy heart will show minimal cardiovascular effects with increasing PEEP levels so long as fluid therapy is adequate. *Increasing PEEP levels in patients with limited cardiac reserves may manifest decreased cardiac output prior to or coinciding with significant increases in arterial P_{O_2}.*

The Three Clinical Goals of PEEP Therapy

1. *To assure tissue oxygenation.* — This demands maintaining an adequate cardiac output. *Any increase in arterial oxygen content accomplished at the expense of cardiac output is potentially detrimental to the organism.*

2. *To accomplish adequate arterial oxygenation at $F_{I_{O_2}}$'s not detrimental to the lung.* — Arterial P_{O_2}'s above 60 mm Hg represent more than 90% oxyhemoglobin saturation. With adequate hemoglobin content, this level assures adequate arterial oxygenation. When this can be accomplished at 40% or less inspired oxygen concentration, the oxygen therapy should not be detrimental to lung "healing."

3. *To optimize lung compliance.* — This will allow spontaneous ventilation (CPAP or IMV/IDV) with minimal work of breathing. If PPV (augmented or control) is necessary, lung pressures will be minimized.

Theoretically all three goals are simultaneously accomplished by reestablishing a near normal FRC and maintaining a proper vascular volume-to-vascular space relationship.

PEEP Therapy Without Pulmonary Artery Catheter

Two preconditions must be met: (1) the diagnosis of ARDS must be reasonably certain, and (2) the cardiovascular system must be clinically judged stable and capable of meeting the metabolic demands of the untreated disease state without threat of decompensation.

The following case studies are presented to clarify general principles of acute respiratory care. They are not complete presentations, nor are they to be interpreted to comprise the entire care required by these patients.

Case Study—CPAP

A 25-year-old previously healthy man was hospitalized for a severe viral pneumonitis and remained stable with oxygen therapy (FI_{O_2} 0.40). On his third hospital day he became increasingly dyspneic, tachypneic, and revealed a refractory hypoxemia to 100% oxygen. His chest x-ray interpretation changed from "resolving interstitial pneumonitis" to a "typical ARDS pattern." Upon transfer to ICU he was noted to be very short of breath, using all accessory muscles and unable to speak more than three words at a time.

*BP	140/100	pH	7.46
P	130	P_{CO_2}	29
RR	40 and regular	P_{O_2}	41
VT	600	FI_{O_2}	0.60
MV	24		

After a careful explanation of the proposed therapy, the patient's nose was appropriately anesthetized and he was intubated via the nasotracheal route. He was placed on a CPAP system with 5 cm H_2O PEEP and 60% inspired oxygen; 15 minutes following intubation:

*BP	140/100	pH	7.44
P	120	P_{CO_2}	31
RR	36	P_{O_2}	45
VT	600	FI_{O_2}	0.60
MV	21.6		

PEEP was increased to 10 cm H_2O; 5 minutes later:

*BP	140/100	pH	7.44
P	120	P_{CO_2}	30
RR	36	P_{O_2}	43
VT	600	FI_{O_2}	0.60
MV	21.6		

PEEP was increased to 15 cm H_2O; 10 minutes later:

*BP	125/90	pH	7.42
P	110	P_{CO_2}	32
R	28	P_{O_2}	58
VT	500	FI_{O_2}	0.60
MV	14		

The patient was observed another 10 minutes during which vital

---

*BP = mm Hg, P = per minute, RR = per minute; VT = ml; MV = L/min; P_{CO_2} = mm Hg, P_{O_2} = mm Hg.

signs, clinical condition, and blood gases remained unchanged. PEEP was then increased to 20 cm H_2O; 10 minutes later:

*BP	125/85	pH	7.37
P	110	Pco_2	35
RR	22	Po_2	110
VT	500	FIo_2	0.60
MV	11		

The patient's breathing was significantly less labored, and he communicated that he felt very much improved; 15 minutes later on 20 cm H_2O PEEP:

*BP	120/75	pH	7.35
P	100	PCO_2	38
RR	22	Po_2	180
VT	450	FIo_2	0.60
MV	9.9		

The FIo_2 was decreased to 0.50; 10 minutes later vital signs were unchanged:

*pH	7.36
PCO_2	38
Po_2	110
FIo_2	0.50

The FIo_2 was decreased to 0.40. Twenty minutes later vital signs were unchanged:

pH	7.36
PCO_2	37
Po_2	73
FIo_2	0.40

Note that within 2 hours of initiation of PEEP therapy the clinical goals were reached, namely:

1. Circulatory and perfusion status remained adequate and stable.
2. Adequate arterial oxygenation at FIo_2 0.40.
3. Work of breathing significantly diminished, patient comfortable and breathing without significant effort.

A total of 350 ml of crystalloid solution was administered intravenously during the 2-hour period.

Case Study—CPPV

A 34-year-old woman was getting out of her parked car when she was hit by a passing auto and suffered multiple fractures of both legs

---

*BP = mm Hg, P = per minute; RR = per minute; VT = ml; MV = L/min; PCO_2 = mm Hg; Po_2 = mm Hg.

and pelvis. She was placed in traction and received three units of blood. For 36 hours she was stable and then suddenly complained of severe shortness of breath. She was noted to be tachypneic, tachycardiac, mildly hypotensive, and intermittently obtunded and agitated. The urine was positive for fat content. Respirations were labored. Urine output was adequate and extremities were warm and dry.

*BP	100/60	pH	7.41
P	110	PCO_2	33
RR	36	PO_2	35
VT	300	FIO_2	0.60
MV	10.8		

100% inspired oxygen increased the arterial PO_2 to 42 mm Hg.

The patient was intubated following ventilation by bag and mask and sedation. Spontaneous respiratory efforts were minimal and she was placed on a volume ventilator with 5 cm H_2O PEEP and given 300 ml I.V. fluid.

**BP	100/60	ETV	900	pH	7.43
P	120	Rate	8	PCO_2	32
RR	0	MV	7.2	PO_2	38
VT	0	Pei	40	FIO_2	0.60
MV	0	PEEP	5		
		ESC	26		

PEEP was increased to 10 cm H_2O and 100 ml I.V. fluid administered; 15 minutes later:

**BP	110/70	ETV	900	pH	7.42
P	120	Rate	8	PCO_2	33
RR	0	MV	7.2	PO_2	41
VT	0	Pei	45	FIO_2	0.60
MV	0	PEEP	10		
		ESC	26		

PEEP was increased to 15 cm H_2O; 10 minutes later:

**BP	110/70	ETV	900	pH	7.42
P	120	Rate	8	PCO_2	33
RR	20	MV	7.2	PO_2	55
VT	100	Pei	45	FIO_2	0.60
MV	2	PEEP	15		
		ESC	30		

Note that spontaneous respirations have returned. Likewise ESC

**BP = mm Hg; P = per minute; RR = per minute; VT = ml; MV = L/min; ETV = ml; Pei = cm H_2O; PEEP = cm H_2O; ESC = ml/cm H_2O; PCO_2 = mm Hg; PO_2 = mm Hg.

and PO_2 have somewhat improved; 100 ml I.V. fluid was administered in past 25 minutes; 15 minutes after last measurements:

**BP	110/70	ETV	900	pH	7.46
P	110	Rate	8	PCO_2	29
RR	20	MV	7.2	PO_2	90
VT	150	Pei	40	FIO_2	0.60
MV	3	PEEP	15		
		ESC	36		

Ventilator rate was decreased to 4 per minute; 10 minutes later:

**BP	120/80	ETV	900	pH	7.42
P	110	Rate	4	PCO_2	33
RR	18	MV	3.6	PO_2	110
VT	250	Pei	40	FIO_2	0.60
MV	4.5	PEEP	15		
		ESC	36		

Spontaneous respirations were without apparent distress. FIO_2 was decreased to 0.50; 15 minutes later:

**BP	120/80	ETV	900	pH	7.42
P	110	Rate	4	PCO_2	33
RR	18	MV	3.6	PO_2	64
VT	250	Pei	40	FIO_2	0.50
MV	4.5	PEEP	15		
		ESC	36		

Urine output was 60 ml in past hour; 150 ml I.V. fluid administered. PEEP increased to 20 cm H_2O; 15 minutes later:

**BP	120/80	ETV	900	pH	7.40
P	110	Rate	4	PCO_2	35
RR	18	MV	3.6	PO_2	95
VT	250	Pei	45	FIO_2	0.50
MV	4.5	PEEP	20		
		ESC	36		

FIO_2 was decreased to 0.40; 10 minutes later:

**BP	120/80	ETV	900	pH	7.41
P	110	Rate	4	PCO_2	34
RR	18	MV	3.6	PO_2	68
VT	250	Pei	45	FIO_2	0.40
MV	4.5	PEEP	20		
		ESC	36		

**BP = mm Hg; P = per minute; RR = per minute; VT = ml; MV = L/min; ETV = ml; Pei = cm H_2O; PEEP = cm H_2O; ESC = ml/cm H_2O; PCO_2 = mm Hg; PO_2 = mm Hg.

Note that within 2 hours of initiation of PEEP therapy, the clinical goals were reached:

1. Circulation and perfusion status adequate and stable.
2. Adequate arterial oxygenation at FIO_2 0.40.
3. Positive-pressure ventilation minimized.

PEEP Therapy with Pulmonary Artery Catheter

Case Study—IMV and PEEP

A 62-year-old man sustained severe upper gastrointestinal bleeding for 36 hours with significant periods of hypotension. He was taken to the operating room where a gastric ulcer was found and the appropriate surgical procedure accomplished. For 24 hours postoperatively he was on IMV of 4 per minute. A typical ARDS developed on the first postoperative day, and prior to PEEP therapy a Swan-Ganz catheter and arterial catheter were placed. The patient was warm and dry with adequate urine output.

***MAP	60	ETV	1100	pH	7.44	A-V$_{O_2}$	3.3
P	120	Rate	4	PCO_2	30	PWP	15
RR	45	MV	4.4	PO_2	40	C.O.	5.0
VT	150	Pei	55	FIO_2	0.70	Q̇s/Q̇T	42
MV	6.75	PEEP	0	P̄v$_{O_2}$	30		
		ESC	20				

PEEP of 5 cm H_2O produced no change over 15 minutes and PEEP was increased to 10 cm H_2O; 10 minutes later:

***MAP	50	ETV	1100	pH	7.40	A-V$_{O_2}$	4.3
P	130	Rate	4	PCO_2	34	PWP	13
RR	45	MV	4.4	PO_2	48	C.O.	4.4
VT	150	Pei	63	FIO_2	0.70	Q̇s/Q̇T	43
MV	6.75	PEEP	10	P̄v$_{O_2}$	31		
		ESC	21				

Note that PEEP has resulted in decreased cardiac output (increased A-V$_{O_2}$ difference) and slight decrease in PWP. A fluid challenge was carried out (see Chapter 27) with 200 ml of crystalloid administered over 10 minutes and then repeated over the following 10 minutes; 15 minutes later:

***MAP (mean arterial pressure) = mm Hg; P = per minute; RR = per minute; VT = ml; MV = L/min; ETV = ml; Pei = cm H_2O; PEEP = cm H_2O; ESC = ml/cm H_2O; PCO_2 = mm Hg; PO_2 = mm Hg; P̄v$_{O_2}$ = mm Hg; A-V$_{O_2}$ = vol%; PWP = mm Hg; C.O. = L/min; Q̇s/Q̇T = %.

***MAP	70	ETV	1100	pH	7.42	A-V$_{O_2}$	3.1
P	110	Rate	4	P$_{CO_2}$	31	PWP	19
RR	40	MV	4.4	P$_{O_2}$	65	C.O.	6.1
V$_T$	200	Pei	58	F$_{I_{O_2}}$	0.70	$\dot{Q}s/\dot{Q}T$	35
MV	8	PEEP	10	P$\bar{v}_{O_2}$	35		
		ESC	23				

PEEP was increased to 15 cm H$_2$O, and another 100 ml I.V. fluid administered; 15 minutes later:

***MAP	75	ETV	1100	pH	7.42	A-V$_{O_2}$	3.4
P	105	Rate	4	P$_{CO_2}$	33	PWP	20
RR	30	MV	4.4	P$_{O_2}$	165	C.O.	6.2
V$_T$	250	Pei	51	F$_{I_{O_2}}$	0.70	$\dot{Q}s/\dot{Q}T$	26
MV	7.5	PEEP	15	P$\bar{v}_{O_2}$	44		
		ESC	31				

F$_{I_{O_2}}$ was incrementally decreased to 0.40, with a resultant Pa$_{O_2}$ of 65 mm Hg.

Summary of Oxygenation Support

The support of oxygenation in ARDS primarily involves the application of PEEP therapy. Of course, appropriate cardiovascular support is essential, and positive-pressure ventilation should be applied to the minimal degree necessary for homeostasis. There are numerous methods for approaching such clinical care, and ours is suggested only as a guideline. However, whatever the methodology, the principles and rationale presented in this chapter must apply. In our experience (1) most patients with ARDS who do not have concomitant C.N.S. disease do best with either IMV or CPAP; (2) over 90% of ARDS patients adequately respond to between 10 and 30 cm of PEEP; (3) the survival rate is dismal for patients requiring above 30 cm H$_2$O PEEP; and (4) less than 10 cm H$_2$O PEEP seldom produces significant responses in adults.

Prophylactic Antibiotics in ARDS

Significant threats to the survival of the ARDS patient are pulmonary infection and generalized sepsis. Many ARDS patients are excel-

---

***MAP (mean arterial pressure) = mm Hg; P = per minute; RR = per minute; V$_T$ = ml; MV = L/min; ETV = ml; Pei = cm H$_2$O; PEEP = cm H$_2$O; ESC = ml/cm H$_2$O; P$_{CO_2}$ = mm Hg; P$_{O_2}$ = mm Hg; P$\bar{v}_{O_2}$ = mm Hg; A-V$_{O_2}$ = vol%; PWP = mm Hg; C.O. = L/min; $\dot{Q}s/\dot{Q}T$ = %.

lent hosts for bacterial superinfection because of their diminished immunologic status and the numerous iatrogenic pathways for bacterial contamination. In addition to possible contamination of urine, intravenous, arterial, and central venous catheters, the placement of an intratracheal tube and respiratory apparatus leads to certain contamination of the tracheobronchial tree.

Although careful and constant evaluation must be maintained for pulmonary bacterial superinfection, there is *no* indication for giving prophylactic antibiotics. No convincing evidence exists that prophylactic antibiotics decrease the incidence of pulmonary bacterial superinfection in these patients, but it appears that they most probably increase the incidence of *gram-negative* superinfection.[496, 503]

Steroid Therapy in ARDS

Appropriate administration of steroid compounds may be of benefit in reversing ARDS of certain etiologies.[443] It has been postulated that there is a decrease in the tendency for white blood cells to adhere to the pulmonary-capillary walls following hemorrhagic shock when the patient is preloaded with methylprednisolone sodium succinate (Solu-Medrol).[444] Also, steroid therapy may enhance surfactant production by stabilizing the cell wall membranes of alveolar type II cells. There has also been reasonable clinical evidence (especially in fat embolization) to show that steroid therapy does play a role in interfering with the pathophysiologic process of ARDS.[445] Obviously, the numerous causes of ARDS explain differences in the clinical disease process, and this may well account for the variability of reaction to various steroid regimens.

Steroid therapy in large doses for short periods of time is well accepted in critical care medicine and immunology. There is little evidence that large doses of steroid compounds administered over short periods ("pulse" doses of less than 48 hours) are significant in depressing the body defense mechanisms or producing electrolyte imbalance. The "classic" side effects of steroid therapy are based on long-term administration rather than on short-term pulse doses.

The use of steroid therapy in ARDS is controversial. We believe it is reasonable to consider early intervention with large doses of methylprednisolone sodium succinate (15 mg/kg, 4–6 times a day) for a period of 24 to 72 hours. Although convincing documentation is still lacking concerning the clinical value of this course, there seems to be reasonable evidence that it may, in fact, play a role without significant harm to the patient.

Diuretic Therapy in ARDS

The increased interstitial water of ARDS is not significantly diminished by diuresis.[411] However, many patients may benefit from diuretics for nonpulmonary reasons.[443] Although intravascular volume must be maintained, fluid overload is detrimental and should be meticulously avoided.

31 • THE POSTSURGICAL PATIENT

The Pulmonary Insult of Surgical Intervention

SURGICAL INTERVENTION is frequently followed by pulmonary disease. This is partly due to the body's increased metabolic responses to trauma (surgical insult), leaving uninvolved and previously normal organ systems (e.g., urinary tract and lungs) vulnerable to infection. However, it is also due to the fact that postoperative abdominal and thoracic surgical patients experience unique predictable pulmonary function alterations. These transient physiologic alterations must be appreciated by the respiratory care practitioner and the physician involved in postoperative care.

Reduction of Vital Capacity

The observation that vital capacity is reduced 50–75% within 24 hours following thoracic or abdominal surgery was first reported in 1927.[446] This observation has been reconfirmed numerous times and has proved to be extremely consistent.[447, 448] Normal adult vital capacity is reported to range between 55 and 85 ml/kg of normal body weight.[41] Thus, any insult causing an acute decrease of up to 75% in vital capacity would leave most normal individuals with a vital capacity greater than 15 ml/kg. As discussed in Chapter 3 and Section III, any acute decrease in vital capacity that remains in excess of 15 ml/kg *should* transiently provide an adequate ventilatory reserve and allow adequate deep breathing and coughing.

The postoperative vital capacity reduction occurs gradually over 12 to 18 hours following the surgical procedure. Therefore, the patient's ventilatory reserve (see Chapter 3) will usually be significantly *less* 12 hours postoperatively than immediately following the surgical procedure. A clinical axiom of respiratory evaluation in the postsurgical patient states: *The vital capacity is maximally reduced 12–18 hours postoperatively and then gradually improves unless complications intervene.* Most patients with an uncomplicated course approach their preoperative vital capacities by the third or fourth postoperative day.[446-448]

Clinical Guidelines

The reproducibility of surgically induced vital capacity reduction has allowed the following clinical guidelines to be developed and they have proved reliable beyond any reasonable doubt:

1. Elective upper abdominal procedures or thoracic procedures involving splitting of the sternum will, within 24 hours, result in a 60–75% decrease in the preoperative vital capacity.

2. Elective lower abdominal or thoracic procedures will, within 24 hours, result in a 30–50% decrease in the preoperative vital capacity.

3. Elective non-thoracoabdominal procedures will usually result in little postoperative vital capacity reduction; however, reductions resulting from anesthesia and narcotics are variable.

Routine Monitoring

The simplest means of clinically monitoring the postoperative severity of vital capacity reduction is to serially observe the respiratory rate. Acute decreases in vital capacity usually result in *rapid* and *shallow* ventilatory patterns (see Chapter 3). When an adult postoperative patient's respiratory rate becomes *progressively* faster in the first 12 hours and approaches 30 per minute, it usually reflects significant loss of ventilatory reserve unless significant pain is present. In such circumstances it is advisable to serially measure vital capacity, tidal volume, and arterial blood gases in addition to performing frequent clinical chest examinations.

The Acute Restrictive Pattern (Fig 31–1)

The predictable postoperative restriction in total lung capacity is believed secondary to the limitation of diaphragm and chest wall muscular activity. In other words, the thorax is limiting the inflation capability of reasonably unaltered lungs. One may anticipate that this would result in minimal diminishment of residual volume,[449-451] since airway closure would tend to maintain residual volume in the basilar areas.[62, 452] Thus, the significant reduction in total lung capacity would be primarily at the expense of the vital capacity. Figure 31–1 represents this type of acute restrictive disease. It might also be anticipated that hypoxemia resulting from this kind of restrictive pulmonary disease would be the result of "shunt effect" (see Chapters 4, 6, and 7) and thereby be responsive to oxygen therapy.[35, 453-457]

Summary

Abdominal and thoracic surgical intervention results in a transient acute restrictive pulmonary abnormality that primarily affects vital capacity. The resulting limitation in ventilatory reserves is reasonably predictable, and the resulting hypoxemia is readily responsive to moderate levels (30–40%) of oxygen therapy.

Pulmonary Complications of Surgical Intervention

Most patients survive the acute restrictive pulmonary insult of elective thoracic and abdominal surgery with few detectable clinical problems.[458] However, cardiopulmonary homeostasis is significantly stressed in many patients and results in complications. These postoperative pulmonary *complications* may be separated into two general categories: acute ventilatory failure and atelectasis/pneumonia. Although the complications are often difficult to clinically differentiate, it is convenient to separate them for purposes of discussion. For simplicity and clarity, variables such as cardiovascular, hepatorenal, and C.N.S. function as well as surgical technique and general medical care are not emphasized in the following discussions; however, these variables must always be considered in an actual clinical evaluation.

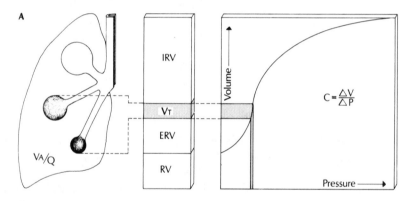

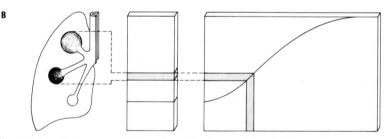

Fig 31–1.—**A** represents the normal relationships between lung volumes, compliance, and V$_A$/Q. **B** represents the changes that occur in the uncomplicated postabdominal or thoracic surgery patient (see text). *IRV* = inspiratory reserve volume; *V$_T$* = tidal volume; *ERV* = expiratory reserve volume; *RV* = residual volume.

Acute Ventilatory Failure

Acute ventilatory failure is defined as the sudden inability of the pulmonary system to adequately meet the metabolic demands of the body in reference to carbon dioxide homeostasis (see Chapter 4). Through blood gas measurements, this condition is clinically detectable by an arterial P_{CO_2} greater than 50 mm Hg in conjunction with a pH below 7.30[35] This may occur secondary to the significant increase in the energy required for adequate physiologic ventilation in the first 24 postoperative hours.[459, 460] As illustrated in Figure 31 – 1; (1) ventilatory reserve (vital capacity) is significantly decreased from normal; (2) lung compliance is less than normal; and (3) ventilation-perfusion relationships are less than optimal.[461, 462]

When vital capacity becomes less than 10 ml/kg for a significant period, the capabilities to provide the energy required for adequate ventilation are greatly decreased[347] (see Chapter 19). In addition, any increase in airway resistance will increase the work of breathing, whereas any cardiovascular, hepatorenal, or C.N.S. abnormality will decrease the patient's ability to meet increased energy requirements for ventilation.

Clinical Guideline

A general guideline and reference point for estimating the probability of ventilatory failure in the first 24 hours is as follows: *For an upper abdominal procedure in a patient with a normal cardiovascular, hepatorenal, and central nervous system, if %FVC + %FEV₁/FVC* is less than 100, there is a 50% chance of that patient experiencing acute ventilatory failure in the first 24 hours.* This rule of thumb reflects the fact that, if the patient is normal in all systems except pulmonary, and that pulmonary disease significantly limits ventilatory reserve, the chances of ventilatory failure caused by the surgical insult are great. Of course, significant disease in any other organ system will *increase* the chances of ventilatory failure.[347]

This becomes an extremely important guideline for major decisions such as (1) maintaining the patient in an intensive care area for the first 24 hours for monitoring purposes; (2) applying early, aggressive bronchial hygiene therapy; and (3) providing elective ventilatory support for the first 24 hours postoperatively.

Atelectasis/Pneumonia

A decreased FRC, decreased vital capacity, and the absence of periodic deep inflations are believed the main factors contributing to re-

---

*Refer to Chapter 3 for detailed explanation.

TABLE 31-1.—INCIDENCE OF POSTOPERATIVE
PULMONARY COMPLICATIONS IN RELATION
TO VARIOUS FACTORS

Abnormal pulmonary function study/Normal	23/1
Abdominal operation/Non-abdominal	4/1
Smoking history/Non-smoker	4/1
Above 60 years/Under 60 years	3/1
Overweight (20%)/Not overweight	2/1

tained secretions and stasis pneumonia[182-186] (Section III). It stands to reason that any intrinsic lung abnormality would tend to exaggerate the process.

The incidence of atelectasis and pneumonia after abdominal and thoracic surgery has been reported to be 12–80%.[193, 448, 457, 458, 461] The disparity is probably explainable by such variables as (1) the surgical procedure undertaken; (2) surgical technique; (3) preoperative condition of the patient; (4) pre- and postoperative care; (5) retrospective versus prospective investigation; and (6) criteria used for diagnosing atelectasis and pneumonia.

Perhaps the most practical way to utilize the available information is to compare the incidence within each study with the various factors believed to influence the incidence of pulmonary complications. Table 31-1 is the compilation of such a comparison[44] and emphasizes that *the single most useful clinical factor for delineating the postoperative patient at high risk for atelectasis and pneumonia is the abnormal expiratory spirogram.* This effective noninvasive bedside measurement has also proved simple and inexpensive.

Classifying the Risk for
Postoperative Pulmonary Complications

The anticipated abdominal or thoracic surgical procedure must be clearly identified. Past medical history of pre-existent lung disease, smoking, sputum production, exercise tolerance, and restrictive and obstructive phenomena must be examined. Information as to pre-existent cardiovascular disease (dyspnea on exertion, orthopnea, paroxysmal nocturnal dyspnea, dependent edema) and evidence of congestive heart failure, angina, and myocardial infarctions must be noted. Any pre-existent renal disease and metabolic disease must be evaluated. Physical examination as to body weight; state of nutrition; color and temperature of the skin; chest configuration; skeletal abnormalities; pattern of ventilation; and auscultatory findings of the chest, including heart tones and murmurs, are essential. General labo-

TABLE 31-2. – CLASSIFICATION OF RISK OF
PULMONARY COMPLICATIONS OF THORACIC
AND ABDOMINAL PROCEDURES

CATEGORY	POINTS
I. Expiratory spirogram	
a. Normal ($\%$FVC + $\%$FEV$_1$/FVC > 150)	0
b. $\%$FVC + $\%$FEV$_1$/FVC = 100–150	1
c. $\%$FVC + $\%$FEV$_1$/FVC < 100	2
d. Preoperative FVC < 20 ml/kg	3
e. Post-bronchodilator FEV$_1$/FVC < 50$\%$	3
II. Cardiovascular system	
a. Normal	0
b. Controlled hypertension, myocardial infarction without sequelae for more than 2 years	0
c. Dyspnea on exertion, orthopnea, paroxysmal nocturnal dyspnea, dependent edema, congestive heart failure, angina	1
III. Nervous system	
a. Normal	0
b. Confusion, obtundation, agitation, spasticity, discoordination, bulbar malfunction	1
c. Significant muscular weakness	1
IV. Arterial blood gases	
a. Acceptable	0
b. Pa$_{CO_2}$ > 50 mm Hg or Pa$_{O_2}$ < 60 mm Hg on room air	1
c. Metabolic pH abnormality > 7.50 or < 7.30	1
V. Postoperative ambulation	
a. Expected ambulation (minimum, sitting at bedside) within 36 hours	0
b. Expected complete bed confinement for at least 36 hours	1

0 points = low risk; 1–2 points = moderate risk; >3 points = high risk.

ratory studies, including ECG and chest x-ray, must be evaluated. *At minimum, a forced expiratory spirogram must be obtained* and, if advisable, complete pulmonary function studies accomplished. If indicated, a blood gas measurement to further evaluate the pulmonary gas exchange should be made.

A reliable system for generally arriving at a risk category for pulmonary complications in the patient undergoing abdominal or thoracic surgery is put forth in Table 31–2. Each of the five categories is evaluated and the patient ascribed a total score from zero to 7. (Only one score is assigned for each variable, making 7 the highest score possible).

Low Risk (0 points)

When the patient receives no points, there should be little expectation that he or she will have pulmonary complications postoperatively. Incentive spirometry may prove useful, but above all the patient must be encouraged to cough and deep breathe frequently. Oxygen therapy is usually not necessary after discharge from the recovery room.

Moderate Risk (1 or 2 points)

These patients have a significant incidence of postoperative complications, i.e., atelectasis, pneumonia, decreased basilar breath sounds, fever of unknown origin, or mild hypoxemia. However, if properly treated, these entities should not prove life threatening. These patients deserve a careful evaluation for postoperative bronchial hygiene (see Chapter 14) and their pulmonary status should be followed carefully by the physician. Incentive spirometry is definitely indicated as a prophylactic measure, and therapeutic measures (see Section III) should be instituted when indicated. Serious consideration should be given to daily vital capacity measurements and arterial blood gas measurements to aid the physician in his pulmonary evaluation. Oxygen therapy is often indicated for several postoperative days.

High Risk (3 or more points)

These patients should be seriously considered for remaining in an intensive care area for 24–48 hours postoperatively. Serial evaluation of cardiopulmonary reserves is indicated, as well as evaluation for aggressive bronchial hygiene therapy.

A preoperative FVC of less than 20 ml/kg places the patient at high risk for acute ventilatory failure in the postoperative period. These patients deserve careful evaluation and may be candidates for elective ventilator support.

Significant preoperative *irreversible* airway obstruction will significantly increase the postoperative work of breathing and diminish bronchial hygiene capability. In our experience, a patient free of pulmonary infection who manifests a postbronchodilator $\%FEV_1/FVC$ of less than 50% should be considered "at high risk" for postoperative pulmonary complication.

It must be stated emphatically that the authors are not presuming that this system can predict a patient's capability to withstand an abdominal or thoracic surgical procedure. Rather, we are stating that the system aids in identifying the patient at moderate and high risk for pulmonary complications. The analysis is dependent upon an adequate preoperative respiratory care evaluation and a thorough understanding of the factors contributing to the incidence of postoperative pulmonary complication.

"High-Risk" Postoperative Respiratory Care

Patients classified as at high risk should be placed in an appropriate intensive care area for at least the first 24 hours. The more limited the patient's reserves, the greater the need for serial blood gas measurements, since they alone provide a reflection of the adequacy of physiologic gas exchange in the pulmonary system. Serial blood gas measurements assure the appropriateness of oxygen therapy, assure that appropriate ventilation is being provided, and provide a reflection of acid-base status. It is our recommendation that indwelling arterial lines be established postoperatively, if not already accomplished before or during the operative procedure. This will assure the availability of serial blood gas samples even in the event of hemodynamic instability.[35]

Frequent measurement of mechanical pulmonary function parameters such as vital capacity, tidal volume, and rate of ventilation is essential. The ventilatory pattern must be serially assessed and compared with blood gas measurements. This will allow a reasonable assessment of the physiologic efficiency of ventilation and will aid in clinical assessment of the work of breathing (see Chapters 3 and 19).

Maintenance of an adequate airway is essential! The decision whether or not to keep an endotracheal tube in place is critical. It is generally advisable in high-risk patients to establish a nasotracheal tube during the operative procedure and leave it in place until the patient meets criteria for extubation. However, in some patients it is important to extubate early, such as the asthmatic to avoid bronchospasm and the severe COPD patient to allow the glottic mechanism to function normally. If the COPD patient must remain intubated, 5 cm H_2O PEEP is suggested (see Chapter 24).

Postoperative ventilator support may be indicated in the patient who shows an inability to maintain an adequate ventilatory state, or it may be initiated on an elective basis in response to increased chances of ventilatory failure. Mechanical support of ventilation in the postoperative patient follows the same general principles outlined for all ventilator care (see Chapters 22 and 23). Though most patients tolerate a control mode satisfactorily, the use of augmented modes of ventilation should be encouraged whenever possible.

Pain relief is essential in the early postoperative period and will greatly affect coughing and deep breathing. The patient who has adequate pain relief will actually breathe more deeply and cough better than the patient who is experiencing significant pain.[463] Thus, pain relief is not only humane; it is physiologically desirable. In the critical care area, narcotics should be administered in small, frequent doses by the intravenous route. Such techniques as lumbar and thoracic epidural catheters may prove desirable for pain relief in certain high-risk patients.

Preoperative Bronchial Hygiene Therapy

Patients with significant retained secretions should have an aggressive preoperative bronchial hygiene program instituted. This often results in significant increases in vital capacity and/or forced expiratory volumes. It is our experience that a preoperative bronchial hygiene program can usually accomplish its goals within 48 hours.

Any preoperative program must include proper preparation for the postoperative bronchial hygiene program. At minimum this should include instructing the patient in breathing exercises, cough methods, and other techniques of enhancing his postoperative ventilatory muscle mechanics. This is the opportune time to familiarize the patient with the expected postoperative course and the techniques, equipment, and procedures planned for postoperative bronchial hygiene therapy.

Preoperative instruction and psychologic reassurance remove a great deal of anxiety and pain from the postoperative period. We have found that these patients appear to have better results from their postoperative bronchial hygiene program because of the preoperative instruction. With well-ordered communication between surgeons, nursing staff, and a smoothly running respiratory therapy department, the indicated preoperative program can be accomplished without causing delay in the surgical schedule.

"Routine" Postoperative Bronchial Hygiene

Postoperative bronchial hygiene therapy has become the vogue in the past years and is presently the subject of much controversy. If perfect postoperative nursing care existed, there would be no need for routine respiratory therapy. It is impossible to justify the expense and personnel time involved in routine postoperative respiratory therapy for low-risk patients; however, neither nursing staffs nor physicians have the time or training to effectively apply appropriate stir-up regimens to *high-risk* patients. The answer obviously lies in the ability to preoperatively distinguish the high-risk from the moderate-risk patient and *appropriately* apply respiratory therapy in the postoperative period.

Remember, therapeutically indicated bronchial hygiene therapy in critically ill patients is dramatic in its results; however, the efficacy of *prophylactic* bronchial hygiene therapy has never been documented! The only possible justification for expensive and time-consuming *prophylactic* bronchial hygiene therapy is in the high-risk postoperative patient, and even in that circumstance it remains controversial.

The rationale for application of incentive spirometry, IPPB, aerosol, and chest physical therapy has been discussed in detail in Section III. Most surgical patients are healthy and undergo nonabdominal procedures, making them low-risk patients needing no more than minimal stir-up regimens (e.g., incentive spirometry, good nursing care, early ambulation). The need and effectiveness of bronchial hygiene therapy in the great majority of surgical patients are readily judged by common sense and a few well-understood guidelines. The need and effectiveness of bronchial hygiene therapy in high-risk patients and those undergoing extensive major surgery must be judged on logical and unbiased grounds. The answer is far from clear!

32 • CHRONIC OBSTRUCTIVE PULMONARY DISEASE

CHRONIC OBSTRUCTIVE PULMONARY DISEASE (COPD) has become the nation's fastest growing health care problem. Bronchitis, emphysema, and asthma have increased over 200% as a cause of death in the past 25 years,[464] and COPD has become the second largest disease entity receiving social security disability.[465] The American Lung Association estimates that over 450,000 new COPD patients are seen each year, and there may be as many as 15,000,000 sufferers in the United States.

In addition to genetic predisposition and many unknown factors, three realities of our modern environment guarantee the continued rise of chronic obstructive pulmonary disease as a health care problem.

1. *Cigarette smoking* has been shown to be a contributing factor in the early development and severity of COPD. This is reflected in the increased incidence of COPD in the female population because of the increasing duration of their heavy cigarette smoking. Despite the clear link between cigarette smoking and pulmonary disease, there is little indication that the younger generation is heeding the warning.

2. *Air pollution* plays a role in the symptomatology and progression of COPD. As the particulate and noxious gaseous components of air in urban areas increase, the problem of chronic obstructive pulmonary disease becomes more apparent.

3. Modern medicine has created an ever-increasing *geriatric population*. As people live longer, the problem of COPD becomes a greater sociologic and medical problem.

Chronic obstructive pulmonary disease is neither of infrequent occurrence nor of small consequence to our society. The costs for treating this disease entity are overwhelming; at present the American taxpayer spends hundreds of millions of dollars on the care of patients with COPD. The incidence, sociologic impact, and expense make it imperative that the discipline of respiratory care address itself to the treatment of the COPD patient. Unfortunately, most of the efforts have been focused on acute hospital care while little energy has been applied to treatment of the chronic state.

Obstructive Pulmonary Disease

Obstructive pulmonary disease has been classically defined as an increased total lung capacity in conjunction with decreased expiratory flow rates.[41] Since the power to inspire is actively provided by the muscles of ventilation, it is much easier to overcome resistance during inhalation than during the passive process of exhalation—especially during forced exhalation. Therefore, a resistance abnormality affects expiration far more than inspiration (see Chapter 20).

Acute Obstructive Disease

There are two common obstructive diseases (bronchitis and asthma) that are intermittent and reversible; between acute episodes there are few pulmonary function abnormalities and the patients are essentially symptom free.

Bronchitis is inflammation of the mucosal lining of the tracheobronchial tree. This inflammatory reaction has the common factors of increased and abnormal glandular secretion, mucosal hyperemia (blood vessel congestion), edema (swelling), ciliary dysfunction, and disruption of the continuity of the mucous blanket. Recurrent or consistent bronchitis leads to chronic changes in the pulmonary mucosa. Bronchitis is caused by such major factors as (1) smoke and air pollution, (2) inhalant allergens, and (3) infections.

Asthma is an acute onset of muscle spasm in the tracheobronchial tree. The smooth muscle linings of the bronchi and bronchioles contract and result in a narrowing of the lumina. The acute bronchospasm is usually quite amenable to pharmacologic treatment. There is also a glandular component to the asthmatic condition in which very thick, copious secretions are produced in the tracheobronchial tree. These tenacious secretions play an important pathophysiologic role in asthma.

The treatment of acute obstructive disease is essentially based on sound internal medicine principles. Appropriate pharmacologic and anti-allergic methods of therapy are the hallmarks of good care. *It is rare for acute obstructive disease to result in acute respiratory failure.* Occasionally infants will manifest respiratory insufficiency with bronchiolitis. Rarely, the asthmatic patient presents in acute respiratory failure (status asthmaticus—see Chapter 34).

Defining COPD in Respiratory Care

The exact definition of COPD and identification of the patient population are controversial at best. However, it is essential to develop a clear definition of the entity referred to as chronic obstructive pulmonary disease, at least as it pertains to respiratory care. The word *chronic* denotes an ever-present and continuing disease entity. There are two major irreversible, degenerative pulmonary processes in COPD: (1) chronic bronchitis and (2) emphysema.

Chronic Bronchitis

Chronic bronchitis has been arbitrarily defined as cough with sputum production during at least 3 months of the year for at least 2 consecutive years.[466] Anatomically, it is a disease of the airways — primarily mucosal hypertrophy; inflammation; and excessive, abnormal mucus production. There are numerous areas where the cilia are absent. Therefore, not only is the mucus abnormal, but the basic transport mechanism (ciliary action) for the mucous blanket is noncontinuous ("skip areas"). *Effective bronchial hygiene is permanently impaired and becomes dependent upon "routine" use of the cough mechanism.*

Emphysema

Emphysema is a nonreversible pulmonary disease causing an obstructive pathology. It is characterized by destruction of interalveolar septal walls and destruction of the connective tissue responsible for much of the elastic recoil of the lung, resulting in large alveolar sacs that have little elastic recoil properties.[466] The resultant increase in residual volume is accompanied by small airway changes leading to increased airway resistance. The distribution of these pathologic features throughout the lung has led to various anatomic descriptions, e.g., centrilobular or panlobular emphysema. These variances will undoubtedly hold more clinical significance as we learn more about the disease's etiology.[467, 468] Emphysema is an irreversible process and therefore is a chronic disease.

COPD (Fig 32-1)

Chronic obstructive pulmonary disease is a *progressive, irreversible,* and *degenerative* process that in respiratory care may be considered a combination of five different disease entities: (1) emphysema; (2) bronchitis; (3) asthma; (4) failure of the right heart; and (5) failure of the left heart. Patients may have any combination of the five entities.

A lifelong asthmatic patient may gradually become a COPD patient with a predominant bronchospastic component. The dramatic relief obtained from bronchodilators steadily diminishes as the emphysematous component becomes dominant. Emphysematous change is believed the universal entity in COPD, but very severe cases almost

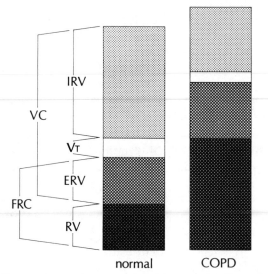

normal   COPD

Fig 32–1. — Comparison of normal total lung capacity and lung volumes with classic COPD. *RV* = residual volume; *ERV* = expiratory reserve volume; *V*$_T$ = tidal volume; *IRV* = inspiratory reserve volume; *VC* = vital capacity; *FRC* = functional residual capacity.

always involve chronic bronchitis and cardiac malfunction. The classic "pink puffer" is the primarily emphysematous patient; he may have some element of chronic left heart failure and some bronchospasm but basically little pulmonary vascular abnormality.

Degenerative and fibrotic perivascular changes lead to increased pulmonary vascular resistance and eventually compromise right ventricular function. This is commonly referred to as *cor pulmonale* (right heart failure secondary to pulmonary disease). The "blue bloater" is primarily the chronic bronchitic with severe cor pulmonale and right heart failure.

The pathophysiology of COPD may eventually result in a failure to meet the body's oxygen requirements. In this event the cardiovascular system compensates by increasing cardiac output. Eventually the myocardial reserves will be exceeded and left heart failure ensues.

This chapter is devoted to the principles of respiratory care as applied to the patient with COPD. Thus, our definition and classification are functional ones based on the pathologies and pathophysiologies amenable to support and treatment with respiratory therapy modalities. Appropriate medical care and support are assumed.

For our purposes COPD may be defined as a progressive, irreversible, and degenerative obstructive process involving (1) impaired lung clearance because of decreased ciliary and mucous blanket function; (2) chronic bronchial inflammation; (3) inflammatory airway obstruction secondary to edema and cellular infiltration; (4) weakened bronchiolar walls and disrupted alveoli; and (5) collapsed small airways on forced expiration. These entities lead to increased airflow resistance on expiration and an increased total lung capacity primarily caused by the increased residual volume.

Diagnosis of Chronic Obstructive Pulmonary Disease

Diagnosis of severe chronic obstructive pulmonary disease is made by medical history, physical examination, and laboratory studies. *Medical history* may include an early complaint of cough and sputum production or intermittent wheezing episodes. Significant cigarette smoking over a reasonable period of time is a common finding. Limitation of normal activity attributable to shortness of breath is usually present. The patient may attribute the start of this problem to a specific event (e.g., pneumonia 3 years ago); however, careful questioning usually reveals in insidious onset of symptoms prior to that event. Bronchitis is specifically delineated by categorization of cough and sputum production.[466]

Physical examination may reveal an increased anteroposterior chest diameter (this is not as common as previously believed). Rounded shoulder posture is almost always found and there is some use of accessory and intercostal muscles. The chest is tympanic to percussion, and the diaphragm has diminished excursion. Ventilatory rate is rapid along with a rapid pulse rate. Breath sounds are distant and wheezes are usually heard during forced expiration.

Pulmonary function studies document the existence of COPD. Increased total lung capacity and functional residual capacity result primarily from an increased residual volume. Timed expiratory flow rates are decreased. Chest x-ray will usually reveal flattened diaphragms, hyperlucent lung fields, and increased vascular markings. Arterial blood gas analysis is seldom involved in the diagnosis but may aid in evaluating the physiologic severity.

External Respiration in COPD

An *increased functional residual capacity* means a constant state of hyperinflation, which decreases the efficiency of air exchange at the alveolar level. The result is decreased alveolar oxygen tensions (responsive hypoxemia-shunt effect — see Chapter 4) and potentially increased alveolar carbon dioxide tensions.

Degenerative alveolar changes (emphysema) result in a diminished area for exchange between alveolar air and pulmonary blood. Thus, a greater portion of the alveolar gas does not exchange with blood. This "wasted" ventilation is termed *deadspace ventilation.* Increased deadspace ventilation requires increased work of breathing.

Bronchitic, asthmatic, and emphysematous pathology lead to *uneven distribution of ventilation.* This creates hypoventilated areas in relation to blood flow, which results in less than optimal oxygenation of the blood perfusing that area of lung. This shunt effect leads to arterial hypoxemia, which causes the cardiopulmonary system to increase work in order to meet the organism's metabolic demands.

Increased work of breathing, decreased efficiency in the distribution of ventilation, and decreased efficiency in the distribution of pulmonary perfusion eventually lead to chronic hypoxemia.

CO_2 Retention in COPD

There is no demonstrable correlation between the severity of COPD and CO_2 retention. It appears that numerous factors are involved, few of them well understood. Central nervous system response to increased carbon dioxide blood levels is complex and variable. Some obese patients have decreased response capability (Pickwickian syndrome), as do some nonobese individuals (primary alveolar hypoventilation syndrome). Recent investigations into these responses during sleep and within families[468, 469] (i.e., genetic factors) have raised fascinating questions, but as yet no answers.

Although these matters are of great intellectual interest and deserve intensive investigation, the respiratory care practitioner needs a practical, comprehensible, and *clinically* applicable schema into which clinical realities may be set and which may provide a foundation for future knowledge. The following theoretic and teleologic discussion is illustrated in such a schema (Fig 32–2). It assumes that cardiac reserves diminish in a progressive manner with time, but the heart maintains a cardiac output adequate to meet metabolic demands in terms of tissue oxygenation.

As depicted in Figure 32–2, the early disease process results in progressive arterial hypoxemia secondary to ventilation-perfusion deterioration (point A). When arterial oxygen tension reaches some minimal level, usually around 60 mm Hg, the peripheral chemoreceptors experience decreased tissue oxygen supply and respond by stimulating both the ventilatory muscles and the myocardium.[24] This stimulation produces the amount of myocardial and ventilatory work necessary to maintain the arterial oxygen tension at a level minimizing chemoreceptor tissue hypoxia.

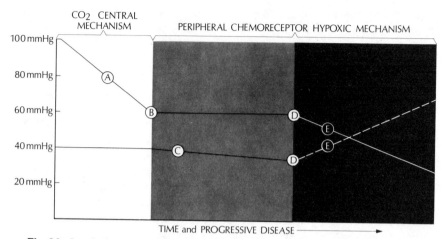

Fig 32–2.—A theory on the pathogenesis of ventilatory failure in chronic obstructive pulmonary disease. *A,* decreasing arterial Po_2 due to early disease process; *B,* peripheral chemoreceptor stimulation begins and becomes the primary drive to breathe; *C,* arterial Po_2 level remains fairly constant, whereas arterial Pco_2 level may decrease to some degree; *D,* theoretic points at which work of breathing is so costly that a decreased arterial Po_2 is unavoidable (see text); *E,* arterial Po_2 begins to decrease and arterial Pco_2 begins to increase. (From Shapiro, B. A., Harrison, R. A., and Walton J. R.: *Clinical Application of Blood Gases* [2d ed.; Chicago: Year Book Medical Publishers, Inc., 1977].)

Maintaining the arterial oxygen tension at a level where the peripheral chemoreceptors are minimally stimulated in the face of progressive disease necessitates increasing ventilatory and myocardial work. The increasing ventilatory work is reflected in Figure 32–2 by a somewhat decreasing arterial carbon dioxide tension at point *C*. The increased ventilatory and myocardial work continues to maintain the minimal arterial oxygen tension that "satisfies" the chemoreceptors.

Point *D* will be reached when the work of breathing uses so much oxygen that increasing total ventilation actually consumes more oxygen than is gained. In other words, physiologic deadspace is so great, shunting so significant, and the work of breathing so inefficient that a further increase in alveolar ventilation (seldom below 35 mm Hg) produces a net loss in arterial oxygen tension. It is essential to understand that at point *D* the organism faces a decrease in arterial oxygen tension, whether ventilation is unchanged, increased, or decreased, for the following reasons:

1. *Unchanged* alveolar ventilation leads to decreased arterial Po_2 because of increasing shunting and shunt effect.

2. *Increased* alveolar ventilation requires a great increase in ventilatory muscle work because the "wasted" ventilation (physiologic deadspace) is large. In addition, the vital capacity is decreased and airway resistance is increased. These factors lead to an oxygen consumption for increased ventilatory work that is greater than the oxygen gained from the increased alveolar ventilation, i.e., a decrease in mixed venous PO_2.

3. *Decreased* alveolar ventilation decreases the oxygen consumed for the work of breathing, but this oxygen gain is not great enough to offset the oxygen loss from the decreased alveolar ventilation.

The organism obviously chooses the alternative that results in the smallest arterial oxygen loss for the least energy expended. As shown at points *E* in Figure 32–2, alveolar ventilation slowly decreases as arterial PO_2 slowly decreases. The cardiopulmonary homeostatic mechanisms dictate that the organism decreases effective ventilation and adjusts to the hypoxemia.[470] It should be recalled that the organism chooses a ventilatory pattern according to work efficiency rather than ventilatory efficiency (see Chapter 3).

Clinical Course of Chronic Obstructive Pulmonary Disease

The respiratory care practitioner's difficulty in understanding the severe COPD patient stems from a hesitancy to accept two essential facts: (1) The COPD patient's base-line state varies from the normal population. This means that a chronic CO_2 retainer must be evaluated from his *own* base-line state rather than from the "normal" PCO_2 of 40 mm Hg. (2) Symptomatology and disability cannot be evaluated in the usual terms of acute medicine. A broad definition of disability is "a significant limitation in the ability to perform common or essential tasks." A patient with pulmonary disability is one who is unable to perform activities of daily living because of pulmonary limitations.[471]

A COPD patient manifests pulmonary disability for the following reasons: (1) The progressive pathology results in increasing disparity between ventilation and perfusion—this leads to increased work of breathing, decreased arterial oxygenation, and increased work of the heart; (2) emphysema, chronic bronchitis, and asthma cause congestion of the pulmonary mucosa as well as dried, retained secretions— these factors lead to increased work of breathing, uneven distribution of ventilation, decreased arterial oxygenation, and increased myocardial work; (3) the patient attempts to avoid physical activity that precipitates shortness of breath or other discomfort—this limitation of activity produces "lazy muscles" that require more oxygen to do less work,[471] and this increased oxygen requirement results in further limitation of activity;[472] (4) the psychologic and emotional overlay is profound—the patient becomes depressed and believes there is no hope; and (5) failure of the right and left heart as well as other nonpulmonary diseases, may compound the symptom complex.

The COPD patient is a chronically ill individual with overwhelming physical and emotional symptoms, is always hypoxemic, and often is a carbon dioxide retainer. His exercise tolerance is diminished, and he depends primarily upon his cardiac reserve to maintain homeostasis.[472] He lives in a hostile environment where he is threatened in his ability to perform ordinary activities of daily living. This may lead to a state of depression that becomes overwhelming. These individuals are often cantankerous, for they have been shuttled from doctor to doctor and from institution to institution and this has led to great frustration. They do not trust the doctors and are usually distrustful of therapists and nurses. Above all, *they are individuals who are hesitant and unwilling to accept their chronic disease.* The respiratory care practitioner comes in contact with this patient in two circumstances: (1) when the patient becomes acutely ill and enters the hospital; and (2) in the setting of pulmonary rehabilitation.

Acute Care of Chronic Obstructive Pulmonary Disease

It is common for the respiratory care practitioner to be confronted with the COPD patient who has an acute decompensation of cardiopulmonary homeostasis. This decompensation is most commonly due to acute pulmonary infection, atelectasis, bronchospasm, or heart failure.[473] In any case, the respiratory care supportive needs fall into two categories: (1) maintenance of adequate bronchial hygiene, and (2) judicious oxygen therapy.

"Aggressive" Bronchial Hygiene Therapy

The COPD patient has a chronically decreased ability to maintain adequate pulmonary hygiene, and therefore retention of secretions is almost certain when an acute insult occurs. Aerosol, IPPB, and chest physical therapy techniques should be used in an attempt to promote and maintain optimal bronchial hygiene (see Section III). Obviously, good systemic hydration is essential.

The airway is important in acute care of the COPD patient. Tracheostomy is usually not necessary, since the placement of a nasotracheal tube is generally adequate for short-term needs. Optimal bronchial hygiene may necessitate intubation. Under these circumstances the risks of airway contamination are worth taking. Remember, it is for the purposes of aspirating the trachea and providing adequate airway care that the endotracheal tube is often indicated. *Intubation should not be performed on the basis of ventilator support alone.*

Quantitation of the effectiveness of bronchial hygiene therapy is frustrating and difficult in these patients. However, when these patients are deteriorating due to retained secretions, the general *improvement* in work of breathing, spirometry, and arterial blood gases is obvious and impressive to any observer. It is essential to serially measure arterial blood gases to assure maintenance of base-line Pco_2 and to avoid severe acidemia (below 7.20). Cardiac and circulatory status must be clinically evaluated.

Oxygen Therapy

The schema in Figure 32–2 clearly demonstrates that maintenance of tissue oxygenation is the primary determinant of ventilatory effort in the CO_2 retainer. Thus, these patients provide an unusual circumstance: the ability to manipulate ventilatory and acid-base status with varying inspired oxygen concentrations. In addition to this built-in "hypoxic" drive mechanism, all COPD patients have very poor distribution of ventilation and, therefore, have a great degree of shunt effect, i.e., alveolar oxygen tension will change significantly with small variations in FI_{O_2} (see Chapter 7).

The prime cardiopulmonary homeostatic response to increased alveolar oxygen tensions will be decreases in ventilatory and cardiac work—not changes in arterial Po_2! The respiratory care practitioner must understand the nuances and sophistications of oxygen therapy for these patients. In the acutely ill patient, the need for high-flow oxygen systems (see Chapter 7) is common; often, it is an inappropriate oxygen apparatus that causes severe problems. Remember, the acutely ill COPD patient is breathing rapidly and shallowly; therefore, small tidal volumes exist in which low-flow delivery systems are often unpredictable and inconsistent.

Chronic Hypercarbia

Chronic hypercarbia secondary to COPD is the classic picture of a "respiratory failure" patient:[467] the Pa_{CO_2} is above 50 mm Hg and the Pa_{O_2} is below 50 mm Hg when the patient is breathing room air. These patients have "adjusted" to an inadequate alveolar ventilation and low Pa_{O_2}. They depend upon the heart's ability to maintain an adequate cardiac output even though the cardiac reserves are limited. The drive to breathe is primarily from oxygen chemoreceptor stimulation. This patient is in precarious homeostatic balance.

A typical example is a 70-year-old man with COPD and chronic hypercarbia. In his base-line state without any acute distress, his vital signs and arterial blood gases are

pH	7.43	BP	160/120	V_T	300 ml
P_{CO_2}	65 mm Hg	P	110/min	MV	9L
P_{O_2}	43 mm Hg	RR	30/min		

It should be noted that the patient has a pH greater than 7.40. This is typical and is believed to be due to water and chloride ion shifts between intracellular and extracellular spaces, occurring as part of the metabolic compensation for the respiratory acidemia.[474, 475]

It must be remembered that this patient breathes primarily in response to chemoreceptor stimuli and *only* hard enough to retain his base-line hypoxemic state. Administering 40% oxygen to this patient will result in a *profound* decrease in the demand for ventilation; i.e., the increased *alveolar* oxygen tension allows the usual arterial oxygen tension to be maintained at even less alveolar ventilation than before oxygen was administered. *The organism will elect to breathe less hard rather than overwhelmingly increase the Pa_{O_2}.* This results in an acute *decrease* in alveolar ventilation (increased Pa_{CO_2} and acidemia).

The vital signs and blood gases of this patient on 40% oxygen may be

pH	7.20	BP	200/40	V_T	200 ml
P_{CO_2}	90 mm Hg	P	140/min	MV	9L
P_{O_2}	60 mm Hg	RR	45/min, shallow		

Oxygen therapy has produced an acute respiratory acidosis! This acute decrease in alveolar ventilation is superimposed on the chronic hypercarbic state. Despite improved arterial oxygen tensions, the acute acidemia and general C.N.S. obtundation now threaten tissue oxygenation to a greater degree than did the pre-existing hypoxemia. *The primary effect of oxygen therapy in a patient with chronic hypercarbia may be the change in ventilatory status.* This is not true in acute ventilatory failure (acute respiratory acidosis) or in other conditions in which the drive to breathe is *not* chemoreceptor stimulation from hypoxemia.

Much confusion and misinformation exist concerning the application of low concentrations of oxygen to support "respiratory failure." A clear understanding of the pathophysiology and pathogenesis of chronic hypercarbia makes the clinical application of oxygen predictable and understandable in its supportive role. Remember, oxygen therapy is never a cure! Proper application of oxygen will, one hopes, support the patient's cardiopulmonary system by improving the ventilatory status as well as the oxygenation status.

The "Low Concentration Oxygen" Technique

The typical patient for the "low concentration oxygen" technique is the "chronic lunger." He suffers from chronic hypercarbia and has acquired an acute disease such as infectious pneumonia. In response to this acute shunt-producing disease, he attempts to increase his ventilatory and myocardial work to maintain the base-line Pa_{O_2}. He finds this detrimental and so, in an attempt to meet the hypoxemic challenge of the increased shunt, he begins to breathe *less*. Tissue hypoxia ensues because of the combination of hypoxemia and acidemia. The C.N.S. obtundation leads to the patient's breathing less and less. This vicious physiologic cycle leads to death. On room air his blood gases and vital signs might be

pH	7.25	BP	200/140	V_T	200 ml
P_{CO_2}	90 mm Hg	P	140/min	MV	9L
P_{O_2}	30 mm Hg	RR	45/min, labored		

If one were to judge the severity of ventilatory failure on Pa_{CO_2} alone, this patient would appear to be in extremis. However, the pH is *not* severely acidemic, which means the *acute* change in alveolar ventilation has not been as great as the 90 mm Hg Pa_{CO_2} would lead one to believe. *The severity of acute ventilatory failure (respiratory acidosis) is judged on the severity of acidemia.*

The patient has a great deal of shunt effect because of his chronic obstructive pulmonary disease. Therefore, very small increases in inspired oxygen concentration will have profound effects on alveolar oxygenation. Increased *alveolar* oxygen tensions will allow this patient to meet the *acute* hypoxemic challenge without the demand for changing ventilation; i.e., he will be able to resume the base-line hypoventilatory state and still maintain his base-line hypoxemic state.

Thirty minutes after 25% oxygen, the measurements might be

pH	7.30	BP	200/140
P_{CO_2}	80 mm Hg	P	130/min
P_{O_2}	40 mm Hg	RR	40/min, labored

The paradox is that this patient's response to oxygen is to increase alveolar ventilation, maintaining arterial oxygen tensions at the highest possible level. *The oxygen therapy has allowed the patient to increase alveolar ventilation back to his base-line level without sacrificing tissue oxygenation.* This leads to decreases in the acidemia and in tissue hypoxia. The improved C.N.S. oxygenation state allows even better alveolar ventilation and, by increasing the F_{IO_2} to 28%, the following measurements are obtained after several hours:

pH	7.35	BP	170/120
P_{CO_2}	70 mm Hg	P	120/min
P_{O_2}	45 mm Hg	RR	35/min

The arterial oxygen content has been significantly increased. Of equal importance is that *the oxygen therapy has manipulated the ventilatory status so that the acute acidemia is corrected.* In addition, the improved arterial P_{O_2} and pH have probably decreased pulmonary artery pressures and thereby improved function of the right heart. This allows the patient to maintain a good cardiopulmonary status for the next 24–36 hours, while the acute infectious pneumonia is being treated.

Proper oxygen therapy allows this patient to maintain his normal tissue oxygenation state *without* demands to increase his ventilatory work. He is thus able to tolerate the acute increase in shunting without requiring ventilator support. If this patient's response to low concentrations of oxygen had not been an improvement in alveolar ventilation and pH, it might have been necessary to institute ventilatory support. Blood gas analysis makes this response obvious within several hours of the patient's presenting with his acute problem, and the decision as to whether or not mechanical support of ventilation will be needed is usually quite evident after this time. High-flow oxygen delivery systems should be used when feasible, because these patients often have irregular and shallow breathing patterns.

Not all chronic hypercarbic patients with an acute shunting disease present with acute hypercarbia superimposed on a chronic hypercarbia. Some patients possess the strength to increase alveolar ventilation and present with acute alveolar hyperventilation superimposed on a chronic hypercarbic state, as the following blood gas measurements show:

pH	7.52
P_{CO_2}	55 mm Hg
P_{O_2}	45 mm Hg

These measurements would be initially interpreted as partially compensated metabolic alkalosis *with hypoxemia*. Whenever such an interpretation is made, one must be alert to the possibility that this may be acute alveolar hyperventilation superimposed on chronic hypercarbia.[35]

The chronic hypercarbic patient who responds to an acute disease by increasing alveolar ventilation responds to supportive oxygen therapy in the same way as any patient with alveolar hyperventilation secondary to hypoxemia. Thus, 24% oxygen in this patient results in an increase in alveolar oxygen tension and a decrease in alveolar ventilation to the base-line state:

$$
\begin{array}{ll}
\text{pH} & 7.45 \\
\text{P}_{CO_2} & 65 \text{ mm Hg} \\
\text{P}_{O_2} & 55 \text{ mm Hg}
\end{array}
$$

Great care must be taken to prevent administration of too much oxygen, which may result in acute hypercarbia.

Intubation and Mechanical Ventilation

Some patients require nasotracheal intubation to accomplish the necessary bronchial hygiene. Although best avoided, intubation at the appropriate time often prevents the need for the ventilator and, therefore, should not be "avoided at all costs." Well-trained therapists are the best means of keeping the necessity for intubation and ventilation to a minimum. It is advisable to apply 5 cm H_2O CPAP to COPD patients who are intubated but spontaneously breathing.

The use of pharmacologic C.N.S. stimulants to improve ventilation in these patients has been suggested. We have not found their use necessary or advisable. In our experience, fewer than 5% of chronic hypercarbic patients that present with reversible nonsurgical acute illness require positive-pressure ventilatory support. Prompt and appropriate medical therapy, oxygen therapy, and bronchial hygiene therapy constitute the most effective regime.

In COPD patients who *do* require ventilator care, it is essential to maintain their base-line P_{CO_2}; otherwise, they become significant weaning problems (see Chapters 22 and 23). A general rule is to maintain the P_{CO_2} level that provides an arterial pH between 7.40 and 7.50. Arterial P_{O_2} levels *above* 60 mm Hg should be avoided, since they will not improve tissue oxygenation and may produce a decreased drive to breathe. Augmented modes of ventilatory support (IMV/IDV) prove very beneficial in most of these patients. *An appropriately maintained chronic hypercarbic patient with a reversible acute disease should not prove to be a difficult weaning problem!*

Pulmonary Rehabilitation

In approaching the care of the *stabilized* COPD patient, it is essential that the principles of rehabilitation medicine be adopted.[471] A chronic disease state means that there is an irreversible circumstance in which the impairment is always present. Acute medicine is devoted to the therapeutics of acute disease. One cannot measure the success or failure of rehabilitation by the criteria of acute medicine.

A rehabilitative program must view the patient as an entire unit—a unit that must function in family and social surroundings.[476] The degree of physiologic *impairment* may be documented by appropriate physiologic measurement. The degree of *disability* that is suffered by a given patient subsequent to a given physiologic impairment is variable. There may be little correlation between impairment and disability, and certainly *there can be a marked improvement in disability without a change in impairment!* This may be best illustrated by a classic problem in rehabilitation medicine, the acute paraplegic. This patient, usually an accident victim, suddenly finds himself paralyzed from the waist down. The impairment is documentable by physical examination and electromyography. The impairment will not change for the rest of the patient's life; i.e., he will not regain the use of lost musculature. However, the individual's disability may be dramatically improved through a rehabilitative program.[477, 478, 482] The patient can be taught to become completely self-sustaining and ambulatory. Thus, *rehabilitation medicine addresses itself to the patient's disability primarily and the patient's impairment secondarily.*

The respiratory care practitioner must deal with the chronic state of COPD in terms of these principles. Improvement of the patient's disability, rather than the futility of his physiologic impairment, must be emphasized. Pulmonary rehabilitation must place the major emphasis on optimal lung function, excellent general medical care, social and psychological services, vocational counseling, and occupational therapy. Only in this milieu can appropriate respiratory therapy be applied.

General Medical Care

The COPD patient demands careful evaluation and treatment of the cardiovascular system. There is a high incidence of generalized arteriosclerotic vascular disease as well as high blood pressure. The chronic pulmonary disease creates heart disease that must be carefully followed and evaluated.[479] The cardiovascular status must be optimal before the rehabilitation program is begun. Both ECG and chest x-ray must indicate that the patient is free of acute disease. A high incidence of pulmonary infection demands rapid recognition and treatment. All medications must be reviewed and regimens stabilized prior to the beginning of a pulmonary rehabilitative program. Adjustment in the medications is frequently necessary during the program.

Emotional Factors

The pulmonary disabled individual has been forced to make numerous emotional adjustments over many years; these adjustments may superficially appear adequate. However, depression, anger, and hostility usually lie beneath the surface. The patient believes that no one realizes his plight and no one (especially the doctor) can help.

Many patients find secondary gains in their disability, gains they may be unwilling to give up.[480] For example, the patient may be living with a son or daughter. He believes he is welcome only because he is "sick" — getting better may appear to him to be a threat to his security. Careful and thorough evaluation of the patient's motivation for improvement is essential. In most cases, this can be adequately accomplished through careful patient interview. Expert psychologic counseling must be readily available whenever needed; otherwise, the entire program will be a lesson in futility! Assessment of patient motivation and emotional stability is required, not only initially, but continuously throughout a pulmonary rehabilitation program.

Social Factors

The patient must function in *his* environment. The importance of a pulmonary rehabilitation program is that the patient be taught to function in his world, *not* in the hospital. This means that pulmonary rehabilitation should be accomplished outside of the hospital as much as possible. In many cases, the home environment and financial problems must be carefully evaluated. Only after these problems are discovered and defined is it possible to approach solutions. An active social service department must be available and involved.

The Day Care Concept

The long-term objective of a pulmonary rehabilitation program must be to educate, train, and equip the patient to properly treat himself in the home environment. Our experience has shown that a high level of home care capability is difficult or impossible to accomplish when the patient has been exposed only to an inpatient course of treatment.

The concept of a day care program is one in which the patient spends 4 to 6 hours a day receiving necessary therapy and learning a practical home program. Each evening at home he tries the program and returns the next day with numerous questions and problems. These are easily solved by trained personnel, but would be extremely frustrating to the patient if left to his own devices. As the program progresses, the patient spends several entire days at home developing a program for home care that is flexible. When he returns to the day care facility, the trained personnel can help him develop a sensible and workable home program.

Psychologic counseling is used to evaluate rehabilitation potential and provide individual or group therapy sessions aimed at resolving behavioral problems, leading to acceptance of disability. Social services are provided to help with environmental conditions and financial problems.

At completion of the day care program, the short-term goal of improving the patient's symptom complex is accomplished. The patient and his family are trained and equipped to continue a good home program. The referring physician receives a complete report on the home care program and recommendations for continuing this care.

Respiratory Therapy in Pulmonary Rehabilitation

Many attempts to provide programs for the pulmonary disabled have been composed basically of careful treatment and evaluation of the cardiovascular status, proper antibiotic therapy, bronchodilator therapy, and some efforts at breathing retraining. Few attempts have been made to establish a facility to apply the techniques of respiratory therapy for chronic care. Much needed are programs that teach the patient to treat himself continuously at home.[481] Most reported failures appear to be caused by lack of emphasis on this factor.

The effectiveness of each technique of respiratory therapy on stabilized COPD is not known, but it appears that proper application of each of them reduces the patient's symptoms and brings relief to him and his family.[482] There is little question that respiratory intensive care saves many lives. Now we must investigate what can be done to help the long-term patient to solve his problems of relentless shortness of breath and progressive disability. An important meeting of experts in the country was held in May 1974 to outline the "state of the art" of respiratory therapy in the stabilized COPD patient.[483] Many more such meetings are needed to attempt to delineate the role of respiratory therapy methods in the stabilized COPD patient.

Complicating the physical elements of pulmonary disability are psychologic, social, and vocational problems. The anxiety caused by air hunger and a belief that one cannot enjoy activities of family and friends are depressing. Employment possibilities are greatly reduced. Consequently, two fundamental life rewards are denied: accomplishment and financial income.

In addition to the medical care and rehabilitative services, the patient needs respiratory therapy. The basic aim of respiratory therapy is to relieve the work of breathing and give the patient immediate and long-term relief. However, unless the patient is taught to administer this therapy himself, and does so, the results will be very short-term. As applied to rehabilitation, respiratory therapy has four basic areas: (1) aerosol and positive-pressure breathing therapy; (2) postural drainage, percussion, and vibration of the chest; (3) breathing exercises and retraining; and (4) oxygen exercise programs.

There are two goals of respiratory therapy in pulmonary rehabilitation: (1) to decrease the work of breathing, and (2) to decrease the oxygen demand for muscular work. To improve the efficiency of ventilation and decrease the work of breathing, airway resistance must be decreased. This can be accomplished by relieving bronchospasm; decreasing mucosal hyperemia and edema; and mobilizing dried, retained secretions — in other words, keeping the tracheobronchial tree clean! These principles have already been discussed in great detail (see Section III).

Bronchial Hygiene Therapy

Home aerosol therapy may be a great adjunct in the bronchial hygiene of many patients. Proper handling of equipment has proved to be both a feasible and helpful parameter at home.[482] Great emphasis must be made on very slow, deep breaths during aerosol therapy and on constant attempts at mobilization of secretions. IPPB and aerosol therapy has proved helpful in COPD patients needing pulmonary rehabilitation, since most of these patients have limited vital capacities and decreased ability to cough effectively.[482] The IPPB therapy is aimed solely at the accomplishment of good, deep breaths and adequate coughing. Appropriate medications, such as bronchodilators and decongestants, may be added to the IPPB. We have found little use for mucolytics in COPD. Many patients on chronic steroid therapy have decreased their oral dosage by the inclusion of steroid in the IPPB. This has accomplished a decrease in side effects (bruising, edema, electrolytes, osteoporosis). It must be emphasized that aerosolized medications are supplemental and are by no means the main reason COPD patients need aerosol and IPPB therapy! Undoubtedly, the greatest problem arises from improper care of equipment, leading to infection. Maintenance of equipment sterility is essential.

Chest Physical Therapy

The methods of chest physical therapy have long been recognized as helpful in the mobilization of secretions. When combined with proper aerosol and IPPB, these methods make bronchial hygiene dramatically effective and beneficial.[484] Such factors as postural drainage, chest percussion and vibration, and appropriate cough instruction have proved helpful in the maintenance of a bronchial hygiene program for the home patient.

Breathing Efficiency

Pathophysiologic changes of COPD, such as increased deadspace, increased intrapulmonary shunting, increased functional residual capacity, increased compliance, and flattened diaphragm, place the patient in a position of acquiring bad habits of posture and ventilation. Posture correction is an essential part of improving the ventilatory efficiency of the COPD patient.[196] They tend to "hunch over," raise the shoulders upward, and push the head and neck forward. These are natural attempts to stabilize the chest wall so that accessory muscles of ventilation have a greater mechanical advantage. This is a profitable short-term mechanism but very detrimental over the long run. The patient must be trained to use good posture and emphasize diaphragmatic breathing.

Breathing retraining is primarily the instruction of diaphragm breathing, but must be repeated until it becomes a natural mode of breathing once again. Breathing exercises are techniques to strengthen the diaphragm and promote proper diaphragmatic breathing. These techniques should be taught and practiced each day at home. They may be combined with general exercises for the arms, legs, and abdomen. Proper application and continued use of these breathing methods result in improved ventilating patterns, improved posture, and improved diaphragm usage. This all leads to less muscular work for adequate physiologic ventilation.[485]

Exercise Programs

Exertion requires muscular work. Oxygen metabolism is required to produce the energy for muscular work.[52] The more in shape a muscle, the less oxygen it consumes for a given amount of work.[196, 472] If oxygen is not available, anaerobic metabolism takes place (see Chapter 6). This produces lactic acidosis, which creates muscle cramping, increased heart rate, and dizziness. The COPD patient has difficulty delivering oxygen to the blood and also has muscles that are out of shape because of the lack of use. Therefore, the limited amount of oxygen available produces little muscular work for the muscular oxygen demands.

An exercise program is instituted to get the muscles back in shape.[486] To speed the progress of the exercise program, the patient may be given oxygen to breathe while exercising. The goal of such an "oxygen exercise" program is to get the patient to do at room air what he can barely do initially breathing oxygen. At the end of the program, the patient usually does not need oxygen to exercise. Oxygen exercise programs seem to be one of the most successful parts of a pulmonary rehabilitation program.[486] The emotional and psychologic uplift of being able to walk upstairs and be active again is of great benefit to the patient. At the present time it is impossible to separate the true physiologic methods of improvement from the psychologic – an academic question at best. Well-designed and executed oxygen exercise programs can be extremely helpful.[196]

Summary

Our experience with pulmonary rehabilitation for 7 years has proved simultaneously exhilarating and depressing. This ambivalence is due to the realization that *many* patients can be significantly helped! However, is that gain reasonably balanced against the failures and fantastic costs in money, personnel, and energy to properly run such a program? Investigations are underway to attempt to answer this perplexing question.

Continuous Home Oxygen Therapy

Despite advances in technology, the continuous use of ambulatory oxygen is clumsy and expensive. It signifies a constant reminder to the patient that he is, in fact, a pulmonary cripple. It is always beneficial to avoid the use of continuous oxygen therapy during periods when it may be psychologically depressing to the patient. It is the authors' opinion that continuous home oxygen therapy is grossly misused and overused in stabilized COPD.

The indications for continuous oxygen therapy are based on specific physiologic needs:[487] (1) The patient who manifests pulmonary hypertension caused by severe hypoxemia is greatly relieved by oxygen therapy. Decreasing the pulmonary artery pressures is beneficial in increasing exercise tolerance and in decreasing the work of the heart. Patients who demonstrate pulmonary hypertension relieved by oxygen therapy benefit from home oxygen therapy. (2) Severe secondary polycythemia may be well controlled by continuous oxygen therapy.

Some patients may require home oxygen for maintaining an exercise program; some may require supplementation for meaningful ambulation. Oxygen should be used where indicated and sensible. It must not be used as a "crutch" or "easy out" by the physician.

33 • ASPIRATION PNEUMONITIS AND SMOKE INHALATION

Aspiration Pneumonitis

ASPIRATION PNEUMONITIS is a major cause of anesthetic mortality.[488] Most of the contributing factors involved in causing anesthetized and postanesthetic patients to be at high risk for aspiration are present in the critically ill (e.g., obtundation, unconsciousness, diminishment of airway protective reflexes. Although the acute respiratory care patient is recognized to be at high risk for aspiration, few data regarding the incidence or impact on morbidity and mortality are available. Suffice it to say that *prevention* of aspiration and appropriate support for aspiration pneumonitis must be prime requisites in acute respiratory care.

Confusion reigns among respiratory care clinicians concerning the definition, clinical course, and preferred treatment of aspiration pneumonitis. The following discussion is designed to provide the respiratory care practitioner with a basis for establishing general rationale for assessment and treatment of aspiration pneumonitis. For further reading, excellent review articles are available.[489, 490, 491]

Defining Aspiration Pneumonitis

Inhalation of pharyngeal contents into the pulmonary tree is defined as *aspiration*. Inhalation of gastric content is referred to as *gastric aspiration*. When particulate matter (solid material) is aspirated, immediate attempts at removal (i.e., bronchoscopy) are indicated. However, the vast majority of gastric aspiration in critically ill patients involves *fluid stomach contents* and, therefore, the remainder of this discussion will assume that particulate matter has not been aspirated.

Inflammation is a generalized tissue reaction to stress from varying agents. *Chemical pneumonitis* is a pulmonary inflammatory reaction secondary to the stress of noxious substances. *Aspiration pneumonitis is most logically defined as chemical pneumonitis resulting from aspiration of fluid gastric content.*

Pathophysiology of Aspiration Pneumonitis

The effects of acid insufflation into the tracheobronchial tree were first described in 1920[492] and have since been voluminously studied.

491

The acute inflammatory reaction begins within several hours and increases in severity until a peak is reached between 12 and 36 hours following aspiration. Assuming that bacterial superinfection does not occur, the inflammation decreases to clinical insignificance by 72 hours post aspiration.

The primary irritant is hydrogen ion concentration.[493] In dog models, pH above 2.50 causes inflammation similar to that from water aspiration, whereas pH below 2.50 causes severe reactions.[494] Although pH governs the *severity* of inflammation, it does not alter its time course. Enzymatic actions of gastric contents have little or no affect on the chemical pneumonitis.

In man, aspiration of fluid with pH below 1.50 results in chemical pneumonitis throughout the entire lung. In dogs, aspiration of fluid below 2.5 in volumes greater than 0.4 ml/kg will produce reactions at the surface of the lung within 12–18 seconds and cause atelectasis at the surface of the lung within 3 minutes.[495]

Diagnosis of Aspiration

Massive aspiration is rarely difficult to diagnose; however, most cases of aspiration are less than massive and are seldom immediately insulting to the patient. Therefore, the diagnosis must be made by clinical evaluations carried out at the time of suspected aspiration. *Regurgitation* is the backward flow of fluid in a physiologic system. *Vomiting* (active regurgitation) involves reverse peristalsis, whereas *passive regurgitation* occurs without peristalsis and may be caused solely by excess pressure in the stomach. *Active vomiting need not be present for aspiration to take place.*[496]

Much credence must be given to clinical observations made at the time of suspected aspiration. Such occurrences are most often associated with an episode of vomiting or severe coughing, except in the comatose patient in whom passive regurgitation and "silent" aspiration are common.[497] Following are general guidelines for clinically evaluating the possibilities of aspiration:

1. The more alert and awake the patient, the more unlikely that aspiration has occurred. The alert patient has intact protective airway reflexes that may cause coughing, breath-holding, cyanosis, and extreme distress. These "protective" mechanisms must never be confused with aspiration; their presence reduces the likelihood of aspiration.

2. Simple testing of the gag, laryngeal, and tracheal reflexes can provide excellent corroborative evidence in evaluating the probability of aspiration.

3. The pH of the suspected aspirant should be assessed along with an estimation of the quantity of aspirant.

4. Clinical evidence of acute respiratory distress following suspected aspiration is highly suggestive. However, the absence of respiratory distress does *not* rule out aspiration.

5. Physical examination of dependent lung segments may reveal coarse rhonchi; however, their absence does *not* rule out aspiration.

6. X-ray evidence of localized infiltrate and/or atelectasis in appropriate lung segments is suggestive of aspiration; however, a negative chest film does *not* rule out aspiration.

In summary, the diagnosis of aspiration depends upon clinical evaluation of the suspected event, plus careful physical examination and chest x-ray interpretation. Although positive findings help to make the diagnosis, their absence never rules out the possibility of aspiration.[488]

Clinical Assessment

The severity of chemical inflammation and the resultant physiologic stress depend primarily on three factors: (1) general patient status, (2) quantity of aspirant, and (3) acidity of aspirant.

General Patient Status

The degree of physiologic stress imposed by an inflammatory reaction is greatly dependent on the reserves of the system prior to insult. Obviously, a small degree of chemical pneumonitis may be quite significant in an elderly or debilitated patient, whereas a great degree of chemical pneumonitis may be less significant in a young, previously healthy patient. The clinical judgment determining the prognosis of an aspiration partly depends on clinical assessment of the patient's over-all status.

Quantity of Aspirant

Large quantities of aspirant will cause obstruction and mucosal irritation regardless of pH. The degree of insult caused by non-acid fluid will depend primarily on the amount of aspirant (see Near Drowning in this chapter).

Acidity of the Aspirant

A pH below 2.50 will cause widespread chemical pneumonitis throughout the lung regardless of the volume aspirated.[498]

Clinical Pathophysiology

Much clinical information has been gathered concerning aspiration pneumonia since Mendelsohn first described the clinical syndrome in 1946.[499] The tachycardia, dyspnea, cyanosis, and expiratory rhonchi described by Mendelsohn are present with *severe* aspiration pneumonia; however, more subtle presentation is the rule.

Inflammation of the Tracheobronchial Tree

The parenchymal inflammatory reaction of gastric aspiration ensues within 0–5 hours.[500] However, the damage to the pulmonary mucosa occurs on contact. This mucosal irritation may elicit a severe *bronchorrhea*, which may be confused with pulmonary edema of cardiac origin. Much of the initial dyspnea and responsive hypoxemia of aspiration pneumonitis is probably secondary to the severe bronchorrhea and bronchospasm that occurs *immediately* following aspiration. Dilution or lavage of the aspirated substance is generally considered ineffective and, in fact, may be harmful.[501]

Parenchymal Effects

Although the aspirant seldom physically reaches the alveolar epithelium, parenchymal reaction is severe when aspirant pH is less than 2.50. Parenchymal effects are primarily those of abnormal alveolar type II cells' metabolic activity,[502] causing a decrease in surfactant production and rapid interstitial exudation and edema. The resulting decreased compliance is mainly responsible for the increased work of breathing, tachypnea, and refractory hypoxemia of severe aspiration pneumonitis.

Hemodynamics

Immediate decreases in systemic blood pressure are common; however, pulmonary wedge pressures and central venous pressure are *not* elevated.[503] It appears that most of the "left heart failure" classically described following aspiration is, in fact, bronchorrhea with resultant dyspnea, tachypnea, and rales that mimic heart failure.

Arterial Blood Gas Abnormalities

Hypoxemia is usually present. Initially the hypoxemia is secondary to bronchospasm and bronchorrhea (responsive) but eventually becomes secondary to decreased FRC and interstitial edema (refractory). Hypercarbia is a dire occurrence and necessitates immediate ventilatory support.

Treatment of Aspiration Pneumonitis

Assurance of an adequate airway and proper oxygenation are the hallmarks of supportive therapy, along with proper fluid, electrolyte, and acid-base balance.

Respiratory Therapy

All patients with aspiration pneumonitis require *oxygen therapy*. The establishment of an artificial airway may be indicated for (1) airway protection, (2) bronchial hygiene, or (3) airway pressure therapy. Positive-pressure ventilation is often necessary, and some evidence exists that PEEP therapy may be beneficial in decreasing morbidity and mortality.[504, 505]

Antibiotic Therapy

Despite the inability to predict bacterial superinfection or what organisms will be involved, many investigators recommend giving prophylactic antibiotics.[506, 507] At best, the effectiveness of such therapy is doubtful. Retrospective studies have revealed little, if any, decrease in the incidence of bacterial superinfection and a preponderance of gram-negative organisms, which often lead to severe, necrotizing pneumonitis with sepsis.[496, 503] In general, antibiotic therapy is contraindicated as a *prophylactic* measure in aspiration pneumonitis.

Steroid Therapy

Although controversial and without conclusive data, the use of corticosteroids in aspiration pneumonitis appears to be rational if several factors are recognized: (1) high doses of steroids administered for less than 48 hours do *not* appear to result in undesirable effects; (2) severe acid aspiration has a very significant mortality, which no therapeutic regimen has been conclusively documented to alter; (3) no experimental evidence is available to dispute the effectiveness of steroids in acid aspiration of pH fluid above 2.50 (a common occurrence in clinical medicine);[508] (4) theoretic considerations of steroids decreasing inflammatory response are substantial; and (5) the administration of steroid anti-inflammatory agents *prior* to onset of a chemical inflammatory process is widely accepted as beneficial.[509, 510]

We recommend that dexamethasone (Decadron) be administered immediately after aspiration. If effective at all, it must be administered in the first 2 hours following aspiration. For the average-sized adult, 20 mg of dexamethasone should be given by intravenous "push" as soon as possible following aspiration. This should be followed by 10 mg of dexamethasone given intravenously at 4- to 6-hour intervals for the first 24–36 hours. If there is no clinical evidence of chemical pneumonitis at the end of 24 hours, steroid therapy should be discontinued. In all patients in whom there are no complications, steroid therapy is discontinued by 48 hours. Experience has shown that there is no need to taper this short-term steroid therapy.

Near Drowning

It is estimated that over 8,000 deaths occur each year from drowning.[511] Near drowning is the event of water submersion after which the victim arrives at a hospital in a "potentially" salvageable condition. Approximately 15% of near drowning victims develop intensive laryngospasm that prevents water aspiration. Such *"dry" drowning* is a true asphyxiation without pulmonary damage.[512] Recovery is excellent if the patient is rescued and treated prior to irreversible hypoxic brain damage.

Eighty-five percent of near drowning victims have significant water aspiration. It is estimated that 90% of these will survive if rescue has occurred prior to hypoxic brain damage and if appropriate therapy is administered.[513]

Pathophysiologic events in human near drowning are (1) hypoxemia; (2) metabolic acidosis; (3) *minimal* changes in electrolytes and hemoglobin; (4) hypovolemic shock in some salt water drownings; and (5) pulmonary edema. It must be realized that many near drownings are associated with alcohol or drug ingestion and that gastric aspiration may have occurred.[514]

A *post-immersion syndrome* may occur within 24 hours: (1) respiratory distress, (2) hypoxemia, (3) pulmonary edema, (4) fever, and (5) leukocytosis. These appear *after* the patient is initially judged clinically stable and unaffected by the near drowning incident. Near drowning patients must be observed in the hospital for 24 hours. It appears safe to state that all patients who have a normal admission chest x-ray should survive with proper therapy.[514]

Fresh water aspiration appears to be of greater consequence than salt water aspiration, since fresh water appears to directly affect alveolar type II cell function. This problem appears to respond to appropriate PEEP therapy.[514]

Metabolic acidosis must be vigorously treated with sodium bicarbonate. Hemodynamic monitoring is important in patients with limited cardiovascular reserves. Prophylactic antibiotics and steroid therapy appear to have little, if any, indication or benefit.

Carbon Monoxide Poisoning

Carbon monoxide (CO) is a natural byproduct of red blood cell destruction and normally is attached to about 1% of the available oxygen-binding sites of hemoglobin.[515] Carbon monoxide attached to hemoglobin is known as carboxyhemoglobin (COHb). Heavy cigarette smokers often have greater than 5% carboxyhemoglobin levels.

Heavy exposure to smoke or auto exhaust may result in carboxyhemoglobin levels well in excess of 25%,[516] a clinical circumstance referred to as *carbon monoxide poisoning*. Such a diagnosis is made primarily by history of exposure and measurement of COHb levels. Patients typically manifest a cherry red color, tachypnea, and tachycardia.

Pathophysiology

Carbon monoxide has an affinity for the hemoglobin molecule that is 200–250 times greater than that of oxygen. A carbon monoxide partial pressure of less than 1 mm Hg may result in a carboxyhemoglobin level of 40% or greater.[517] The rate of dissociation of carbon monoxide from hemoglobin is *extremely* slow; thus, carbon monoxide poisoning produces an acute decrease in blood oxygen content that is not readily reversed. In addition, high levels of COHb cause the oxyhemoglobin dissociation curve to shift markedly to the left, i.e., the greater the concentration of carboxyhemoglobin, the greater the hemoglobin affinity for oxygen molecules. In practical terms, this means that tissue will be better oxygenated when 50% of the hemoglobin is absent (anemia) than when 50% of the hemoglobin has carbon monoxide attached.[517]

Acute carbon monoxide poisoning may result in varying degrees of brain cell hypoxia. All therapeutic measures must be instituted as soon as possible to minimize the hypoxic effect of CO poisoning. There are no known *direct* toxic effects of carbon monoxide.

Respiratory Care

Primarily the CO-poisoned patient must be removed from the atmosphere containing the carbon monoxide while airway patency and ventilation are assured. Secondly, the patient must receive 100% oxygen as soon as possible. The high blood oxygen tension will speed the dissociation of carbon monoxide from hemoglobin. In our experience, the COHb level decreases by one half each hour that 100% oxygen is given, as long as the cardiopulmonary system is stable. The increasing oxygen content of arterial blood greatly accelerates the clearance of carbon monoxide from hemoglobin. It is not acceptable to give low concentrations of oxygen while the COHb level is over 20%. When *immediately* available, the hyperbaric chamber appears appropriate for severe CO poisoning.

Smoke Inhalation

Exposure to fire and smoke is not an uncommon occurrence in urban areas, and the respiratory care practitioner must be aware of immediate supportive steps. *Carbon monoxide exposure must be assumed!*

There are two concerns in the patient who has been exposed to smoke and heat: (1) inhalation of incomplete products of combustion (carbon particles) and toxic fumes, both of which lead to chemical tracheobronchitis and pneumonia; and (2) thermal injury, which leads to mucosal sloughing, bronchorrhea, and pulmonary edema.[518]

Carbonaceous Inhalation

Carbonaceous inhalation is diagnosed by the presence of carbon particles in the mouth, pharynx, and sputum. The foreign body reaction, in addition to toxic fume inhalation, may lead to a chemical pneumonitis similar to that discussed for aspiration pneumonia. Prime attention must be given to airway patency, ventilation, and oxygenation. *Steroid therapy* is indicated, along with oxygen and bronchial hygiene therapy. Prophylactic antibiotics are contraindicated.

Thermal Injury

Immediate concern in thermal injury must be for glottic and laryngeal edema leading to airway obstruction. Tracheostomy is often needed and may be preferable to an endotracheal tube, which may do significant damage to the already traumatized glottis.

Pulmonary edema is the most severe sequela of thermal lung injury and is usually fatal. Supportive care is primarily airway care and airway pressure therapy.

34 • COMMON ENTITIES IN ACUTE RESPIRATORY CARE

The Unconscious Patient

COMMON TO ALL patients with loss of consciousness is the danger of *inadequate* airway patency, *inadequate* airway protective mechanisms, *inadequate* lung inflation, and *inadequate* arterial oxygenation. Thus, all acutely unconscious patients should have thorough and serial respiratory care evaluations to *prevent* these problems rather than to have them recognized in extremis. *Upper airway obstruction* is a very common phenomenon that is potentially life threatening; its recognition and therapy are discussed in Chapter 15. *Obtundation of airway protective mechanisms* may lead to aspiration, a significant threat to the survival of the unconscious patient (see Chapter 33). The airway protective reflexes are discussed in Chapter 15.

The unconscious patient tends to have shallow respirations and a loss of chest wall tone. This leads to acute decreases in functional residual capacity (see Chapter 20) with eventual atelectasis and pneumonia. Appropriate assessment of ventilatory reserve (see Chapter 19) is essential in these patients in order to support ventilation and oxygenation prior to the need for resuscitation. All acutely unconscious patients demand the skills and expertise of the respiratory care practitioner!

Drug Overdose

The overwhelming majority of intentional overdose in the United States is with sedative, hypnotic, and tranquilizing drugs.[519] If there is no underlying terminal disease and the patient arrives in the hospital without hypoxic brain damage, survival should be better than 90%.[371] However, mortality as high as 25% is still reported; therefore, careful management is crucial. Numerous studies throughout the world consistently intimate one obvious fact: no single form of treatment is more important to survival than appropriate airway management and cardiopulmonary support.

Airway protection is the hallmark of care for these patients. Tracheal intubation is indicated when airway protection is questionable. We follow a simple principle: the patient who will allow laryngoscopic visualization should be intubated. If gastric lavage is contemplated and obtundation is present, intubation of the trachea should be accomplished. However, the benefit of gastric lavage is questionable, since at best it may accomplish a lessened comatose period in conjunction with adequate supportive care. No evidence exists that gastric lavage decreases mortality. In fact, it appears that it may decrease morbidity in only 10% of patients.[371] Our recommendation is that gastric lavage be carried out on patients who are fully alert and awake or already intubated. There appears to be little justification for lavage if intubation is required only for the express purpose of gastric lavage.

Once airway care is instituted, airway pressure therapy, bronchial hygiene therapy, and cardiovascular supportive therapy are applied as indicated. Extubation should be accomplished only after the patient has fulfilled the necessary criteria (see Chapter 16) for *at least* 2 hours. All attempts must be made to document the drugs ingested so that the C.N.S. depressive course and other organ system toxicities may be anticipated.

In our experience, fewer than 5% of overdose patients manifest hypotension or myocardial irritability when adequate ventilation, oxygenation, acid-base balance, and fluid therapy are provided.

Increased Intracranial Pressure

Prevention of brain hypoxia is the essence of acute respiratory care. Oxygenation of brain depends on maintaining adequate cerebral perfusion. Regional blood flow through the brain is a complex subject, particularly in the presence of local disease or injury. However, autoregulatory mechanisms in the brain are excellent and provide reasonably adequate regional blood flow under all but the most severe stresses.

When cerebral blood flow is threatened due to increased intracranial pressure (ICP), it is reasonable to conceive of the problem on a

TABLE 34-1.—MAJOR FACTORS AFFECTING
CEREBRAL BLOOD FLOW

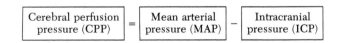

| Cerebral perfusion pressure (CPP) | = | Mean arterial pressure (MAP) | − | Intracranial pressure (ICP) |

1. ICP >20 mm Hg is harmful to brain cell survival regardless of cerebral blood flow.
2. Globally, a CPP >60 mm Hg assures adequate cerebral blood flow.

Normal MAP = 90 mm Hg (80–100); normal ICP = <10 mm Hg.

"global" basis, assuming that autoregulatory mechanisms are functioning. On this assumption, the major relationship regarding cerebral blood flow is illustrated in Table 34 – 1. Thus, when one is confronted with a patient with increased intracranial pressure, it is essential to provide excellent arterial oxygenation and optimal mean arterial pressure (MAP). Although pharmacologic means of decreasing ICP are available (e.g., diuretics, barbiturates), an immediate and widely used method is acute alveolar hyperventilation.

Acute Alveolar Hyperventilation

Sudden increases in C.S.F. and brain pH result in *cerebral arteriolar constriction*. Sudden changes in C.S.F. and brain pH are usually secondary to sudden changes in arterial P_{CO_2}, since the CO_2 will rapidly equilibrate between blood and C.S.F. The blood brain barrier does not allow bicarbonate ions to readily equilibrate, leaving the C.S.F. with little buffering capacity. For this reason, the CO_2 change in C.S.F. results in a greater pH change than occurs in blood. Thus, *a sudden drop in arterial P_{CO_2} will decrease the vascular space (vasoconstriction) within the cranium and thereby tend to relieve the acutely increased intracranial pressure due to cerebral edema.*[520, 521] This should result in an overall improvement in cerebral perfusion.

As effective and dramatic as alveolar hyperventilation is in decreasing acute increases in ICP, it is time limited! *Maintaining alveolar hyperventilation for over 24 hours will result in C.S.F. equilibration in both pH and volume.*[522] Therefore, ICP will be returned to prehyperventilation status even if the arteriolar constriction persists.

We believe that mechanical hyperventilation for purposes of decreasing intracranial pressure should be limited to short periods (definitely less than 24 hours). After the acute emergency is dealt with, ICP should be controlled by other means and eucapneic ventilation restored. In our experience this has the advantages of (1) avoiding the necessity for "stepwise" increases in P_{CO_2} when ventilator discontinuance is desired;[371] (2) avoiding the metabolic acidosis resulting from a long-standing respiratory alkalosis; (3) providing an immediate decompression therapy if ICP suddenly rises during the illness; and (4) providing maximal cerebral blood flow.

Measurement of intracranial pressure has proved valuable in allowing diuretic and barbiturate therapy to control ICP. Under these circumstances the ventilation should be maintained eucapneic and airway suction accomplished only with maximal sedation. Adequate cardiovascular and pulmonary support is paramount (see Sections VI and VII).

Brain Resuscitation and Brain Death

Much investigation and concern have recently been devoted to the subject of brain resuscitation following hypoxic insult, head trauma, and non-global C.N.S. disease. Discussion of the present state of knowledge is not within the scope of this text. The reader is referred to recent literature for this information.[522, 523]

Acute High Spinal Cord Injury

With improvement in emergency evacuation systems, paramedic on-the-scene supportive care, and improved respiratory care capability in community hospitals, the short-term survival of patients with high cervical spinal cord trauma is dramatically increasing. Although the prospect for long-term survival and rehabilitation is excellent for paraplegics, the outlook for quadraplegics is far less encouraging.

Nerve roots constituting the phrenic nerve are mainly from C3, C4, and C5, although some fibers from C2 and C6 usually are present. Cervical trauma often results in spinal cord edema and vasoconstriction, rendering the phrenic nerve inoperable for several days to several weeks. It is not uncommon for a patient with cervical trauma to present as a total quadraplegic (ventilator dependent) and regain phrenic nerve function within several weeks. Thus, initial aggressive support must be given these patients because the extent of permanent damage is not clear for several weeks post trauma.

Our 5-year experience in a regional trauma center for spinal cord injury has allowed us to develop the following clinical guidelines for respiratory care of high cervical cord injury:

1. Dependence upon ventilatory assistance after the patient's neck is stabilized carries a totally dismal 2-year post-hospital survival rate and essentially prevents meaningful rehabilitation. Thus, all attempts must be made to wean the patient from the ventilator!

2. In the first several months, maintenance of an adequate *nutritional* status is paramount. Early nasogastric feedings, gastrostomy, or intravenous hyperalimentation is essential!

3. Tracheostomy should be performed at the earliest elective time.

4. "Stabilized" spontaneously breathing quadraplegics with vital capacities of less than 10 ml/kg (normal body weight) should be maintained with a tracheal button or fenestrated tube (see Chapter 16) for the first year or until the rehabilitative process is near completion. Our experience is that these patients are severely stressed when confronted with minor infections. Without an available suction port, their incidence of acute respiratory failure (ARF) in the first year approaches

100%; with the suction port available, the incidence of ARF appears less than 50%.

5. Following stabilization of the acute injury, aggressive *prophylactic* bronchial hygiene therapy is disappointing. Incentive spirometry does as well prophylactically as aggressive chest physical therapy (CPT), aerosol, and IPPB therapy; however, these methods are very effective for *therapeutic* indications, e.g., atelectasis, pneumonia and secretions (see Chapter 14).

Blunt Chest Trauma

The thorax is commonly involved in trauma.[524] The patient often presents with minimal initial findings despite significant injury. Thoracic trauma is notorious for hiding life-threatening pathology, since symptoms are commonly insidious in onset. Often the trauma is not recognized until cardiopulmonary collapse occurs. In addition, chest wall trauma can lead to significant pulmonary pathology several days following the traumatic episode. It is incumbent upon the respiratory care practitioner to be alert for signs of thoracic trauma and pursue clinical evaluation of these with a high index of suspicion.

Chest Wall Splinting

Nonpenetrating wounds to the thorax cause bruising and possibly rib fracture, which result in pain on movement of the chest wall. In response, a reflex tightening of thoracic musculature ensues to avoid painful chest wall movement. This phenomenon is referred to as chest wall splinting. Such immobilization leads to poor ventilation of lung in the area of splinting and ultimately may result in atelectasis and pneumonia.

Chest wall splinting is seldom significant in otherwise healthy patients. In such circumstances, the splinting may be partially relieved by mild analgesics. With encouragement, the patient will cough and breathe deeply to aid prevention of atelectasis. If atelectasis results or the patient experiences intolerable pain, intercostal nerve block or thoracic epidural analgesia may be indicated to relieve the pain and allow respiratory therapy techniques to be applied. It should be remembered that uncomplicated rib fractures heal within several weeks and present no particular life-threatening problem. *Don't overtreat chest wall splinting!*

Flail Chest

Double fracture of three or more adjacent ribs *may* result in chest wall instability that prevents subatmospheric pressures from developing in the pleural space; i.e., the chest wall will "sink in" (flail) during inspiration. In respiratory care, the term flail chest implies an unstable area of the thoracic cage in which paradoxical chest wall movement results in the underlying lung receiving inadequate ventilation. Thus, the diagnosis of flail chest in respiratory care is made by clinical observation only! The chest x-ray may document the fractures, but chest wall splinting may well lend stability to the area. *The only way the diagnosis of flail chest requiring respiratory care support can be made is by observation of the unstable paradoxical chest wall.*

Pathophysiology

The pleural space underlying the unstable chest wall may not maintain appropriate inspiratory subatmospheric pressures, with the underlying lung becoming unventilated while perfusion continues. The resultant "shunt" will lead to arterial hypoxemia, which may stimulate increased ventilatory efforts. These increased efforts may result in greater flailing; thereby, the vicious cycle of increasing atelectasis is established and perpetuated. The atelectasis eventually leads to pneumonia.

When a flail chest occurs in conjunction with *lung contusion*, the two processes are synergistic. Although they often occur together,[525] we shall discuss them separately.

Small areas of flail will seldom prove of life-threatening consequence to otherwise healthy patients; however, *large* areas of flailing will lead to significant morbidity and mortality.[526] Prior to modern respiratory care, the mortality of a unilateral severe flail chest was greater than 80%; with ventilator stabilization, the *survival* rate is believed greater than 80%.[527] Reported higher mortality is apparently secondary to C.N.S. and abdominal trauma, not due to the flail chest.[524, 528]

However, *morbidity* of flail chest has not been decreased as dramatically as has the mortality.[529] This is partially due to the fact that positive-pressure ventilation in a patient who has suffered chest trauma runs a high risk of causing pneumothorax.[530] The medical judgment must be made as to whether the risk of atelectasis and pneumonia is greater than the risk of pneumothorax.

Treatment

Small areas of flailing may be successfully treated with adequate pain relief and bronchial hygiene therapy to assure expansion of the underlying lung. This course of therapy requires good pain relief and a cooperative patient. Significant areas of flailing require both stabilization of the chest wall to allow bone healing and prevention of atelectasis. In our opinion controlled volume ventilation best accomplishes these goals, since in our experience, a *severe* flail chest requires a *minimum* of 5 days of mechanical ventilation to allow adequate rib stabilization. However, other authors report good results with augmented ventilation and PEEP.[525]

Improper or over-vigorous closed chest massage may result in "sternal flailing." This seldom requires volume ventilation for stabilization and must not be a criterion for "routine" ventilator care. Such a patient should be evaluated for ventilatory support the same as any other patient (see Chapter 22).

Lung Contusion

Although lung contusion is not clearly defined, it generally refers to the phenomenon of interstitial pulmonary bleeding following chest trauma.[531] Lung contusion rarely produces symptomatology in the first few hours following trauma, but may result in significant hypoxemia and decreased compliance in the first several days following chest trauma.[533] Severe lung contusion presents on chest x-ray as a totally "white lung" and has been referred to as the "white lung syndrome."[534]

When lung contusion is unilateral, it seldom causes life-threatening cardiopulmonary embarrassment since the hypoxemia is reasonably supported by appropriate oxygen therapy.[535] When lung contusion is bilateral or unilateral in conjunction with a flail chest, it is often life threatening and requires airway pressure support.[536] The major requirement for airway pressure support appears to be the poor lung compliance.

The combination of lung contusion and flail chest has probably led to overtreatment with volume ventilation and fluids, resulting in a worsening of the contusion.[530] In addition, the patient may no longer need the ventilator for his flail chest when the contusion clears.[525] Sound clinical judgment and serial cardiopulmonary evaluation will provide the proper approach for each patient. Do not overtreat unilateral lung contusion or minimal flail chest!

Pulmonary Embolism

The true incidence of the pulmonary embolic phenomenon is not clear. The general belief that the phenomenon is very common stems from postmortem examinations, which suggest an incidence as high as 60%. These figures may be clinically applicable to elderly, chronically ill, malnourished, and postsurgical patients, but certainly not to the population as a whole.[537]

The diagnosis of pulmonary embolus is uncertain and difficult, and is missed as often as it is misdiagnosed. The problem of diagnosis is compounded in patients manifesting acute respiratory failure.[538] To the respiratory care practitioner, pulmonary embolus remains an enigma and an elusive entity. The basic principles of respiratory care must be applied and the diagnosis of pulmonary embolus never taken as a certainty unless documented by pulmonary angiography.

Status Asthmaticus

Rarely, an adult asthmatic undergoes an acute exacerbation that is unresponsive to aggressive medical therapy. In such a circumstance, the thick mucous secretions have become the major hindrance to maintaining adequate external respiration.[539] The hallmark of status asthmaticus to the respiratory care practitioner is *carbon dioxide retention.* Suggested therapy is as follows:

1. Forty-eight to seventy-two hours of *controlled* positive-pressure ventilation. Very heavy sedation with morphine sulfate is advised to assure unconsciousness and eventual reversibility. Pharmacologic paralyzation is advised to assure optimal chest wall compliance and tolerance of bronchial hygiene therapy.

2. Tapering and discontinuance of bronchodilating drugs during this period, with maintenance of steroid, antibiotic, and fluid therapy.

3. Placement of a large, stable endotracheal tube so that thick tenacious secretions can be mobilized without obstructing the airway.

4. Frequent aerosol and chest physical therapy (CPT). Within 24 hours the mobilization of secretions should become copious.

5. Following 2–3 days of "sleep," bronchial hygiene, and minimal bronchodilating drugs, the patient should be awakened (reverse morphine and relaxant) and extubated immediately.

The disease is usually pharmacologically controllable after these steps; however, occasionally the process must be repeated in 3 to 7 days.

Adult Cystic Fibrosis

The disease entity cystic fibrosis is worthy of special note because it is the major *chronic* lung disease of childhood and young adults. The chronicity involves the need for continuous respiratory care.

Cystic fibrosis (mucoviscidosis) is a triad of (1) chronic pulmonary disease, (2) pancreatic deficiency, and (3) high chloride content in sweat. It may be thought of as a disease of exocrine glands, which includes the mucous and serous glands of the pulmonary mucosa.

The pathology is essentially bronchial obstruction with infection. *Primary involvement of lung parenchyma is minimal.* Autopsy findings typically are bronchiolitis; bronchitis; plugs of tenacious yellow-green mucus clinging to bronchi; bronchiectasis; patchy atelectasis; extensive pneumonitis; and numerous, small pulmonary abscesses.[540]

The clinical course shows repeated pulmonary infections, hypoxemia, and difficulty maintaining bronchial hygiene. This eventually leads to pulmonary hypertension, cor pulmonale, and death. Carbon dioxide retention occurs late in the disease and is commensurate with the onset of heart failure.[541] In our experience, most patients die within 1 year of the onset of significant CO_2 retention.

Respiratory care involves judicious and appropriate use of antibiotic and oxygen therapy. Bronchial hygiene is essential and must involve aggressive chest physical therapy (CPT) techniques in a continuous home program. Ultrasonic aerosol proves beneficial to bronchial hygiene in the vast majority of patients. More controversial is the use of IPPB, mucolytics, and decongestants.

Our experience has shown that continuous home therapy is best composed of ultrasonic aerosol and CPT. Acute infections with impending decompensation must be treated in the hospital with oxygen and antibiotics. During these episodes we believe the cough is best augmented by IPPB; the addition of mucolytics to the aerosol may be beneficial.

Pediatric Respiratory Care

The medical specialty of pediatrics evolved because the small child and especially the infant cannot be treated as "little adults." Separation of pediatric patients into age groups is arbitrary. We shall use the following guidelines: (1) the *newborn* is from birth to 48 hours; (2) the *premature* is a newborn under 5½ pounds; (3) the *neonate* is from 2 days to 2 weeks of age; (4) the *infant* is from 2 weeks to 2 years of age; (5) the *preschooler* is from 2 years to 5 years; and (6) the *child* is from 5

TABLE 34–2.—NORMAL RANGES OF VITAL SIGNS
IN PEDIATRICS

	AGE	WEIGHT (LB)	RR	PULSE	BP (SYSTOLIC)
Newborn . .	First 48 Hours	6–9	40	120–140	50–90
Neonate . . .	2 Days–2 Weeks	6–10	40	120	75–85
Infant	2 Weeks–2 Years	8–25	25–30	120	80–90
Preschool . .	2 Years–5 Years	25–45	20	100–110	80–100
Child.	5 Years–Puberty	45–80	16–20	85–100	120

years to puberty. Table 34–2 shows the normal ranges of vital signs for these age groups.

Although there are differences in respiratory care requirements between the child and the adult, these differences are primarily of technique and behavior rather than physiology. We shall limit our discussion of pediatric respiratory care to the age group under 2 years and compare the significant anatomic, physiologic, and pharmacologic differences with those of the adult. The role of oxygen therapy and bronchial hygiene techniques and the disease entities peculiar to the newborn and the infant will be discussed. The principles of pediatric respiratory intensive care are beyond the scope and intent of this text.[542]

Pulmonary Anatomy

The infant tongue is larger in proportion to the body size than in the adult; therefore, extending the neck and moving the jaw forward may not relieve soft tissue airway obstruction. An oral airway is often necessary. In comparison to the adult, there is a tremendous amount of lymphoid tissue in the pharynx; this, together with a large tongue, makes lymphoid hyperplasia extremely threatening to upper airway patency. The infant epiglottis is extremely large, U-shaped (rather than V-shaped), and very susceptible to trauma. The infant larynx lies higher in the neck than in the adult. The narrowest portion of the larynx and trachea is found at the level of the cricoid ring in the infant as opposed to the glottis in the adult.

All of these factors make the presence of edema or infection serious threats to upper airway patency. The respiratory care practitioner must be aware of the great increase in airway resistance and the increased likelihood of obstruction in the infant.

At birth, the bifurcation of the trachea is at the level of the third thoracic vertebra and by 12 years is at the level of the sixth thoracic vertebra. The tracheal diameter increases about threefold from birth to maturity, being approximately 6 mm in diameter at birth, 12 mm at age 6, and 18 mm at adulthood. Airway infection or inflammation will be of greater significance in the infant than the adult.

The neonate's ribs are more horizontal than the adult's and, therefore, provide little leverage to increase AP diameter. Ventilation is much more dependent upon diaphragmatic breathing in the early years of life than in the adult. In the newborn, the sternum is extremely soft and offers little stability to the chest wall.[543]

Pulmonary Physiology

The neonate is instinctively a nose-breather, breathing through the mouth only when crying. Anatomic deadspace increases steadily as size increases—the rule of 1 ml per pound of body weight holds throughout life. Obviously, absolute increases in deadspace are of greater disadvantage to the smaller patient than the adult.

Metabolism

Infants have higher metabolic rates than adults. Peak metabolic rate is from 6 to 18 months of age and then steadily declines until a second peak at puberty. At birth, the basal oxygen requirement is 6 ml/kg per minute; in the adult, it is 4 ml/kg per minute. Thus, there is a greater oxygen requirement per body mass in the infant than in the adult.

Cardiopulmonary Reserve

An infant has a greater cardiovascular reserve than an adult. The nondiseased infant has a resilient cardiovascular system capable of meeting significant degrees of stress. The pulmonary system has little reserve in the normal infant because of (1) poor stability of the chest wall; (2) a large heart; and (3) a large abdomen pushing up the diaphragm. Infants have little ability to increase tidal volumes in relation to adults; therefore, infants prefer to increase ventilatory rate rather than depth of ventilation. Healthy newborns can double their ventilatory rate from 30–60 per minute without any appreciable difference in the work of breathing.[544]

Surface Areas

The smaller the patient, the greater the *relative* surface area. A newborn has 9 times greater surface area per unit body weight than the adult; by 6 years of age the difference is only twofold. Skin plays an important role in heat regulation and fluid balance. The infant has much more rapid fluid utilization than the adult. Approximately 80% of the newborn's total body weight is water, compared with 55–60% in adults. In the infant, extracellular fluid is the greater part of the total body water; intracellular fluid is the greater part of total body water in the adult. Since it is the extracellular fluid that is rapidly utilized for metabolic function, the infant has a rapid turnover of this fluid, making dehydration and fluid-overloading a significant problem. In addition, decreased bicarbonate and buffer activity makes acid-base balance easier to upset.

Pharmacology

Infants and children do not react to drugs in proportion to age, weight, or any other known relationship. The response to any medication may be different in intensity, action, side-effects, or toxicity. Altered response may be due to the type of medication, the maturity of the central nervous system, the metabolic activity of the child, or enzymatic and endocrine activity. In addition, the effects of many medications vary with the emotional state of the child. It must *never* be assumed that infants should take simply smaller doses of the same medications!

Our guidelines for aerosol *bronchodilators* are as follows: isoproterenol (Isuprel) — maximum infant dose, 0.65 mg per treatment or ⅛ ml of 1:200 isoproterenol diluted in 2.5 ml of normal saline. These dosages are doubled for the older child. For *decongestion* we recommend racemic epinephrine — a maximum of ¼ ml in 2.5 ml of normal saline per treatment. The effectiveness of *mucolytics* in infants is unknown. With the exception of cystic fibrosis or lung abscess there appears to be little rationale for the use of proteolytics or mucolytics. It has been our experience that with the exception of the cystic fibrotic patient, good hydration and aerosol therapy are far superior to the administration of mucolytic agents.

Delivery of Respiratory Therapy

Technical differences in the application of respiratory care exist between the infant and the adult. The sick neonate, premature infant, or small infant requires a temperature-regulated, oxygen-controlled environment. An infant with a respiratory problem needs isolation, warmth, and humidity. It was established many years ago that the lowest mortality in infants is found when they are placed in a neutral-thermal environment. An infant's body metabolism is lowest when the infant's skin temperature is maintained between 36°C. and 37°C. At this temperature the infant has the lowest oxygen consumption. Cooling or overheating will increase body oxygen consumption.[545]

Because the infant must be accessible for routine nursing care and monitoring, it is difficult to control the temperature, oxygen atmosphere, and humidity. Although many pieces of equipment have been introduced, the incubator has proved itself the most dependable. Numerous new techniques, such as heat shields and heat hoods, are being tried and may well prove to be excellent environmental control devices. However, at present, the incubator is still the standard device for infant care.

Oxygen Therapy

Of prime concern to the respiratory care practitioner is maintaining appropriate oxygen therapy for the infant and neonate. There is nothing that can assure consistency except the monitoring of arterial blood gases in coordination with clinical assessment. Most blood gas samples are obtained by capillary stick in the infant.

Masks are poorly tolerated by infants, and temperature and humidity obviously cannot be controlled by mask. Thus, incubators or oxygen tents are still the means of choice for infant oxygen therapy. The premature, newborn, and neonate may require incubator care with supplemental use of oxygen hoods for specifically controlled inspired oxygen concentrations.[542]

Aerosol Therapy

There is more need for therapy techniques that reduce airway hyperemia and edema in the infant than in the adult. Because airway edema is a greater potential insult in the infant, decongestants are more frequently used. Mist-tent therapy is more effective for infants and small children than is mask therapy. Studies on particle deposition in the lower respiratory tract in tent therapy have shown that as little as 5% of the nebulized fluid entering the tent was retained by the subject in the lower respiratory tract; most was deposited in the upper airway and swallowed.[546] It has been suggested that the value of mist-tent therapy in infants is not that of particle deposition, but that of guaranteeing a high humidity in inspired air—thus decreasing the evaporative loss via the respiratory tract and decreasing the likelihood of dry, retained secretions.

Distilled water is used in tent therapy, since salt water solutions are irritating to the eyes and can potentially cause electrolyte imbalance. Perhaps the greatest danger with aerosol therapy is the wetting and initial mobilizing of secretions without sufficient attention to helping the infant mobilize the mucus, either by suctioning or stimulating a cough.

IPPB Therapy

The technical difficulties of applying IPPB therapy in the infant are obvious. However, the main reason for not using IPPB therapy in infants to any great extent is actually not the technical difficulty but the fact that there is little indication for its use. The only advantage of IPPB therapy seems to be the effective delivery of topical vasoconstrictor drugs for decongestion. There is good clinical evidence to support the contention that many patients with infectious croup can be appropriately treated without the need for a tracheostomy or endotracheal intubation when racemic epinephrine is properly delivered by IPPB.[547] In the asthmatic or the cystic fibrotic patient, we have no evidence that there is any advantage to the administration of bronchodilators by IPPB. The administration of bronchodilators is as effective by aerosol spray or intravenous administration as by IPPB.[548] In older children, IPPB therapy can play the same role as in adults by increasing the effectiveness of the cough and improving the distribution of ventilation.

Above all, the general rule for the effectiveness of respiratory therapy techniques is the same in infants as it is in adults. It is dependent upon the skill with which the therapist accomplishes the treatment! Much depends on the cooperation of the patient and this becomes an art in the infant and small child. For example, an infant must be cuddled to become familiar with the therapist before a treatment begins. Therapists must play with the older children and attempt to make the treatment a game. Above all, they must gain the confidence of the child.

Chest Physical Therapy

Chest physical therapy is extremely effective in infants and children once the therapist gains the cooperation and confidence of the patient. Because of the infant's size, manipulation into various drainage positions is easy. Pediatric chest physical therapy techniques are discussed in Chapter 12.

Pediatric Disease Entities

The infant pulmonary system is extremely vulnerable to infection. Forty-two percent (42%) of all hospital admissions for children under the age of 2 are for respiratory problems.[542] There are several disease entities found in the pediatric age group that demand particular attention and skill from the respiratory care practitioner.[549]

Infectious Croup

Laryngotracheal bronchitis is termed infectious croup in the infant.[547] It is an acute inflammation of the upper respiratory tract and large airways. The most common pathogen is parainfluenza virus. It is commonly seen between the ages of 6 months and 3 years, with the infant often exhibiting signs of laryngeal and sublaryngeal obstruction (see Chapter 17).

The inflammatory swelling results in respiratory distress of varying degrees. The infant may exhibit hoarseness; a barking cough; stridor; labored breathing; intercostal, sternal, and substernal retractions. A reasonable differential diagnosis would include diphtheroid croup, foreign body aspiration, retropharyngeal abscess, upper airway trauma, tumor, and congenital malformations.

Aerosol and appropriate oxygen therapy seem to be universally accepted supportive elements in the treatment of croup. Substitution of I.V. for oral fluids is necessary in the more severe cases. The use of antibiotics, steroids, and decongestants is controversial; all have been used under various circumstances but their effects on the mortality and morbidity of croup are unclear. Racemic epinephrine or other appropriate decongestants applied topically have been reported to have dramatic effects. When obstructive symptoms are severe, intubation and tracheostomy may be necessary.

Acute Epiglottitis

Acute epiglottitis is usually caused by the organism *Hemophilus influenzae* and is characterized by an extremely rapid onset of upper airway obstruction. The child is almost always febrile and usually has a low-pitched stridor. As the swollen epiglottis pushes up into the hypopharynx, a complete obstruction may occur. Acute epiglottitis is mainly distinguished from croup by the fact that it is a supraglottic obstruction rather than laryngeal or sublaryngeal. Treatment is primarily that of assuring a patent airway.

Bronchiolitis

Bronchiolitis is a viral infection that causes swelling of bronchiolar mucosa and the production of mucosal exudates, leading to obstruction of the small airways. It affects mainly the 6-month to 2-year age group. The early symptoms are usually a "cold," which may soon be accompanied by a cough, increased restlessness, and a rapid ventilatory rate, which begins to interfere with feedings. Bronchiolar inflammation is probably no more common in the infant than the adult but causes far greater symptomatology because small degrees of inflammation result in great increases in airway resistance in infant tracheobronchial trees.

Supportive treatment is primarily that of appropriate use of oxygen and aerosol therapy. One must be careful in sedating these children because the restlessness may well be due to severe arterial hypoxemia and tissue hypoxia. In a patient who may be fatigued secondary to increased work of breathing, sedation may result in apnea. Rarely, a patient with bronchiolitis will require intubation and mechanical ventilation while the inflammation subsides.

Cystic Fibrosis

Cystic fibrosis is a hereditary disease in which there is dysfunction of all or most of the exocrine glands. Clinical manifestations of the disease include a chronic pulmonary disease, pancreatic insufficiency, and gastrointestinal symptomatology. Interestingly, the electrolytes are elevated in the sweat because of malfunction of these exocrine glands.

The pulmonary disease of cystic fibrosis is characterized by chronic infection resulting in small airway obstruction. Bronchiectasis usually accompanies the bronchitic component. The frequent infections usually precipitate hospital admission.

Children with cystic fibrosis produce copious amounts of thick, tenacious secretions. The respiratory therapy consists of aerosol and chest physical therapy, which must be carried out in the home as well as the hospital. The benefit of nightly mist-tent therapy is widely disputed but seems to be of some benefit for the infant. Oxygen therapy should be administered cautiously and judiciously, as in any chronic obstructive pulmonary disease patient.

Psychologic support of this chronically diseased child and his family is imperative. All attempts should be made to maintain a normal growth process and home environment despite the time-consuming respiratory therapy regimens. In the severely symptomatic cystic child, avoiding pulmonary infection, maintaining adequate nutrition and proper gastrointestinal function are a challenge. The respiratory care practitioner is a vital member of the health care team in the treatment of the patient with cystic fibrosis.

Respiratory Distress of the Newborn
(Idiopathic RDS, Hyaline Membrane Disease)

Acute restrictive disease in the newborn is similar to the adult respiratory distress syndrome (see Chapter 30). It is believed that the lack of surfactant production in infant RDS is due to the immaturity of the alveolar type II cell. The infant lungs become progressively stiffer and the functional residual capacity decreases; lung compliance drops to 20–25% of normal. The work of breathing becomes greater along with a profound hypoxemia that is unresponsive to oxygen therapy. Histologic examination is similar to that for the adult respiratory distress syndrome.

Respiratory distress syndrome occurs in 1% of live births and has an incidence as high as 33% in premature births. The cardinal signs are a ventilatory rate above 60, nasal flaring, intercostal and subcostal retractions. An expiratory "grunt" is common and peripheral edema with systemic hypotension is found frequently. In the early disease state the arterial Pco_2's are below normal with progressive hypoxemia. Carbon dioxide retention is an extremely grave sign and is indicative of a far-advanced RDS. If the infant has an increased Pco_2, he will need ventilator support as well as positive end-expiratory pressure. The chest x-ray findings are similar to those of the adult, showing a granular, honeycomb alveolar pattern with air bronchograms.

The treatment of choice is early intervention with continuous positive-airway pressure (CPAP).[550] Ventilator support is avoided if at all possible because of the high mortality of infants on ventilators. In most cases, early intervention with CPAP will allow reasonable arterial oxygen tensions with inspired oxygen concentrations of less than 60%. It must be remembered that the normal newborn has an arterial Po_2 of between 40 and 70 mm Hg. The establishment of continuous positive airway pressure should (1) increase the functional residual capacity; (2) decrease the work of breathing; and (3) increase arterial oxygenation (Chapter 24). Careful attention must be paid to the infant's thermal environment since the increased oxygen consumption related to sub- or above-normal body temperatures will further compromise the amount of oxygen available to vital organ systems.[551]

Retrolental Fibroplasia

Retrolental fibroplasia occurs primarily in premature infants in whom the retinal arteries have not developed fully. Arterial Po_2's above 150 mm Hg for as little as 4 hours may cause malformation of these arteries and lead to blindness. This malformation is probably due to arteriolar vasoconstriction that occurs with arterial Po_2's above 100 mm Hg.[542] Even after the excessive oxygen therapy has been discontinued, an infant who has been exposed to high Po_2's is not out of danger. As the infant matures, new vessels may grow in a disorderly manner, causing scarring and retinal detachment.

The general rule is to keep the inspired oxygen concentration below 40% in the newborn. With the normal degree of alveolar collapse and poor expansion of newborn lung, an inspired oxygen concentration of 40% will seldom result in arterial Po_2's above 100 mm Hg. (It is desirable to monitor the newborn's blood gases and to keep the arterial Po_2 below 80 mm Hg if long-term oxygen therapy is required.)

Remember, it is not the concentration of oxygen exposed to the eyeball that causes retrolental fibroplasia, but rather the *arterial* Po_2. Infants who are hypoxemic must be provided with oxygen therapy; 100% oxygen administered to a severely cyanotic baby will not result in retrolental fibroplasia because arterial Po_2's are not above 100 mm Hg.

Summary

The basic principles of adult respiratory care may apply to the pediatric patient, with the exception of the techniques and specific differences discussed in this chapter. One must remember that it takes a great deal of training, skill, and knowledge to apply respiratory therapy successfully to the neonate and infant. Those respiratory care practitioners with special interest and training in pediatrics should be the ones involved in the specialized care of these small children.

ANNOTATED GUIDE TO REFERENCES

REFERENCES

1. Ellis, H., and Meharty, M.: *Anatomy for Anaesthetists* (2d ed.; St. Louis: C. V. Mosby Co., 1973).
2. Deweese, D., and Saunders, W.: *Textbook of Otolaryngology* (4th ed.; St. Louis: C. V. Mosby Co., 1973).
3. Gray, H.; Goss, C. M. (ed.): *Gray's Anatomy* (27th ed.; Philadelphia: Lea & Febiger, 1959).
4. Bates, D. V., and Christie, R. V.: *Respiratory Function in Disease* (2d ed.; Philadelphia: W. B. Saunders Co., 1971).
5. Macklem, P., and Mead, J.: Resistance of central and peripheral airways measured by a retrograde system, J. Appl. Physiol. 22:395, 1967.
6. Nunn, J. F.: *Applied Respiratory Physiology: With Special Reference to Anaesthesia* (New York: Butterworth & Co., Ltd., 1969).
7. Niden, A.: Bronchiolar and large alveolar cell in pulmonary phospholipid metabolism, Science 158:1323, 1967.
8. Kapanci, Y., et al.: Ultrastructure and morphometric studies, Lab. Invest. 20:101, 1969.
9. Weibel, E., and Gil, J.: Structure-Function Relationships at the Alveolar Level, in West, J. B. (ed.): *Bioengineering Aspects of the Lung* (New York: Marcel Dekker, 1977), pp. 1–81.
10. Staehlin, L. A.: Structure and function of intercellular junctions, Int. Rev. Cytol. 39:191, 1974.
11. Gil, J., and Reiss, O.: Isolation and characterization of lamellar bodies and tubular myelin from rat lung homogenates, J. Cell Biol. 58:152, 1973.
12. Fisher, A. B.: Functional evaluation of lung mitochondria, Chest 67:245, 1975.
13. Meyer, B. J., et al.: Interstitial fluid pressure. V. Negative pressure in the lungs, Circ. Res. 22:263, 1968.
14. Yoffey, J. M., and Courtice, F. C.: *Lymphatics, Lymph and the Lymphomyeloid Complex* (London: Academic Press, 1970).
15. Kinmonth, J. B., and Taylor, G.: Spontaneous rhythmic contractility in human lymphatics, J. Physiol. (Lond.) 133: 1956.
16. Leak, L. V.: The Fine Structure and Function of the Lymphatic Vascular System, in Das Lymphgefassystem, *Hb. Allg. Pathol.* (Berlin: Springer, 1972).
17. Schipp, R.: In Colleite, J. M., et al. (eds.): *New Trends in Basic Lymphology* (Basil: Brikhauser, 1967), pp 50–57.
18. Schneeberger, E. E., and Karnovsky, M. J.: Substructure of intercellular junctions in free-fractured alveolar-capillary membranes of mouse lung, Circ. Res. 38:104, 1976.
19. Taylor, A. E., and Gaar, K. A.: Estimation of equivalent pore radii of pulmonary capillary and alveolar membranes, Am. J. Physiol. 218:1133, 1970.

20. Slonim, N., et al.: *Respiratory Physiology* (2d ed.; St. Louis: C. V. Mosby Co., 1971).
21. Sorokin, S.: Properties of alveolar cells and tissues that strengthen alveolar defenses, Arch. Intern. Med. 126:450, 1970.
22. Mackenzie, M. B., et al.: The shape of the human adult trachea, Anesthesiology 49:48, 1978.
23. Egan, D.: *Fundamentals of Respiratory Therapy* (2d ed.; St. Louis: C. V. Mosby Co., 1973).
24. Comroe, J. H., Jr.: *Physiology of Respiration* (2d ed.; Chicago: Year Book Medical Publishers, Inc., 1974).
25. Burton, A. C.: *Physiology and Biophysics of the Circulation* (Chicago: Year Book Medical Publishers, Inc., 1965).
26. Wood, J. E.: The venous system, Sci. Am. 218:86, 1968.
27. Conn, H. L., Jr., and Horwitz, O.: *Cardiac and Vascular Disease* (Philadelphia: Lea & Febiger, 1971).
28. Singer, D. H., et al.: Pharmacology of cardiac arrhythmias, Prog. Cardiovasc. Dis. 11:488, 1969.
29. Goldman, M. J.: *Principles of Clinical Electrocardiography* (8th ed.; Los Altos, Calif.: Lange Medical Publications, 1973).
30. Marriott, H. J. L.: *Practical Electrocardiography* (5th ed.; Baltimore: Williams & Wilkins Co., 1974).
31. Braunwald, E., et al.: Mechanics of contraction of the normal and failing heart, N. Engl. J. Med. 277:910, 1967.
32. Starling, E. H.: *Linacre Lecture on the Law of the Heart* (London: Longmans-Green & Co., 1918).
33. Green, H. O.: Circulation: Physical Principles, in Glosser (ed.): *Medical Physics*, Vol. I (Chicago: Year Book Medical Publishers, Inc., 1944).
34. Mountcastle, V. B.: Medical Physiology, vol. 1 (12th ed.; St. Louis: C. V. Mosby Co., 1968).
35. Shapiro, B. A., Harrison, R. A., and Walton, J. R.: *Clinical Application of Blood Gases* (2d ed.; Chicago: Year Book Medical Publishers, Inc., 1977).
36. Clements, J.: Surface tension in lungs, Sci. Am. 207:121, 1962.
37. von Neergaard, K.: Neue Auffassungen über einen Grundbegriff der Atemmechanik. Die Retraktionskaft der Lunge, abhangig von der Oberflächenspannung in der Alveolen, Z. Gesamte Exper. Med. 66:373, 1929.
38. Macklin, C.: The pulmonary alveolar mucoid film and the pneumonocytes, Lancet 1:1099, 1954.
39. Pattle, R.: Surface Tension and the Lining of the Lung Alveoli, in Caro, C. (ed.): *Advances in Respiratory Physiology* (London: Edward Arnold & Co., 1966).
40. Briscoe, W., et al.: Alveolar ventilation at very low tidal volumes, J. Appl. Physiol. 7:27, 1954.
41. Comroe, J. H., et al.: *The Lung* (2d ed.; Chicago: Year Book Medical Publishers, Inc., 1962).
42. Hyatt, R. E., et al.: The flow-volume curve, Am. Rev. Respir. Dis. 107:191, 1973.
43. Cotes, J. E.: *Lung Function: Assessment and Application in Medicine* (3d ed.; Philadelphia: J. B. Lippincott Co., 1975).

44. Bendixen, H. H., et al.: *Respiratory Care* (St. Louis: C. V. Mosby Co., 1965).
45. Petty, T. L.: *Intensive and Rehabilitative Respiratory Care* (Philadelphia: Lea & Febiger, 1971).
46. Earle, R. H.: Evaluation of respiratory dysfunction (lung volumes: expiratory flow rates: distribution of ventilation: gas transfer), Ann. Clin. Lab. Sci. 3:277, 1973.
47. FitzGerald, M. X., et al.: Evaluation of "electronic" spirometers, N. Engl. J. Med. 269:1283, 1973.
48. McIlroy, M., et al.: The effect of added elastic and non-elastic resistances on the pattern of breathing in normal subjects, Clin. Sci. 15:337, 1956.
49. Bartlett, R., et al.: Oxygen cost of breathing, J. Appl. Physiol. 12:413, 1958.
50. Peters, R.: The energy cost (work) of breathing, Ann. Thorac. Surg. 7:51, 1969.
51. Otis, A.: The work of breathing, Physiol. Rev. 34:449, 1954.
52. Simonson, E. (ed.): *Physiology of Work Capacity and Fatigue* (Springfield, Ill.: Charles C Thomas, Publisher, 1971).
53. Campbell, E., et al.: Simple methods of estimating oxygen consumption and efficiency of the muscles of breathing, J. Appl. Physiol. 11:303, 1957.
54. Cherniack, R. M.: The oxygen consumption and efficiency of the respiratory muscles in health and emphysema, J. Clin. Invest. 38:494, 1959.
55. Johansen, S., et al.: Ventilatory reserve in the dog during partial curarization, Anesthesiology 33:322, 1970.
56. Safar, P., et al.: Critical care medicine, Chest 59:535, 1971.
57. Weil, M., et al.: The new practice of critical care medicine, Chest 59:473, 1971.
58. Mushin, W. W., et al.: *Automatic Ventilation of the Lungs* (Oxford: Blackwell Scientific Publications, 1959).
59. Hunter, A. R.: The Classification of Respirators, Anesthesia 16:231, 1961.
60. Kirby, R. R., et al.: Mechanical Ventilation, in Burton, G. B., et al. (ed.): *Respiratory Care: A Guide to Clinical Practice* (Philadelphia: J. B. Lippincott Co., 1977).
61. McPherson, S. P.: *Respiratory Therapy Equipment* (St. Louis: C. V. Mosby Co., 1977).
62. West, J. B.: *Ventilation/Blood Flow and Gas Exchange* (2d ed.; Philadelphia: F. A. Davis Co., 1970).
63. Warrell, D. A., et al.: Pattern of filling in the pulmonary capillary bed, J. Appl. Physiol. 32:346, 1972.
64. Ravin, M. B., et al.: Contribution of thebesian veins to the physiologic shunt in anaesthetized man, J. Appl. Physiol. 21:1148, 1965.
65. Riley, R., and Cournand, A.: Analysis of factors affecting partial pressures of oxygen and carbon dioxide in gas and blood in lung: theory, J. Appl. Physiol. 4:77, 1951.
66. Riley, R. L., and Permutt, S.: Venous admixture component of the $AaPO_2$ gradient, J. Appl. Physiol. 35:430, 1973.
67. Weil, M., et al.: Symposium on critical care medicine, Mod. Med. 39:82, 1971.

68. Buckingham, W. B., et al.: *A Primer of Clinical Diagnosis* (New York: Harper & Row, 1971).
69. Brooke, S. M.: *Integrated Basic Science* (St. Louis: C. V. Mosby Co., 1962).
70. Cherniack, R. M., et al.: *Respiration in Health and Disease* (2d ed.; Philadelphia: W. B. Saunders Co., 1972).
71. Slonim, N. B., et al.: *Pediatric Respiratory Therapy* (New York: Glenn Education Med. Services, Inc., 1974).
72. Squire, L. F.: *Fundamentals of Roentgenology* (Cambridge: Harvard University Press, 1974).
73. Comroe, J. H.: Some Theories of the Mechanism of Dyspnea in Breathlessness, in Howell, J. B. L., and Campbell, E. J. (eds.): *Breathlessness* (Oxford: Blackwell Scientific Publications, 1966).
74. Campbell, E. J.: Breathlessness and Breathing, in Howell, J. B. L., and Campbell, E. J. (eds.): *Breathlessness* (Oxford: Blackwell Scientific Publications, 1966).
75. Howell, J. B. L.: Respiratory Sensations in Pulmonary Disease, in Patter, R. (ed.): *Breathing* (London: J. & A. Churchill, Ltd., 1970).
76. Bendixen, H. H., et al.: Measurement of inspiratory force in anesthetized dogs, Anesthesiology 23:315, 1962.
77. Lavoisier: Sur les altérations qui arrivent à l'air dans plusiers circonstances oú se trouvent les hommes réunis en société, Mémoires de Médecine en Histoire de la Société de Médecine 5:569 (1782–1783, read in 1785).
78. Priestley, J.: *The Discovery of Oxygen,* Alembic Club Reprints (Chicago: University of Chicago Press, 1906).
79. Bert P.: *Barometric Pressure: Researches in Experimental Physiology,* Translated by Hitchcock, M. A., and Hitchcock, F. A. (Columbus, Ohio: Longs College Book Co., 1943).
80. Gilbert, D. L.: The role of pro-oxidants and antioxidants in oxygen toxicity, Radiat. Res. [Suppl.] 3:44, 1963.
81. Chance, B., et al.: Intracellular oxidation-reduction states *in vivo,* Science 137:499, 1962.
82. MacHattie, L., and Rahn, H.: Survival of mice in absence of inert gas, Proc. Soc. Exp. Biol. Med. 104:772, 1960.
83. DuBois, A. B., et al.: Pulmonary atelectasis in subjects breathing oxygen at sea level or at simulated altitude, J. Appl. Physiol. 21:828, 1966.
84. Markello, R., et al.: Assessment of ventilation-perfusion inequalities by arterial-alveolar nitrogen differences in intensive-care patients, Anesthesiology 37:4, 1972.
85. Benesch, R., et al.: Effect of organic phosphates from the human erythrocyte on the allosteric properties of hemoglobin, Biochem. Biophys. Res. Commun. 26:162, 1967.
86. Finch, C., and Lenfant, C.: Oxygen transport in man, N. Engl. J. Med. 286:407, 1972.
87. Bryan-Brown, C. W., et al.: Consumable oxygen: Availability of oxygen in relation to oxyhemoglobin dissociation, Crit. Care Med. 1:17, 1973.
88. Severinghaus, J. W.: Blood gas calculator, J. Appl. Physiol. 21:1108, 1966.
89. Brewer, G. J., and Eaton, J. W.: Erythrocyte metabolism: Interaction with oxygen transport, Science 171:1205, 1971.

90. Laver, M.: An Arthurian legend, Anesthesiology 40:523, 1974.
91. Shappell, S. D., and Lenfant, C.: Adaptive, genetic, and iatrogenic alterations of the oxyhemoglobin-dissociation curve, Anesthesiology 37:127, 1972.
92. Jöbsis, F. F.: Basic processes in cellular respiration, in Fenn, W. O., and Rahn, H. (eds.): Handbook of Physiology (Baltimore: Waverly Press, 1964).
93. Cohen, P.: The metabolic function of oxygen and biochemical lesions of hypoxia, Anesthesiology 37:148, 1972.
94. Robin, E. D.: Dysoxia: Abnormal tissue oxygen utilization, Arch. Intern. Med. 137:905, 1977.
95. Burton, C. W.: Measurement of inspired and expired oxygen and carbon dioxide, Br. J. Anaesth. 41:723, 1969.
96. Elliott, S. E., et al.: A modified oxygen gauge for the rapid measurement of PO_2 in respiratory gases, J. Appl. Physiol. 21:1672, 1966.
97. Dripps, R. D., Eckenhoff, J. E., and Vandam, L. D.: Introduction to Anesthesia (5th ed.; Philadelphia: W. B. Saunders Co., 1977).
98. Wylie, W. D., and Churchill-Davidson, H. C.: A Practice of Anaesthesia (3d ed.; Chicago: Year Book Medical Publishers, Inc., 1978).
99. Smith, J. L.: The influence of pathological conditions on active absorption of oxygen by the lungs, J. Physiol. 22:307, 1897.
100. Smith, J. L.: The pathological effects due to increase of oxygen tension in the air breathed, J. Physiol. 24:19, 1899.
101. Winter, P., et al.: The toxicity of oxygen, Anesthesiology 37:210, 1972.
102. Kistler, G. S., et al.: Development of fine structural damage to alveolar and capillary lining cells in oxygen-poisoned rat lungs, J. Cell Biol. 32: 605, 1967.
103. Kapanci, Y., et al.: Pathogenesis and reversibility of the pulmonary lesions of oxygen toxicity in monkeys. II. Ultrastructural and morphometric studies, Lab. Invest. 20:101, 1969.
104. Yamamoto, E., et al.: Resistance and susceptibility to oxygen toxicity by cell types of the gas blood barrier of the rat lung, Am. J. Pathol. 59:409, 1970.
105. Haugaard, N.: Cellular mechanism of oxygen toxicity, Physiol. Rev. 48: 311, 1968.
106. Davies, H. C., and Davies, R. E.: Biochemical Aspects of Oxygen Poisoning, in Field, J. (ed.): Handbook of Physiology, Sect. 3, vol. 2, Respiration, Am. Physiol. Soc. (Baltimore: Williams & Wilkins Co., 1965).
107. Gerschman, R.: Biological Effects of Oxygen, in Dickens, F., and Neil, E. (eds.): Oxygen in the Animal Organism, (New York: Macmillan Publishing Co., 1964).
108. Ashbaugh, D. G.: Oxygen toxicity in normal and hypoxemic dogs, J. Appl. Physiol. 31:664, 1971.
109. Bean, J. W.: Reserpine, chlorpromazine and the hypothalamus in reactions to oxygen at high pressure, Am. J. Physiol. 187:389, 1956.
110. Suter, P. M., et al.: Shunt, lung volume and perfusion during short periods of ventilation with oxygen, Anesthesiology 43:617, 1975.
111. McAslan, T. C., Matjasko-Chin, J., Turney, S. Z., and Cowley, R. A.: Influence of inhalation of 100% oxygen on intrapulmonary shunt in severely traumatized patients, J. Trauma 13:811, 1973.

112. Douglas, M. E., et al.: Changes in pulmonary venous admixture with varying inspired oxygen, Anesth. Analg. 55:688, 1976.
113. Clark, J. M., and Lambertsen, C. J.: Pulmonary oxygen toxicity: A review, Pharmacol. Rev. 23:37, 1971.
114. Wanner, A.: State of the art: Clinical aspects of mucociliary transport, Am. Rev. Respir. Dis. 116:73, 1977.
115. Ziment, I.: Mucokinesis — The methodology of moving mucus, Respir. Ther. 4:15, 1974.
116. Friedman, M., et al.: A new roentgenographic method for estimating mucous velocity in airways, Am. Rev. Respir. Dis. 115:67, 1977.
117. Dalhamn, T.: Studies on tracheal ciliary activity, Am. Rev. Respir. Dis. 89:870, 1964.
118. Bleeker, J. D., and Hueksma, P. E.: A simple method to measure the ciliary beat of respiratory epithelium, Acta Otolaryngol. 74:426, 1971.
119. Iravani, J., et al.: Mucociliary function in the respiratory tract as influenced by physicochemical factors, Pharmacol. Ther. 2:471, 1976.
120. McDowell, E. M., et al.: Abnormal cilia in human bronchial epithelium, Arch. Pathol. Lab. Med. 100:429, 1976.
121. Lopez-Vidriero, M. T., and Reid, L.: Bronchial mucus in health and disease, Br. Med. Bull. 34:63, 1978.
122. Dulfand, M. J. (ed.): Sputum: Fundamentals and Clinical Pathology (Springfield, Ill.: Charles C Thomas, 1973).
123. Santa Cruz, R., et al.: Tracheal mucus velocity in normal man and patients with obstructive lung; effects of Terbutaline, Am. Rev. Respir. Dis. 109:459, 1974.
124. Ferris, B. G., Jr., and Pollard, D. S.: Effect of deep and quiet breathing on pulmonary compliance in man, J. Clin. Invest. 39:143, 1960.
125. Egbert, L. D., et al.: Intermittent deep breaths and compliance during anesthesia in man, Anesthesiology 24:57, 1963.
126. Leith, D. E.: Cough, Phys. Ther. 48:439, 1968.
127. Camner, P., et al.: Tracheobronchial clearance and chronic obstructive lung disease, Scand. J. Respir. Dis. 54:272, 1973.
128. Sara, C., et al.: Humidification by nebulization, Med. J. Aust. 1:174, 1965.
129. Altschule, M.: Water vapor in the nasopharynx, Med. Sci. Jan., 1966.
130. Benson, D., et al.: Systemic and pulmonary changes with inhaled humid atmospheres, Anesthesiology 30:199, 1969.
131. Allan, D.: Application of the Ultrasonic Nebulizer in Infants and Children, Proceedings of the First Conference on Clinical Applications of the Ultrasonic Nebulizer, Chicago, 1966.
132. Liese, W., et al.: Humidification of respired gas by nasal mucosa, Ann. Otol. Rhinol. Laryngol. 83:330, 1973.
133. Ahlgren, E. W., et al.: Pseudomonas aeruginosa infection potential of oxygen humidifier devices, Respir. Care 22:383, 1977.
134. Pierce, A., et al.: Bacterial contamination of aerosols, Arch. Intern. Med. 131:156, 1973.
135. Whitby, K., et al.: Response of single particle optical counters to non-ideal particles, Environ. Sci. Techn. 1:801, 1967.
136. Vitols, V.: Theoretical limits of errors due to anisokinetic sampling of particulate matter, J. Air Pollut. Control Assoc. 16:79, 1966.
137. Stöber, W., et al.: Size-separating precipitation of aerosols in a spinning spiral duct, Environ. Sci. Techn. 3:1280, 1969.

138. Lovejoy, F., et al.: Aerosols, bronchodilators, and mucolytic agents, Anesthesiology 23:460, 1962.
139. Davies, C., et al.: Impingement of particles on a tranverse cylinder, Proc. R. Soc. Lond. [Biol.] 234:269, 1956.
140. Davies, C., et al.: The trajectories of heavy solid particles in a two dimensional jet of ideal fluid impinging normally upon a plate, Proc. Phys. Soc. B64:889, 1951.
141. Miller, W.: Fundamental principles of aerosol therapy, Respir. Care 17: 295, 1972.
142. Mitchell, R.: Retention of aerosol particles in the respiratory tract, Am. Rev. Respir. Dis. 82:627, 1960.
143. Cheney, F., et al.: Effects of ultrasonically-produced aerosol on airway resistance in man, Anesthesiology 29:1099, 1968.
144. Modell, J.: Experimental studies in chronic exposure to ultrasonic nebulized aerosols, J. Asthma Res. 5:223, 1968.
145. Litt, S. D.: The Babington Nebulizer, a new principle for generation of therapeutic aerosols, Respir. Care 17:414, 1972.
146. Abramson, H. (ed.): *Proceedings of the Second Conference on Clinical Applications of the Ultrasonic Nebulizer* (Somerset, Pa.: DeVilbiss Co., 1968). Also published in J. Asthma Res. 5:213, 1968.
147. Cherniack, R. M.: Intermittent positive pressure breathing in management of chronic obstructive disease: Current state of the art, Am. Rev. Respir. Dis. 110:188, 1974.
148. Pierce, A. K., et al.: Conference on a scientific basis of respiratory therapy, Am. Rev. Respir. Dis. 110, 1974.
149. Murray, J. F.: Review of the state of the art of intermittent positive pressure breathing therapy, Am. Rev. Respir. Dis. 110:193, 1974.
150. Dohi, S., and Gold, M.: Comparison of two methods of postoperative respiratory care, Chest 73:592, 1978.
151. Shim, C., et al.: The effect of inhalation therapy on ventilatory function and expectoration, Chest 73:6, 1978.
152. Noehren, T.: Is positive pressure breathing overrated? Chest 57:507, 1970.
153. Cournand, A., et al.: Physiologic studies of the effects of intermittent positive-pressure breathing on cardiac output in man, Am. J. Physiol. 152:162, 1948.
154. Price, H. L., et al.: Some respiratory and circulatory effects of mechanical respirators, J. Appl. Physiol. 6:517, 1954.
155. Werko, L.: Influence of positive-pressure breathing on the circulation in man, Acta Med. Scand. [Suppl.] 193:1, 1947.
156. Ziment, I.: Why are they saying bad things about IPPB?, Respir. Care 18:677, 1973.
157. Noehren, T. H., et al.: Intermittent positive pressure breathing (IPPB/I) for the prevention and management of postoperative pulmonary complication, Surgery 43:658, 1958.
158. Wilson, R. H. L., et al.: IPPB: A clinical evaluation of its use in certain respiratory diseases, Calif. Med. 87:161, 1957.
159. Terry, P. B., et al.: Collateral ventilation in man, N. Engl. J. Med. 298:10, 1978.
160. Gray, F. D., and MacIver, S. R.: The use of inspiratory positive pressure breathing in cardiopulmonary diseases, Br. J. Tuberc. 52:2, 1958.

161. Sheldon, G. P.: Pressure breathing in chronic obstructive lung disease, Medicine 42:197, 1963.
162. Torres, G., et al.: The effects of intermittent positive pressure breathing on intrapulmonary distribution of inspired air, Am. J. Med. 29:946, 1960.
163. Jameson, G. A., et al.: Some effects of mechanical respirators upon respiratory gas exchange and ventilation in chronic pulmonary emphysema, Am. Rev. Respir. Dis. 80:510, 1959.
164. Torres, G. E., et al.: The effect of IPPB on intrapulmonary mixing in pulmonary emphysema, Clin. Res. 7:303, 1959.
165. Cohen, A. A., et al.: The effect of IPPB and of bronchodilator drugs on alveolar nitrogen clearance in patients with chronic obstructive pulmonary emphysema, Am. Rev. Respir. Dis. 83:340, 1961.
166. Taguchi, J. T.: IPPB: An evaluation of its use in aerosol therapy of chronic pulmonary emphysema, Am. J. Med. Sci. 238:153, 1959.
167. Froeb, H. F.: On the relief of bronchospasm and the induction of alveolar hyperventilation, Dis. Chest 38:483, 1960.
168. Goldberg, I., et al.: The effect of nebulized bronchodilator delivered with or without IPPB on ventilatory function in chronic obstructive emphysema, Am. Rev. Respir. Dis. 91:13, 1965.
169. Leslie, A., et al.: Intermittent positive pressure breathing, J.A.M.A. 160:1125, 1956.
170. O'Donohue, W. J.: Inhalation therapy in modern medicine, South. Med. J. 66:586, 1973.
171. Wu, N., et al.: A comparative evaluation of the effects of intermittent positive pressure breathing alone, nebulized bronchodilators, in patients with chronic bronchopulmonary disease, Clin. Res. Proc. 2:106, 1954.
172. Smart, R. H., et al.: Intermittent positive pressure breathing in emphysema of chronic lung diseases, J.A.M.A. 150:1385, 1952.
173. Cullen, J. H., et al.: An evaluation of the ability of intermittent positive pressure breathing to provide effective hyperventilation in severe pulmonary emphysema, Am. Rev. Tuberc. 76:33, 1957.
174. Armstrong-Davison, M. H.: Treatment of postoperative pulmonary atelectasis, Br. Med. J. 1:468, 1947.
175. Keown, K. K.: A method of removing tracheobronchial secretions by the production of effective coughing, Anesth. Analg. (Cleve.) 39:570, 1960.
176. Radigan, L. R., and King, R. D.: A technique for the prevention of postoperative atelectasis, Surgery 47:184, 1960.
177. Schwartz, S. J., et al.: Deadspace rebreathing tube for prevention of atelectasis, J.A.M.A. 163:1248, 1967.
178. Adler, R. H., et al.: Postoperative rebreathing aid, Am. J. Nurs. 68:1287, 1968.
179. Bartlett, R. H., et al.: The physiology of yawning and its application to postoperative care, Surg. Forum 21:222, 1970.
180. Mead, J., and Collier, C.: Relation of volume history to respiratory mechanics in anesthetized dogs, J. Appl. Physiol. 14:689, 1959.
181. McCutcheon, F. H.: Atmospheric respiration and complex cycles in mammalian breathing mechanisms, J. Cell Physiol. 41:291, 1953.
182. Laver, M. V., et al.: Lung volume compliance with arterial oxygen tensions during controlled ventilation, J. Appl. Physiol. 19:725, 1964.
183. Caro, C. G., et al.: Some effects of restriction of chest cage expansion on

pulmonary function in man: An experimental study, J. Clin. Invest. 39: 573, 1960.

184. Egbert, L. D., and Bendixen, H. H.: Effect of morphine on breathing pattern: A possible factor in atelectasis, J. A.M.A. 188:485, 1964.

185. Bartlett, R. H.: Post-traumatic pulmonary insufficiency, in Cooper, P., and Nyhus, L. (eds.): *Surgery Annual* (New York: Appleton-Century-Crofts, 1971).

186. Lee, A. B., et al.: Effects of abdominal operation on ventilation and gas exchange, J. Natl. Med. Assoc. 61:164, 1969.

187. Bendixen, H. H., et al.: Atelectasis and shunting during spontaneous ventilation in anesthetized patients, Anesthesiology 25:297, 1964.

188. Anthonisen, N. R.: Effect of volume and volume history of the lungs on pulmonary shunt flow, Am. J. Physiol. 207:239, 1964.

189. Ferris, B. G., Jr., and Pollard, D. S.: Effect of deep and quiet breathing on pulmonary compliance in man, J. Clin. Invest. 39:143, 1960.

190. Bartlett, R. H., et al.: The yawn maneuver: Prevention and treatment of postoperative pulmonary complications, Surg. Forum 22:196, 1971.

191. Ward, R. J., et al.: An evaluation of postoperative respiratory maneuvers, Surg. Gynecol. Obstet. 123:51, 1966.

192. Ravin, M. B.: Value of deep breaths in reversing postoperative hypoxemia, NY State J. Med. 66:244, 1966.

193. Thoren, L.: Postoperative pulmonary complications: Observations on their prevention by means of physiotherapy, Acta Chir. Scand. 107:193, 1954.

194. Shapiro, B. A., and Moran, K.: Unpublished data.

195. Eddy, O. M.: The team approach, Respir. Ther. 55, 1974.

196. Frownfelter, D. L.: *Chest Physical Therapy and Pulmonary Rehabilitation* (Chicago: Year Book Medical Publishers, Inc., 1978).

197. Frownfelter, D. L.: Massage in Chest Physical Therapy, in Wood, E. C. (ed.): *Beard's Massage, Principles and Techniques* (2d ed.; Philadelphia: W. B. Saunders Co., 1974).

198. Cochrane, G. M., et al.: Effects of sputum mobilization on pulmonary function, Br. Med. J. 2:1181, 1977.

199. Lagerson, J.: The cough — Its effectiveness depends on you, Respir. Care 18:434, 1971.

200. Barach, A. L., and Segal, M. S.: The indiscriminate use of IPPB, J.A.M.A. 231:1141, 1975.

201. Wilson, R., et al.: Acute respiratory failure: Diagnostic and therapeutic criteria, Crit. Care Med. 2:293, 1974.

202. Derenne, J. P., et al.: The respiratory muscles: Mechanics, control and pathophysiology, Parts I & II, Am. Rev. Respir. Dis. 118:119, 1978.

203. Knott, J., et al.: *Proprioceptive Neuromuscular Facilitation* (2d ed.; New York: Harper & Row, 1968).

204. Brompton Hospital: *Physiotherapy for Medical and Surgical Thoracic Conditions* (3d ed. rev.; 1967).

205. Kimbel, P.: Physical therapy for COPD patients, Clin. Notes Respir. Dis. Spring:3, 1970.

206. Thacker, W. C.: *Special Problems in Postural Drainage and Respiratory Control* (3d ed.; Chicago: Year Book Medical Publishers, Inc., 1973).

207. Goodman, L., and Gilman, A. (eds.): *The Pharmacological Basis of Therapeutics* (3d ed.; New York: Macmillan Publishing Co., 1965).

208. Middleton, E.: Autonomic imbalance in asthma with special reference to beta adrenergic blockage, Adv. Intern. Med. 18:177, 1972.
209. Butcher, R.: Role of cyclic AMP in hormone actions, N. Engl. J. Med. 279:1378, 1968.
210. Ziment, I.: The pharmacology of airway dilators, Respir. Care 19:51, 1974.
211. Nicholson, D., et al.: A re-evaluation of parenteral aminophylline, Am. Rev. Respir. Dis. 108:241, 1973.
212. Geddes, B., et al.: Respiratory smooth muscle relaxing effect of commercial steroid preparations, Am. Rev. Respir. Dis. 107:395, 1973.
213. Milne, J., et al.: Long-term study of disodium cromoglycate in treatment of severe extrinsic or intrinsic bronchial asthma in adults, Br. Med. J. 4:383, 1972.
214. Hyde, J.: Cromolyn prophylaxis for chronic asthma, Ann. Intern. Med. 78:966, 1973.
215. Webb, W., et al.: Clinical evaluation of a new mucolytic agent, acetylcysteine, J. Thorac. Cardiovasc. Surg. 44:330, 1962.
216. Rumble, L.: The use of nebulized steroids, J. Med. Assoc. Ga. 53:314, 1964.
217. Lifschitz, M., et al.: Safety of kanamycin aerosol, Clin. Pharmacol. Ther. 12:91, 1969.
218. Graham, W. G., and Bradley, D. A.: Efficacy of chest physiotherapy and intermittent positive-pressure breathing in the resolution of pneumonia, N. Engl. J. Med. 299:624, 1978.
219. Blanc, V. F.: The complications of tracheal intubation: A new classification with a review of the literature, Anesth. Analg. (Cleve.) 53:2, 1974.
220. Applebaum, E. L., and Bruce, D. L.: *Tracheal Intubation* (Philadelphia: W. B. Saunders Co., 1976).
221. Hollander, A. R.: *Office Practice of Otolaryngology* (Philadelphia: F. A. Davis Co., 1965).
222. Montgomery, W. W.: *Surgery of the Upper Airway System* (Philadelphia: Lea & Febiger, 1973).
223. Greenbaum, J. M., et al.: Esophageal obstruction during oxygen administration, Chest 65:188, 1974.
224. Benson, D. M., et al.: Inadequacy of prehospital emergency care, Crit. Care Med. 1:130, 1973.
225. Bryson, T. K., et al.: The esophageal obturator airway, Chest 74:537, 1978.
226. Owens, Thomas, J. B.: A follow-up of children treated with prolonged nasal intubation, Can. Anaesth. Soc. J. 14:543, 1967.
227. Arens, J. F., et al.: Maxillary sinusitis, a complication of nasotracheal intubation, Anesthesiology 40:415, 1974.
228. Warner, W. A.: Laryngeal band: Possible relation to prolonged nasotracheal intubation, Anesthesiology 28:466, 1967.
229. Head, J. M.: Tracheostomy in the management of respiratory problems, N. Engl. J. Med. 264:587, 1961.
230. Meade, J. W.: Tracheostomy — Its complications and their management, N. Engl. J. Med. 265:519, 1961.
231. Mulder, D. S., et al.: Complication of tracheostomy: Relationship to long-term ventilatory assistance, J. Trauma 9:389, 1969.

232. Selecky, P. A.: Tracheostomy: A review of present-day indications, complications, and care, Heart Lung 3:272, 1974.
233. Bergstrom, O., et al.: Mediastinal emphysema complicating tracheostomy, Arch. Otolaryngol. 71:628, 1960.
234. Beatraus, W. P.: Tracheostomy: Its expanded indications and its present status, Laryngoscope 78:3, 1968.
235. Davis, J. B., et al.: Hemorrhage as a postoperative complication of tracheostomy, Ann. Surg. 144:893, 1956.
236. Cooper, J. D., et al.: Analysis of problems related to cuffs on intratracheal tubes, Chest [Suppl.]62:215, 1972.
237. Sykes, M. K., et al.: *Respiratory Failure* (Philadelphia: F. A. Davis Co., 1969).
238. Bonanno, P. C.: Swallowing dysfunction after tracheostomy, Ann. Surg. 174:29, 1971.
239. Harley, H. R. S.: Ulcerative tracheoesophageal fistula during treatment by tracheostomy and intermittent positive pressure ventilation, Thorax 27:338, 1972.
240. Stetson, J. B., et al.: Causes of damage to tissues by polymers and elastomers used in fabrication of tracheal devices, Anesthesiology 33:635, 1970.
241. Cunliffe, A. C., et al.: Hazards from plastics sterilized by ethylene oxide, Br. Med. J. 2:575, 1967.
242. Guess, W. L., et al.: Tissue reactions to organotin-stabilized polyvinyl chloride (PVC) catheters, J.A.M.A. 204:508, 1968.
243. Hodgkin, J., et al.: Respirator weaning, Crit. Care Med. 2:96, 1974.
244. Rendell-Baker, L., et al.: The hazards of ethylene oxide, Anesthesiology 30:349, 1969.
245. Stetson, J. B., et al.: Ethylene oxide degassing of rubber and plastic materials, Anesthesiology 44:174, 1976.
246. Stetson, J. B. (ed.): *Prolonged Endotracheal Intubation,* International Anesthesiology Clinics, vol. 8 (Boston: Little, Brown and Co., 1970).
247. Safar, P.: *Respiratory Therapy* (Philadelphia: F. A. Davis Co., 1965).
248. Tonkin, J. P., et al.: The effect on the larynx of prolonged endotracheal intubation, Med. J. Aust. 2:581, 1966.
249. *National Nosocomial Infections,* D.H.E.W. Publication, no. (CDC 75-8257). First and Second Quarters: 173, 1974.
250. Jawetz, E., et al.: *Review of Medical Microbiology* (Los Altos, Calif.: Lange Medical Publications, 1972).
251. Perkins, J. J.: Surgical Scrubs and Preoperative Skin Disinfection, in *Principles and Methods of Sterilization in Health Sciences* (2d ed.; Springfield, Ill.: Charles C Thomas, 1969).
252. Heller, M. L., et al.: Polarographic study of arterial oxygenation during apnea in man, N. Engl. J. Med. 264:326, 1961.
253. Urban, B. J., et al.: Avoidance of hypoxemia during endotracheal suction, Anesthesiology 31:473, 1969.
254. Naigow, D., and Powaser, M.: The effects of different endotracheal procedures on arterial blood gases in a controlled experiment model, Heart Lung 6:808, 1977.
255. Shim, C., et al.: Cardiac arrhythmias resulting from tracheal suctioning, Ann. Intern. Med. 71:1149, 1969.

256. Sloan, H. E.: Vagus nerve in cardiac arrest, Surg. Gynecol. Obstet. 91: 257, 1950.
257. Miller, W.: Complications of Tracheostomy and Prolonged Mechanical Ventilation, in Moyer, J. H., and Oaks, W. W. (eds.): *Pre- and Postoperative Management of the Cardiopulmonary Patient* (New York: Grune & Stratton, Inc., 1970).
258. Baier, H., et al.: Effect of airway diameter, suction catheters and the bronchofiberscope on airflow in endotracheal and tracheostomy tubes, Heart Lung 5:235, 1976.
259. Jung, R. C., and Cottlieb, L. S.: Comparison of tracheobronchial suction catheters in humans, Chest 69:179, 1976.
260. Sackner, M. A., et al.: Pathogenesis and prevention of tracheobronchial damage with suction procedures, Chest 64:284, 1973.
261. Bryant, L. R., et al.: Reappraisal of tracheal injury from cuffed tracheostomy tubes, J.A.M.A. 215:625, 1971.
262. Trout, C. A., et al.: A standard pre-cut fenestrated tacheostomy tube, Respir. Care 17:173, 1972.
263. Nelson, E. J.: A prosthesis for tracheostomy stomas, Inhalation Ther. 14: 91, 1969.
264. Baron, S. H., et al.: Laryngeal sequelae of endotracheal anesthesia, Ann. Otol. Rhinol. Laryngol. 60:769, 1961.
265. Jordon, W. S., et al.: New therapy for postintubation laryngeal edema and tracheitis in children, J.A.M.A. 212:585, 1970.
266. Deming, M. V., et al.: Steroid and antihistaminic therapy for postintubation subglottic edema in infants and children, Anesthesiology 22:933, 1961.
267. Klainer, A. S.: Surface alterations due to endotracheal intubation, Am. J. Med. 58:674, 1975.
268. Myerson, M. C.: Granulomatous polyps of the larynx following intratracheal anesthesia, Arch. Otolaryngol. 62:182, 1955.
269. Gibson, P.: Pathology and repair of tracheal stenosis following tracheostomy and intermittent positive pressure breathing, Thorax 25:6, 1967.
270. Aloulker, P.: Respiratory accidents due to stricture of the laryngotracheal lumen following tracheostomy, Acta Chir. Belg. 59:553, 1960.
271. Friman, L., et al.: Stenosis following tracheostomy, Anaesthesia 31:479, 1976.
272. Aass, A. S.: Complication of tracheostomy and long term intubation: A follow-up study, Acta Anaesthesiol. Scand. 19:127, 1975.
273. Pearson, F. G., et al.: Tracheal stenosis complicating tracheostomy with cuffed tubes, Arch. Surg. 97:380, 1968.
274. Andrews, M. J., et al.: Incidence and pathogenesis of tracheal injury following cuffed tube tracheostomy with assisted ventilation: Analysis of a two-year prospective study, Ann. Surg. 173:249, 1971.
275. Geffin, B., et al.: Stenosis following tracheostomy for respiratory care, J.A.M.A. 216:1984, 1971.
276. Webb, W. R., et al.: Surgical management of tracheal stenosis, Ann. Surg. 179:819, 1974.
277. Pearson, F. G., et al.: A prospective study of tracheal injury complicating tracheostomy with cuffed tubes, Ann. Otol. Rhinol. Laryngol. 77:1, 1968.
278. Cooper, J. D., et al.: The evaluation of tracheal injury due to ventilatory assistance through cuffed tubes, Ann. Surg. 169:334, 1969.

279. Stiles, P. J.: Tracheal lesions after tracheostomy, Thorax 2:1, 1967.
280. Johnson, J. B., et al.: Tracheal stenosis following tracheostomy: A conservative approach to treatment, J. Thorac. Cardiovasc. Surg. 53:206, 1967.
281. Lindholm, D. F.: Prolonged endotracheal intubation (a clinical investigation with specific reference to its consequences for the larynx and the trachea and to its place as an alternative to intubation through a tracheostomy), Acta Anaesthesiol. Scand. [Suppl.] 33:1969.
282. Cross, D. E.: Recent developments in tracheal cuffs, Resuscitation 2:77, 1973.
283. Ching, N. P., et al.: The contribution of cuff volume and pressure in tracheostomy tube damage, J. Thorac. Cardiovasc. Surg. 62:402, 1971.
284. Carroll, R., et al.: Intratracheal cuffs: Performance characteristics, Anesthesiology 31:275, 1969.
285. Crawlery, B. E., and Cross, D. E.: Tracheal cuffs: A review and dynamic pressure study, Anaesthesia 30:4, 1976.
286. Carroll, R. G., et al.: Proper use of large diameter, large residual volume cuffs, Crit. Care Med. 1:153, 1973.
287. Cooper, J. D., et al.: Experimental production and prevention of injury due to cuffed tracheal tubes, Surg. Gynecol. Obstet. 129:1235, 1969.
288. King, R., et al.: Tracheal tube cuffs and tracheal dilation, Chest 67:458, 1975.
289. Hedden, M., et al.: Tracheoesophageal fistula following prolonged artificial ventilation via cuffed tubes, Anesthesiology 31:281, 1969.
290. Geffin, B.: Reduction of tracheal damage by the prestretching of inflatable cuffs, Anesthesiology 31:462, 1969.
291. Wandless, J. G., et al.: Prestretched cuffs on tracheostomy tubes, Br. J. Anaesth. 44:222, 1972.
292. Kamen, J. M., et al.: A new low-pressure cuff for endotracheal tubes, Anesthesiology 34:482, 1971.
293. Lederman, D. S., et al.: A comparison of foam and air-filled endotracheal tube cuffs, Anesth. Analg. (Cleve.) 53:521, 1974.
294. Magovern, G., et al.: The clinical and experimental evaluation of a controlled-pressure intratracheal cuff, J. Thorac. Cardiovasc. Surg. 64:747, 1972.
295. Carroll, R. G.: Evaluation of tracheal tube cuff design, Crit. Care Med. 1:45, 1973.
296. Carroll, R. G., et al.: Recommended performance specifications for cuffed endotracheal and tracheostomy tubes, Crit. Care Med. 1:155, 1973.
297. Perkins, J. F., Jr.: Historical Development of Respiratory Physiology, in The Handbook of Physiology, Respiration, vol. 1 (Washington, D.C.: American Physiological Society, 1964).
298. Harrison, R. A.: Principles of Internal Medicine (8th ed.; New York: McGraw-Hill Book Co., 1977).
299. Harrison, R. A.: Mass Spectrometer in Critical Care. Unpublished data.
300. Heldt, G. P., and Peters, R. M.: A simplified method to determine functional residual capacity during mechanical ventilation, Chest 74:492, 1978.
301. Wilson, R., et al.: Determinations of blood flow through nonventilated

portions of the normal and diseased lung, Am. Rev. Tuberc. 68:177, 1953.
302. Shapiro, B.: . . . to clear an airway, Emergency Med. 6:134, 1974.
303. Ramachandran, P. R., and Fairly, H. B.: Changes in functional residual capacity during respiratory failure, Can. Anaesth. Soc. J. 17:359, 1970.
304. Whitefield, A. G., et al.: Total lung volume and its subdivisions study in physiologic norms: Basic data, Brit. J. Soc. Med. 4:1, 1950.
305. Shapiro, B. A., et al.: Case study: Myasthenia gravis, Respir. Care 19: 460, 1974.
306. Waters, R. M.: Simple methods for performing artificial respiration, J.A.M.A. 123:559, 1943.
307. Emerson, H.: Artificial respiration in treatment of edema of the lungs, Arch. Intern. Med. 3:368, 1909.
308. Drinker, P., and Shaw, L. A.: An apparatus for the prolonged administration of artificial respiration. I. A design for adults and children, J. Clin. Invest. 7:229, 1929.
309. Lassen, H. C. A.: A preliminary report on the 1952 epidemic poliomyelitis in Copenhagen with special reference to the treatment of acute respiratory insufficiency, Lancet 1:37, 1953.
310. Engström, C. F.: The clinical application of prolonged controlled ventilation, Acta Anaesthesiol. Scand. [Suppl.] XIII, 1963.
311. Don, H., et al.: Airway closure, gas trapping and the functional residual capacity during anesthesia, Anesthesiology 6:533, 1972.
312. Motley, H. L., et al.: Observations on the clinical use of positive pressure, J. Aviation Med. 18:417, 1947.
313. Froese, A. B., and Bryan, A. C.: Effects of anaesthesia and paralysis on diaphragmatic mechanics in man, Anesthesiology 41:242, 1974.
314. Henning, R. J., et al.: The measurement of the work of breathing for the clinical assessment of ventilator dependence, Crit. Care Med. 5:264, 1977.
315. Dammann, J. F., and McAslan, T. C.: Optimal flow pattern for mechanical ventilation of the lungs, Crit. Care Med. 5:128, 1977.
316. Bursztein, S., et al.: Reduced oxygen consumption in catabolic states with mechanical ventilation, Crit. Care Med. 6:162, 1978.
317. Jansson, L., and Jonson, B.: A theoretical study of flow patterns of ventilation, Scand. J. Respir. Dis. 53:237, 1972.
318. Knelson, J. H., et al.: Effect of respiratory pattern on alveolar gas exchange, J. Appl. Physiol. 29:278, 1970.
319. Watson, W. E.: Observations on physiologic deadspace during intermittent positive pressure respiration, Br. J. Anaesth. 34:502, 1962.
320. Otis, A. B., et al.: Mechanical factors in distribution of pulmonary ventilation, J. Appl. Physiol. 8:427, 1956.
321. Lyager, S.: Ventilation/perfusion ratio during intermittent positive pressure ventilation, Acta Anesthesiol. Scand. 14:211, 1970.
322. Downs, J. B., et al.: Intermittent mandatory ventilation: A new technique for weaning patients from mechanical ventilation, Chest 64:331, 1973.
323. Lyager, S.: Influence of flow pattern on the distribution of respiratory air during intermittent positive pressure ventilation, Acta Anaesthesiol. Scand. 12:191, 1968.

324. Maffeo, W., and Dammann, J. F.: Influence of Ventilation Parameters on Mechanical Ventilation of the Lungs, *Proc. 9th Annual Model and Simulation Conference*, Vogt, W. G., and Mickle, M. M. (eds.) (Pittsburgh, 1978).

325. Bergman, N. A.: Effects of varying respiratory waveforms on gas exchange, Anesthesiology 28:390, 1967.

326. Herzog, P., and Norlander, O. P.: Distribution of alveolar volumes with different types of positive pressure gas flow, Opusc. Med. 13:27, 1968.

327. Don, H., et al.: The effects of anesthesia and 100% oxygen on the functional residual capacity of the lungs, Anesthesiology 32:521, 1970.

328. Burger, E., et al.: Airway closure: Demonstration by breathing 100% oxygen at low lung volumes and by N_2 washout, J. Appl. Physiol. 25:139, 1968.

329. Bryan, A. C.: Comments of a devil's advocate, Am. Rev. Respir. Dis. 110: 143, 1974.

330. Downs, J. B., et al.: Intermittent mandatory ventilation, Arch. Surg. 109: 519, 1974.

331. Shapiro, B., Civetta, J., Schlobohm, R., and Synder, R.: A four center comparison of respiratory care support. Presented at the SCCM National Meeting (Miami, Fla., 1978).

332. Shapiro, B. A., et al.: Intermittent demand ventilation (IDV): A new technique for supporting ventilation in critically ill patients, Respir. Care 21:521, 1976.

333. Giebisch, G., et al.: The extrarenal response to acute acid base disturbances of respiratory origin, J. Clin. Invest. 34:231, 1955.

334. Lowenstein, E., et al.: Cardiovascular response to large doses of intravenous morphine in man, N. Engl. J. Med. 281:1389, 1969.

335. Wong, K., et al.: The cardiovascular effects of morphine sulfate with oxygen and with nitrous oxide in man, Anesthesiology 38:542, 1973.

336. Henneg, R., et al.: The effects of morphine on the resistance and capacitance vessels of the peripheral circulation, Am. Heart J. 72:242, 1966.

337. Lappas, D., et al.: Filling pressures of the heart and pulmonary circulation of the patient with coronary-artery disease after large intravenous doses of morphine, Anesthesiology 42:153, 1975.

338. Lowenstein, E.: Morphine "anesthesia"—A perspective, Anesthesiology 35:563, 1971.

339. Kallos, T., et al.: Interaction of the effects of nalozone and oxymorphone on human respiration, Anesthesiology 36:278, 1972.

340. Lindholm, C. E., et al.: Flexible fiberoptic bronchoscopy in critical care medicine. Diagnosis, therapy, and complications, Crit. Care Med. 2:250, 1974.

341. Feldman, N. T., and Huber, G. L.: Fiberoptic bronchoscopy in the intensive care unit, Int. Anesthesiol. Clin. 14:31, 1976.

342. Dammann, J. F., et al.: Optimal flow pattern for mechanical ventilation of the lungs. 2. The effect of a sine versus square wave flow pattern with and without an end-inspiratory pause on patients, Crit. Care Med. 6:293, 1978.

343. Fulheihan, S. F., et al.: Effect of mechanical ventilation with end-inspiratory pause on blood gas exchange, Anaesth. Analg. 55:122, 1976.

344. Dolfuss, R., et al.: Regional ventilation of the lung studied with boluses of xenon, Respir. Physiol. 2:234, 1967.
345. Klocke, R. A., and Farhi, E. L.: Simple method for determination of perfusion ventilation ratio of the underventilated element (the slow compartment) of the lung, J. Clin. Invest. 43:2227, 1964.
346. Petty, T.: P.S., don't forget the intensive respiratory care unit, Dis. Chest 56:276, 1969.
347. Pontoppidan, H., et al.: Medical progress: Acute respiratory failure in the adult, N. Engl. J. Med. 287:743, 1972.
348. Buist, A. S., et al.: A comparison of conventional spirometric tests and the tests of closing volume in an emphysema screening center, Am. Rev. Respir. Dis. 107:735, 1973.
349. Rodarte, J. R., et al.: New tests for the detection of obstructive pulmonary disease: Critical review, Chest 72:762, 1977.
350. Solomon, D. A.: Are small airways tests helpful in the detection of early airflow obstruction? Chest 74:567, 1978.
351. Cosio, M., et al.: The relations between structural changes in small airways and pulmonary function tests, N. Engl. J. Med. 298:1277, 1978.
352. Burki, N. K., et al.: Variability of the closing volume measurement in normal subjects, Am. Rev. Respir. Dis. 112:209, 1975.
353. Craig, D. B., and McCarthy, D. S.: Airway closure and lung volumes during breathing with maintained airway positive pressures, Anesthesiology 36:540, 1972.
354. Colgan, F. J., et al.: The cardiorespiratory effects of constant and intermittent positive pressure breathing, Anesthesiology 36:444, 1972.
355. Falke, K. J., et al.: Ventilation with end-expiratory pressure in acute lung disease, J. Clin. Invest. 51:2315, 1972.
356. Kumar, A., et al.: Continuous positive-pressure ventilation in acute respiratory failure. Effects on hemodynamics and lung function, N. Engl. J. Med. 283:1430, 1970.
357. Leftwich, E. I., et al.: Positive end-expiratory pressure in refractory hypoxemia. A critical evaluation, Ann. Intern. Med. 79:187, 1973.
358. Powers, S. R., et al.: Physiologic consequences of positive end-expiratory pressure (PEEP) ventilation, Ann. Surg. 178:265, 1973.
359. Wyche, M. Q., Jr., et al.: Effects of continuous positive pressure breathing on functional residual capacity and arterial oxygenation during intraabdominal operations: Studies in man during nitrous oxide and d-tubocurarine anesthesia, Anesthesiology 38:68, 1973.
360. Suter, P. M., et al.: Effect of tidal volume and positive end expiratory pressure on compliance during mechanical ventilation, Chest 73:158, 1978.
361. Hammon, J. W., Jr., et al.: The effect of PEEP on regional ventilation and perfusion in the normal and injured primate lung, J. Thorac. Cardiovasc. Surg. 72:680, 1976.
362. Berk, J. L., et al.: The use of dopamine to correct the reduced cardiac output resulting from positive end expiratory pressure, Crit. Care Med. 5:269, 1977.
363. Askanazi, J., et al.: Prevention of pulmonary insufficiency through prophylactic use of PEEP and rapid respiratory rates, J. Thorac. Cardiovasc. Surg. 75:267, 1978.

364. Hobelmann, C. F., Jr., et al.: Mechanics of ventilation with positive end expiratory pressure, Ann. Thorac. Surg. 24:68, 1977.

365. Virgilio, R. W.: Personal communication.

366. Civetta, J.: Personal communication.

367. Garrard, C. S., and Shah, M.: The effects of EPAP on FRC in normal subjects, Crit. Care Med. 6:320, 1978.

368. Kirby, R. R., et al.: High level positive end expiratory pressure (PEEP) in acute respiratory insufficiency, Chest 67:156, 1975.

369. Schmidt, G. B., et al.: EPAP without intubation, Crit. Care Med. 5:207, 1977.

370. Lucas, C. E., et al.: Natural history and surgical dilemma of "stress" gastric bleeding, Arch. Surg. 102:266, 1971.

371. Hedley-Whyte, J., et al.: *Applied Physiology of Respiratory Care* (Boston: Little, Brown and Co., 1976).

372. Harris, S. K., et al.: Gastrointestinal hemorrhage in patients in a respiratory intensive care unit, Chest 72:301, 1977.

373. Jama, R. H., et al.: Incidence of stress ulcer formation associated with steroid therapy in various shock states, Am. J. Surg. 130:328, 1975.

374. Johnson, E. R., and Hedley-Whyte, J.: CPPV and portal flow in dogs with pulmonary edema, J. Appl. Physiol. 33:385, 1972.

375. Drury, D. R., et al.: The effects of continuous pressure breathing on kidney function, J. Clin. Invest. 26:945, 1947.

376. Baratz, R. A., et al.: Plasma antidiuretic hormone and urinary output during CPPB in dogs, Anesthesiology 34:510, 1971.

377. Baratz, R., et al.: Urinary output and plasma levels of antidiuretic hormone during intermittent positive-pressure breathing in the dog, Anesthesiology 32:17, 1970.

378. Hall, S. V., et al.: Renal hemodynamics and function with continuous positive pressure ventilation in dogs, Anesthesiology 41:452, 1974.

379. Apuzzi, M. L., et al.: Effect of PEEP ventilation on intracranial pressure in man, J. Neurosurg. 46:227, 1977.

380. Gallagher, T. J., et al.: Terminology update: Optimal PEEP, Crit. Care Med. 6:323, 1978.

381. Suter, P., et al.: Optimum end expiratory airway pressure in patients with acute pulmonary failure, N. Engl. J. Med. 292:284, 1975.

382. Menkes, H. A., and Traystman, R. J.: Collateral ventilation: State of the art, Am. Rev. Respir. Dis. 116:287, 1977.

383. Bonner, J. T.: Clinical use of the pulmonary artery (Swan-Ganz) catheter, Anesthesiol. Rev., July, 1977.

384. Civetta, J. M., et al.: Disparate ventricular function in surgical patients, Surg. Forum 22:136, 1971.

385. Maclaren-Toussaint, G. P., et al.: CVP and PWP in critical surgical illness. A comparison, Arch. Surg. 109:255, 1974.

386. Swan, H. J.: Balloon flotation catheters—their use in hemodynamic monitoring in clinical practice, J.A.M.A. 233:865, 1975.

387. Swan, H. J., et al.: Catheterization of the heart in man with use of a flow-directed balloon-tipped catheter, N. Engl. J. Med. 283:447, 1970.

388. Gilbertson, A. A.: Pulmonary artery catheterization and wedge pressure measurement in the general intensive care unit, Br. J. Anaesth. 46:97, 1974.

389. Shin, B., et al.: Pitfalls of Swan-Ganz catheterization, Crit. Care Med. 5: 125, 1977.
390. Lozman, J., et al.: Correlation of pulmonary wedge and left atrial pressure, Arch. Surg. 109:270, 1974.
391. Shapiro, M. H., et al.: Errors in sampling pulmonary artery blood with a Swan-Ganz catheter, Anesthesiology 40:291, 1974.
392. Cassisy, S. S., et al.: Cardiovascular effects of PEEP in dogs, J. Appl. Physiol. 44:743, 1978.
393. Geer, R. T.: Interpretation of pulmonary artery wedge pressure when PEEP is used, Anesthesiology 46:383, 1977.
394. Downs, J. B.: A technique for direct measurement of intrapleural pressure, Crit. Care Med. 4:207, 1976.
395. Agostoni, E.: Mechanics of the pleural space, Physiol. Rev. 52:57, 1972.
396. Powers, et al.: Physiologic consequences of positive end expiratory pressure ventilation, Ann. Surg. 178:265, 1975.
397. Quist, J., et al.: Hemodynamic responses to mechanical ventilation with PEEP, Anesthesiology 42:45, 1975.
398. Davison, R., et al.: The validity of determinations of pulmonary wedge pressure during mechanical ventilation, Chest 73:352, 1978.
399. Berryhill, R. E., et al.: Pulmonary vascular pressure readings at the end of exhalation, Anesthesiology 49:365, 1978.
400. MacDonnell, K. F., et al.: Comparative hemodynamic consequences of inflation hold, PEEP, and interrupted PEEP, Ann. Thorac. Surg. 19:552, 1975.
401. Katz, A. M.: Application of the Starling resistor concept to the lungs during CPPV, Crit. Care Med. 5:67, 1977.
402. Fick, A.: Ueber die Messung des Blutquantums, in dem Herzventrike In. Sitzungsb. der phys.-med., Ges. zu Wurzburg: 36, 1870.
403. Forster, R. E.: Exchange of gases between alveolar air and pulmonary capillary blood: Pulmonary diffusing capacity, Physiol. Rev. 37:391, 1959.
404. Berggren, S. M.: The oxygen deficit of arterial blood caused by nonventilating parts of the lung, Acta Physiol. Scand. (Suppl. 11) 4:9, 1942.
405. Harrison, R. A., et al.: Unpublished data.
406. Woods, M., et al.: Practical considerations for the use of a pulmonary artery thermister catheter, Surgery 79:469, 1976.
407. Branthwatte, M. A., et al.: Measurement of cardiac output by thermal dilution in man, J. Appl. Physiol. 24:434, 1968.
408. Wessel, H. U., et al.: Limitations of thermal dilution curves for cardiac output determinations, J. Appl. Physiol. 30:643, 1971.
409. Zierler, K. L.: Circulation Times and the Theory of Indicator Dilution Methods for Determining Blood Flow and Volume, in *Handbook of Physiology, Circulation,* vol. 1 (Washington, D.C.: American Physiological Society, 1962).
410. Perutz, M. F.: Stereochemistry of cooperative effects in haemoglobin, Nature 228:726, 1970.
411. Robin, E. D., et al.: Medical progress: Pulmonary edema, Parts 1 & 2, N. Engl. J. Med. 288:239, 1973.
412. Dikshit, K., et al.: Hemodynamic effects of furosemide in cardiac failure, N. Engl. J. Med. 288:1087, 1973.

413. Mason, D. T., et al.: New developments in the understanding of the actions of the digitalis glycosides, Prog. Cardiovasc. Dis. 11:443, 1969.
414. Starling, E. H.: On the absorption of fluids from the connective tissue spaces, J. Physiol. 19:312, 1896.
415. Daluz, P. L., et al.: Pulmonary edema related to changes in colloid osmotic and PWP in patients after acute myocardial infarction, Circulation 51:350, 1975.
416. Morissette, M., et al.: Reduction in COP associated with progression of cardiopulmonary failure, Crit. Care Med. 3:115, 1975.
417. Staub, N. C.: Pulmonary edema. Physiologic approaches to management, Chest 74:559, 1978.
418. Ashbaugh, D., et al.: Acute respiratory distress in adults, Lancet 2:319, 1967.
419. Petty, T., et al.: The adult respiratory distress syndrome, Chest 60:233, 1971.
420. Nash, G., et al.: Pulmonary lesions associated with oxygen therapy and artificial ventilation, N. Engl. J. Med. 276:368, 1967.
421. Yahav, J., et al.: Pulmonary function following ARDS, Chest 74:247, 1978.
422. Katzenstein, A. A., et al.: Diffuse alveolar damage: The role of oxygen, shock, and related factors, Am. J. Pathol. 85:210, 1976.
423. Mead, J., et al.: Relationship of volume history of lungs to respiratory mechanics in anesthetized dogs, J. Appl. Physiol. 14:669, 1959.
424. Lakshminarayan, S., et al.: Prognosis after recovery from ARDS, Am. Rev. Respir. Dis. 113:7, 1976.
425. Fallat, R. J., et al.: Lung function in long term survivors from severe RDS, Am. Rev. Respir. Dis. 113:181, 1976.
426. Rotman, H. H., et al.: Long term physiologic consequences of the ARDS, Chest 72:190, 1977.
427. Campiche, M. A., et al.: An electron microscope study of the fetal development of human lung, Pediatrics 32:976, 1963.
428. Clements, J., et al.: Pulmonary surface tension and the mucous lining of the lungs: Some theoretical considerations, J. Appl. Physiol. 12:262, 1958.
429. Collier, C., et al.: Alterations of surfactant in oxygen poisoning, Dis. Chest 48:233, 1965.
430. Willwerth, B., et al.: The role of functional demand on the development of pulmonary lesions during hemorrhagic shock, J. Thorac. Cardiovasc. Surg. 54:658, 1967.
431. Acute Pulmonary Injury and Repair (The Adult Respiratory Distress Syndrome): The 16th Aspen Lung Conference, Chest[Suppl. 65 and 66]: 1974.
432. Effros, R. M., et al.: Comparison of single transit and equilibration studies of 22 Na+ distribution in the lung, Chest 71:296, 1977.
433. Barber, R., et al.: Oxygen toxicity in man, N. Engl. J. Med. 283:1478, 1970.
434. Joffe, N.: Pulmonary oxygen toxicity in the adult, Radiology 93:460, 1969.
435. Balentine, J.: Pathologic effects of exposure to high oxygen tensions. A review, N. Engl. J. Med. 275:1038, 1966.

436. Nash, G., et al.: Pulmonary lesions associated with oxygen therapy and artificial ventilation, N. Engl. J. Med. 276:368, 1967.
437. Barber, R. E., et al.: Oxygen toxicity in man: A prospective study in patients with irreversible brain damage, N. Engl. J. Med. 283:1478, 1970.
438. Singer, M. M., et al.: Oxygen toxicity in man: A prospective study in patients after open heart surgery, N. Engl. J. Med. 283:1473, 1970.
439. Ashbaugh, D. G., et al.: PEEP: Physiology, indications, and contraindications, J. Cardiovasc. Surg. 65:165, 1973.
440. Civetta, J. M., et al.: Optimal PEEP and IMV in the treatment of acute respiratory failure, Respir. Care 2:551, 1975.
441. Kirby, R. R., et al.: Cardiorespiratory effects of high PEEP, Anesthesiology 43:533, 1975.
442. Robotham, J. L., et al.: Effect of PEEP in left-ventricular performance, Am. Rev. Respir. Dis. 115:371, 1977.
443. James, P., et al.: Experience with steroids, albumin, and diuretics in progressive pulmonary insufficiency, South. Med. J. 65:945, 1972.
444. Wilson, J., et al.: Pulmonary cellular changes prevented or altered by methylprednisolone sodium succinate, Fed. Proc. 30:686, 1971.
445. Werksberger, J., et al.: Fat embolism: The effect of corticosteroids on experimental fat embolism in the rat, Surgery 64:134, 1968.
446. Churchill, E., et al.: The reduction in vital capacity following operation, Surg. Gynecol. Obstet. 44:483, 1927.
447. Lee, A. B., et al.: Effects of abdominal operation on ventilation and gas exchange, J. Natl. Med. Assoc. 61:164, 1969.
448. Hamilton, W. K., et al.: Postoperative respiratory complications, Anesthesiology 25:607, 1964.
449. Caro, C. G., et al.: Some effects of restriction of chest cage expansion on pulmonary function in man: An experimental study, J. Clin. Invest. 39: 573, 1960.
450. Honatt, W., et al.: Pulmonary function changes following repair of heart lesions with the aid of extracorporeal circulation, J. Thorac. Cardiovasc. Surg. 43:649, 1962.
451. Agostoni, E., et al.: Effects of uneven elastic loads on breathing pattern of anesthetized and conscious men, Respir. Physiol. 30:153, 1977.
452. Okinaka, A. J.: Closure of pulmonary air spaces following abdominal surgery, Surg. Gynecol. Obstet. 121:1282, 1965.
453. Diament, M. L., and Palmer, K.: Postoperative changes in gas tensions of arterial blood and in ventilatory function, Lancet 2:180, 1966.
454. Gordh, T., et al.: Pulmonary function in relation to anesthesia and surgery evaluated by analyses of oxygen tension of arterial blood, Acta Anaesthesiol. Scand. 2:15, 1958.
455. Knudson, J.: Duration of hypoxaemia after uncomplicated upper abdominal and thoraco-abdominal operations, Anaesthesia 25:372, 1970.
456. Georg, J., et al.: The mechanism of hypoxaemia after laparotomy, Thorax 22:282, 1967.
457. Wightman, J.: A prospective survey of the incidence of postoperative pulmonary complications, Br. J. Surg. 55:85, 1968.
458. Hansen, G., et al.: Pulmonary complications, ventilation and blood gases after upper abdominal surgery, Acta Anaesthesiol. Scand. 21:211, 1977.

459. Lewis, F. J., and Welch, J. A.: Respiratory mechanics in postoperative patients, Surg. Gynecol. Obstet. 120:305, 1965.

460. Karlson, K. E., et al.: Influence of thoracotomy on pulmonary mechanics: Association of increased work of breathing during anesthesia and postoperative pulmonary complications, Ann. Surg. 162:973, 1965.

461. Latimer, R. G., et al.: Ventilatory patterns and pulmonary complications after upper abdominal surgery determined by pre-operative and postoperative computerized spirometry and blood gas analysis, Am. J. Surg. 122:622, 1971.

462. Peters, R. M., and Stacy, R. W.: Automatized clinical measurement of respiratory parameters, Surgery 56:44, 1964.

463. Egbert, L., et al.: Effect of morphine on breathing pattern, J.A.M.A. 188: 485, 1964.

464. U.S. Department of Health, Education, and Welfare, National Center for Health Statistics, 1950–1969.

465. Chronic Respiratory Disease Control Program, Public Health Service Publications, nos. 1529 and 1802 (Arlington, Va.: National Center for Chronic Disease Control, 1968).

466. American Thoracic Society: Definition and classification of chronic bronchitis, asthma and pulmonary emphysema, a statement, Am. Rev. Respir. Dis. 85:762, 1962.

467. Hugh-Jones, P., and Whimster, W.: The etiology and management of disabling emphysema, State of the art, Am. Rev. Respir. Dis. 117:343, 1978.

468. Muren, O.: Clinical pathological correlation of chronic obstructive pulmonary disease (COPD), M.C. Va. Quarterly 9:121, 1973.

469. Mountain, R., et al.: Hypoventilation in obstructive lung disease, the role of familial factors, N. Engl. J. Med. 298:521, 1978.

470. Eichenholz, A., et al.: Pattern of compensatory response to hypercapnia in patients with chronic obstructive pulmonary disease, J. Lab. Clin. Med. 68:265, 1966.

471. Rusk, H.: Rehabilitation Medicine (2d ed.; St. Louis: C. V. Mosby Co., 1964).

472. Adams, et al.: Long term physiologic adaptations to exercise with special reference to performance and cardiorespiratory function in health and disease, Am. J. Cardiol. 33:765, 1974.

473. Williams, H.: Ventilatory failure, Medicine 45:317, 1966.

474. Robin, E. D.: Abnormalities of acid-base regulation in chronic pulmonary disease, with special reference to hypercapnia and extracellular alkalosis, N. Engl. J. Med. 268:917, 1963.

475. Boddy, K., et al.: Total body and exchangeable potassium in chronic airways obstruction: A controversial area? Thorax 33:62, 1978.

476. U.S. Department of Health, Education, and Welfare: Chronic Bronchitis and Emphysema: The Application of Physical Medicine and Rehabilitation, Public Health Service Publications, no. 1529.

477. Miller, W.: Rehabilitation of patients with chronic obstructive lung disease, Med. Clin. North Am. 51:349, 1967.

478. Petty, T., et al.: A comprehensive care program for chronic airway obstruction, Ann. Intern. Med. 70:1109, 1969.

479. Webster, J., et al.: Chronic bronchitis and emphysema, Postgrad. Med. 50:113, 1971.
480. Luparello, T.: For some illness pays, Med. Insight, p. 24, Jan., 1974.
481. Petty, T.: Does treatment for severe emphysema and chronic bronchitis really help? (A response), Chest 65:124, 1974.
482. Shapiro, B. A., et al.: Rehabilitation in chronic obstructive pulmonary disease: A two-year prospective study, Respir. Care 22:1045, 1977.
483. Proceedings of the Conference on the Scientific Basis of Respiratory Therapy, Temple University Conference Center at Sugarloaf, Philadelphia, May 2–4, 1974, Am. Rev. Respir. Dis. 110:1–203, 1974.
484. March, H.: Appraisal of postural drainage for chronic obstructive pulmonary disease, Arch. Phys. Med. Rehabil. 52:528, 1971.
485. Motley, H.: The effects of slow deep breathing on the blood gas exchange in emphysema, Am. Rev. Respir. Dis. 88:484, 1963.
486. Woolf, C.: A rehabilitation program for improving exercise tolerance of patients with chronic lung disease, Can. Med. Assoc. J. 106:1289, 1972.
487. Petty, T., et al.: Clinical evaluation of prolonged ambulatory oxygen therapy in chronic airway obstruction, Am. J. Med. 45:242, 1968.
488. Cameron, J., et al.: Aspiration pneumonia: Magnitude and frequency of the problem, J.A.M.A. 219:1194, 1972.
489. Arms, R., et al.: Aspiration pneumonia, Chest 65:136, 1974.
490. Awe, W., et al.: The pathophysiology of aspiration pneumonitis, Surgery 60:232, 1966.
491. Wynne, T. W., and Modell, J. H.: Respiratory aspiration of stomach contents, Ann. Intern. Med. 87:466, 1977.
492. Winternitz, M. C., et al.: Effect of intrabronchial insufflation of acid, J. Exp. Med. 32:199, 1920.
493. Teabeaut, J. R., II: Aspiration of gastric contents; experimental study, Am. J. Pathol. 28:51, 1952.
494. Bosomworth, P. P., and Hamelberg, W.: The etiologic and therapeutic aspects of aspiration pneumonitis: Experimental study, Surg. Forum 13: 158, 1962.
495. Hamelberg, W., and Bosomworth, P. P.: Aspiration pneumonitis: Experimental and clinical observation, Anesth. Analg. (Cleve.) 43:669, 1964.
496. Cameron, J. L., et al.: Aspiration pneumonia. Clinical outcome following documented aspiration, Arch. Surg. 106:49, 1973.
497. Heroy, W.: Unrecognized aspiration, Ann. Thorac. Surg. 8:580, 1969.
498. Bosomworth, P., et al.: Aspiration of gastric juice—Physiologic alterations, Anesthesiology 26:241, 1965.
499. Mendelsohn, C. L.: The aspiration of stomach contents into the lungs during obstetric anesthesia, Am. J. Gynecol. Obstet. 52:191, 1946.
500. Dines, D. E., et al.: Aspiration pneumonitis: Mendelson's syndrome, J.A.M.A. 176:229, 1961.
501. Bannister, W. K., et al.: Therapeutic aspects of aspiration pneumonitis, Anesthesiology 22:440, 1961.
502. Greenfield, L. J., et al.: Pulmonary effects of experimental graded aspiration of hydrochloric acid, Ann. Surg. 170:74, 1969.
503. Lewis, R. T., et al.: Cardiorespiratory studies in critical illness, Arch. Surg. 103:335, 1971.

504. Chapman, R. L., et al.: The ineffectiveness of steroid therapy in treating aspiration of hydrochloric acid, Arch. Surg. 108:858, 1974.
505. Chapman, R. L., Jr., et al.: Effect of continuous positive-pressure ventilation and steroids on aspiration of HCl (pH 1.8) in dogs, Anesth. Analg. 53:556, 1974.
506. Tinstman, T. C., et al.: Postoperative aspiration pneumonia, Surg. Clin. North Am. 53:859, 1973.
507. Arms, R. A., et al.: Aspiration pneumonia, Chest 65:136, 1974.
508. Downs, J. B., et al.: An evaluation of steroid therapy in aspiration pneumonitis, Anesthesiology 40:129, 1974.
509. Lewinski, A.: Evaluation of methods employed in the treatment of the chemical pneumonitis of aspiration, Anesthesiology 26:37, 1965.
510. Wilson, J.: Treatment or prevention of pulmonary cellular damage with pharmacologic doses of corticosteroid, Surg. Gynecol. Obstet. 134:675, 1972.
511. U.S. Department of HEW, Public Health Service. Vital Statistics of the United States, 1969, vol. 2. *Mortality,* Part A. Rockville, Md.: National Center for Health Statistics, 1974.
512. Mortiz, A.: Chemical methods for the determination of death by drowning, Physiol. Rev. 24:70, 1944.
513. Modell, J. H.: *The Pathophysiology and Treatment of Drowning and Near Drowning* (Springfield, Ill.: Charles C Thomas, 1971).
514. Modell, J. H., et al.: Clinical course of 91 consecutive near-drowning victims, Chest 70:231, 1976.
515. Maisels, J., et al.: Endogenous production of carbon monoxide in normal and erythroblastotic newborn infants, J. Clin. Invest. 50:1, 1971.
516. Aronow, W., et al: Effect of heavy freeway traffic on cardiopulmonary function in angina, Chest 63:358, 1972.
517. Ayres, S., et al.: Carboxyhemoglobin and the access to oxygen, Arch. Environ. Health 26:8, 1973.
518. Garzon, A., et al.: Respiratory mechanics in patients with inhalation burns, J. Trauma 10:57, 1970.
519. Arieff, A., and Friedman, E.: Coma following non-narcotic drug overdosage. Management of 208 adult patients, Am. J. Med. Sci. 266:405, 1973.
520. Phelps, M. E., et al.: Correlation between $PaCO_2$ and regional cerebral blood volume by x-ray fluorescence, J. Appl. Physiol. 35:274, 1973.
521. Wollman, H., et al.: Effects of extremes of respiratory and metabolic alkalosis on cerebral blood flow in man, J. Appl. Physiol. 24:60, 1968.
522. Special Symposium Issue: Brain resuscitation, Crit. Care Med. 6:199, 1978.
523. Black, P.: Brain death, parts 1 & 2, N. Engl. J. Med. 299:338, 1978.
524. Ashbaugh, D. G., et al.: Chest trauma. Analysis of 685 patients, Arch. Surg. 95:546, 1967.
525. Cullen, P., et al.: Treatment of patients with flail chest by intermittent mandatory ventilation and PEEP, Crit. Care Med. 3:45, 1975.
526. Reid, J. M., and Baird, W. L.: Crushed chest injury: Some physiological disturbances and their correction, Br. Med. J. 1:1105, 1965.
527. Avery, E., et al.: The treatment of crushing injuries to the chest (methods old and new), Am. J. Surg. 93:540, 1957.

528. Perry, J. F., et al.: Chest injury due to blunt trauma, J. Thorac. Cardio-vasc. Surg. 49:684, 1965.
529. Sankaran, S., and Wilson, R. F.: Factors affecting prognosis in patients with flail chest, J. Thorac. Cardiovasc. Surg. 60:402, 1970.
530. Shackford, S. R., et al.: The management of flail chest, a comparison of ventilatory and non-ventilatory treatment, Am. J. Surg. 132:759, 1976.
531. Williams, J., et al.: Pulmonary contusion secondary to non-penetrating chest trauma, Am. J. Roentgenol. 91:284, 1964.
532. Harrison, R. A., et al.: Reassessment of the assumed A-V oxygen content difference in the shunt calculation, Anesth. Analg. (Cleve.) 54:198, 1975.
533. Fulton, R. L., and Peter, E. T.: The progressive nature of pulmonary contusion, Surgery 67:499, 1970.
534. Wiot, J. F.: The radiologic manifestations of blunt chest trauma, J.A.M.A. 231:500, 1975.
535. Garzon, A. A., et al.: Severe blunt chest trauma. Studies of pulmonary mechanics and blood gases, Ann. Thorac. Surg. 2:629, 1966.
536. Roscher, R., et al.: Pulmonary contusion: Clinical experience, Arch. Surg. 109:508, 1974.
537. Robin, E. D.: Overdiagnosis and overtreatment of pulmonary embolism: The emperor may have no clothes, Ann. Intern. Med. 87:775, 1977.
538. Neuhas, A., et al.: Pulmonary embolism in respiratory failure, Chest 73: 4, 1978.
539. Shapiro, B. A., et al.: Case study: Status asthmaticus, Respir. Care 19: 130, 1974.
540. Doershuk, C., et al.: Cystic fibrosis: Comprehensive management, Post-grad. Med. 40:550, 1966.
541. Davis, P. B., et al.: Seventy-five adults with cystic fibrosis, Am. Rev. Respir. Dis. 115:278, 1977.
542. Lough, M. D., et al.: *Pediatric Respiratory Therapy* (Chicago: Year Book Medical Publishers, Inc., 1974).
543. Smith, R. M.: *Anesthesia for Infants and Children* (3d ed.; St. Louis: C. V. Mosby Co., 1968).
544. Wilton, T. N. P.: *Neonatal Anesthesia* (London: Wilmer Brothers, Ltd., Blackwell Scientific Publications, 1965).
545. Jones, R. S., et al.: *Care of the Critically Ill Child* (London: William Clowes & Sons, Ltd., 1971).
546. Bau, S. K., et al.: The measurement of fluid deposition in humans follow-ing mist tent therapy, Pediatrics 48:605, 1971.
547. Adair, J. C., et al.: Ten years' experience with IPPB in the treatment of acute laryngotracheal bronchitis, Anesth. Analg. (Cleve.) 50:649, 1971.
548. Chang, N., et al.: The effect of nebulized bronchodilator administration with or without IPPB on ventilatory function in children with cystic fibrosis and asthma, Am. Rev. Respir. Dis. 106:867, 1972.
549. Kendig, E. L. (ed.): *Disorders of the Respiratory Tract in Children* (Philadelphia: W. B. Saunders Co., 1968).
550. Gregory, G. A., et al.: Treatment of the idiopathic respiratory-distress syndrome with continuous positive airway pressure, N. Engl. J. Med., 284:1133, 1971.
551 Avery, M. E.: *The Lung and Its Disorder in the Newborn Infant* (2d ed.; Philadelphia: W. B. Saunders Co., 1969).

552. Johnson, M. C., et al.: Bronchopulmonary hygiene in cystic fibrosis, Am. J. Nurs. 69:320, 1969.
553. Matthews, J. W., et al.: A therapeutic regimen for patients with cystic fibrosis, J. Pediatr. 65:558, 1964.
554. Downs, J. B., et al.: Comparison of assisted and controlled mechanical ventilation in anesthetized swine, Crit. Care Med. 7:5, 1979.
555. Cohen, R., and Overfield, E.: The diffusion component of arterial hypoxemia, Am. Rev. Respir. Dis. 105:532, 1972.

INDEX